Congenital Anomalies: Diagnosis and Treatment

Congenital Anomalies: Diagnosis and Treatment

Editor: Elsa Hunt

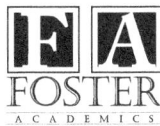

FA
FOSTER
A C A D E M I C S

www.fosteracademics.com

www.fosteracademics.com

FA
FOSTER
ACADEMICS

Cataloging-in-Publication Data

Congenital anomalies : diagnosis and treatment / edited by Elsa Hunt.
 p. cm.
Includes bibliographical references and index.
ISBN 978-1-63242-778-6
1. Abnormalities, Human. 2. Abnormalities, Human--Diagnosis.
3. Abnormalities, Human--Treatment. 4. Pediatrics. I. Hunt, Elsa.
RG626 .C66 2019
618.32--dc23

Foster Academics,
118-35 Queens Blvd., Suite 400,
Forest Hills, NY 11375, USA

ISBN 978-1-63242-778-6 (Hardback)

Contents

Preface

Congenital anomalies, also known as birth defects are the conditions present at birth that affects the intellectual, developmental or physical health of an infant. Such disabilities can range from mild to severe. Functional disorders, which affect the function of a body part, may include degenerative disorders and metabolic disorders. Structural disorders manifest as problems with the shape of a body part. Congenital anomalies can arise from chromosomal or genetic disorders, infections during pregnancy and due to exposure to certain chemicals or drugs. Such abnormalities may be visible at birth, or can be detected before birth through prenatal tests and through screening tests after birth. Their treatment varies according to the type of defect and its severity. Treatment may encompass medicational, surgical and therapeutical interventions. Assistive technology can also aid in providing a better quality of life to such individuals. This book includes some of the vital pieces of work being conducted across the world, on various topics related to congenital anomalies. The topics included herein on the diagnosis and treatment of congenital anomalies, are of utmost significance and bound to provide incredible insights to readers. The extensive content of this book provides the readers with a thorough understanding of the subject.

This book is the end result of constructive efforts and intensive research done by experts in this field. The aim of this book is to enlighten the readers with recent information in this area of research. The information provided in this profound book would serve as a valuable reference to students and researchers in this field.

At the end, I would like to thank all the authors for devoting their precious time and providing their valuable contribution to this book. I would also like to express my gratitude to my fellow colleagues who encouraged me throughout the process.

Editor

1

Thoracic Anomalies

Cringu Ionescu

Abstract

The antenatal and postnatal prognosis for fetuses with chest noncardiac anomalies varies widely, depending of the type of lesion present. An important issue is to establish an accurate prenatal diagnosis, which allows an appropriate counseling of the couple, fetal karyotyping and eventually in utero fetal therapy, if possible. Also, another important feature is preparation for delivery in a tertiary center or an appropriate perinatal institution, able to provide care to the immediate neonatal consequences in such cases. The ultrasound exam is not only crucial in the diagnosis of such lesions, but also important in the serial antenatal follow up, some of them being progressive, and having the potential to lead to compromise of cardiac function and eventually to fetal death. Thus, the sonographer has an important role in the management of such difficult cases. Currently, perinatal centers provide multidisciplinary teams, with maternal fetal specialists, neonatologists, pediatric surgeons, all involved in counseling parents about the outcome and the management options for a fetus with a diagnosis of thoracic anomalies. Although the precise prenatal diagnosis is often possible, this does not necessarily ensure improvement of the postnatal outcome, due to associated pulmonary hypoplasia.

Keywords: thoracic anomalies, congenital cystic adenomatoid malformation (CCAM), bronchopulmonary sequestration (BPS), CCAM-BPS hybrid form, congenital diaphragmatic hernia (CDH), bronchogenic cyst, congenital high airway obstruction syndrome (CHAOS)

1. Introduction

The thoracic anomalies represent a group of abnormalities that can be found either in the lung parenchyma or mediastinum. The thoracic cavity has a conical shape and is delimited at the posterior level by the sternum, at the superior level by the clavicle, at the lower level by the diaphragm, and at the lateral level by the ribs. In the thorax, the organs that are examined by the ultrasound are: the lungs, the heart and the mediastinum. The thoracic anomalies chapter refers to pulmonary and mediastinal fetal abnormalities, the cardiac abnormalities being a separate chapter. Congenital bronchopulmonary malformation comprises a group of abnormalities that are represented by the following entities: congenital cystic adenomatoid malformation (CCAM), bronchopulmonary sequestration (BPS), CCAM-BPS hybrid form, congenital diaphragmatic hernia (CDH), bronchogenic cyst, congenital high airway obstruction syndrome (CHAOS) and pulmonary hypoplasia/agenesis. Currently, it is recommended for the term bronchopulmonary anomalies to be used instead of congenital cystic adenomatoid malformation (CCAM) or bronchopulmonary sequestration (BPS), because it includes better the diagnosis given by the ultrasound, the prognosis and the therapeutic attitude. However, for teaching purposes, we will continue to keep the separate terms for each entity in part. The thoracic-pulmonary anomalies incidence is the following: CCAM—BPS around 40%, CDH around 40% and hydrothorax and other anomalies around 10% [1, 2].

The ultrasound investigation of the thorax is based on emphasizing of the following parameters:

- The size and shape of the rib cage,

- The aspect of the ribs, the pulmonary echogenicity,

- The mediastinal shift absence/presence,

- The diaphragm curvature.

The standard echographic image for assessing the fetal thoracic anatomy is represented by the four-chamber view image of the fetal heart. If a thoracic lesion is evident in this section, then it is necessary to subsequently use the midsagittal, parasagittal and coronal sections. In the midsagittal and parasagittal view, the presence of the diaphragm and the net delimitation between the thorax and the abdomen can be identified. The objectives, in case a congenital bronchopulmonary malformation is detected, are as follows:

- The description of the pulmonary anomaly

- The exclusion of other associated anomalies

- Establishing the prognosis

- Determining the effectiveness of the fetal therapy

According to the European Respiratory Society, we need to keep in mind the following aspects [1]:

- The bilaterality/unilaterality of the lesion,

- The localization (lateral or central),

- The cystic or hyperechoic characteristic,

- Cysts (number size, content), the presence or absence of a nutritive vessel,

- Presence of hydrothorax,

- Mediastinal shift.

Thus, taking all these elements into account, we can classify the various thoracic anomalies as following:

- Unilateral hyperechoic lesions: CDH right sided, CCAM type III, BPS

- Unilateral anechoic lesions: CDH left sided, CCAM type I, unilateral fetal hydrothorax, bronchogenic cyst.

- Bilateral hyperechoic lesions: laryngeal atresia-CHAOS (congenital airway obstruction syndrome)

- Bilateral anechoic lesions: bilateral fetal hydrothorax

- Median hyperechoic lesions: mediastinal teratoma or hemangioma

- Median anechoic lesion: CDH

Depending on the location of the chest masses, we should consider the following possibilities:

- Left hemithorax: CCAM, CDH, BPS

- Right hemithorax: CDH, CCAM, BPS bronchogenic cyst, teratoma, hamartoma

- Anterior mediastinum: teratoma, thymoma

- Posterior mediastinum: teratoma, neuroblastoma, esophageal duplication

- Diaphragm: CDH

With the advantage of three-dimensional ultrasound (3D-US), we often can clarify the diagnosis of lung abnormalities. We can use 3D rendering, or reconstruction of the coronal plane, or minimal rendering mode, 3D with TUI (tomographic ultrasound image). With these ultrasound applications, it is possible to establish: liver position, liver outline, diaphragm outline, relationship between liver, pulmonary tissue and heart, presence of thoracic hypoplasia.

2. Congenital cystic adenomatoid malformation of the lung (CCAM)

2.1. Definition and incidence

Congenital cystic adenomatoid malformation of the lung (CCAM) is a lesion that is characterized by the presence of a mass of multicystic pulmonary tissue and is accompanied by bronchial proliferation. Its occurrence can be explained by:

- The lack of maturation of the bronchial tissue during the pseudoglandular stage of pulmonary development, which is between the 5th and 6th week of gestation [2]

- Focal pulmonary dysplasia with hamartomatous development at the terminal bronchioles [2]

- Secondary to the airway obstruction [3]

The estimated incidence is of 1 in 25,000 births, up to 1 in 30,000 births [4]. Most ultrasound detected CCAM lesions are unilateral and only 2–3% of them are bilateral and they are more frequently encountered in male fetuses [5]. In the case of unilateral lesions, a single lobe is usually involved and in rare situation it is the whole lung. Vascularization of the multicystic mass comes from a branch of the pulmonary artery. Recently, Stocker has classified CCAM in 5 types, depending on the group of airways involved: Type 0, the lesion is bronchial. Type 1, the lesion is bronchial/bronchiolar. Type 2, the lesion is bronchiolar. Type 3, the lesion is bronchiolar/alveolar. Type 4, the lesion is peripheral [6, 7]. A more practical classification is that which considers the ultrasound antenatal aspect, proposed by Adzick [8] and which describes the lesions as macrocystic or microcystic. Thus, CCAM has the following classification: Macrocystic type I with single or multiple cysts larger than 2 cm in diameter, CCAM type 2 with multiple cysts smaller than 2 cm and larger than 0.5 cm in diameter and type 3 with multiple cysts, less than 5 mm in size and with a hyperechogenic aspect. By advancing Adzick's classification, a simpler ultrasound classification was established by Wilson [9]. Thus, the ultrasound appearance is a cystic variant and a solid (or microcystic) variant. The cystic variant is multilocular lesions with cysts of various sizes from a few millimeters to 10 cm. The solid microcystic variant comprises a hyperechogenic mass.

2.2. Ultrasound diagnosis

CCAM ultrasound diagnosis is used for pointing out a cystic or solid lung tumor growth with the absence of systemic Doppler vasculature (**Figure 1**).

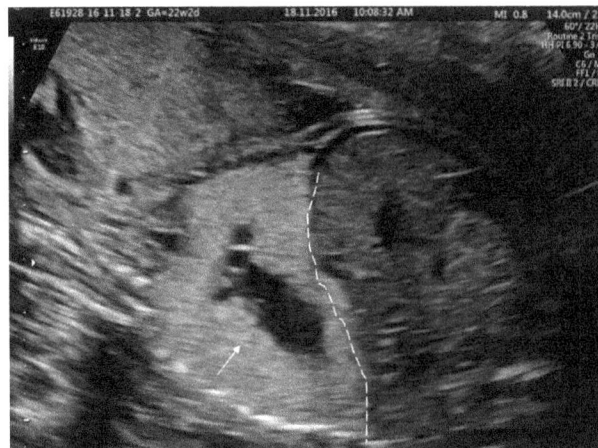

Figure 1. CCAM microcystic, parasagittal view: arrow—lung mass, line—diaphragm.

It is possible to highlight the vascular flow of the lesion that comes from a branch of the pulmonary artery. The use of color Doppler is mandatory to highlight the absence of systemic vasculature and the presence of pulmonary vasculature for CCAM. From the ultrasound point of view, CCAM will be classified in macrocystic and microcystic (**Figures 2–4**).

Both the macrocystic form and the microcystic form can cause fetal hydrops and mediastinal shift (**Figure 5**).

The macrocystic types are rarely accompanied by fetal hydrops. The size of the lesion determines whether a fetus will develop hydrops or not [9]. Large scale macrocystic lesions cause mediastinal shift and cardiac decompensation, accompanied by increased venous central pressure, followed by the appearance of the fetal hydrops (**Figure 6**).

What is important to emphasize, is that the degree of the mediastinal shift has no predictive value for the appearance of the hydrops.

It should be underlined that there are CCAM hybrid lesions which refer to the presence of both pulmonary and systemic circulation that originates directly from the descending aorta [10].

The ultrasound differential diagnosis will consider the following: congenital diaphragmatic hernia (CDH), bronchopulmonary sequestration (BS), pericardial teratoma, enteric or bronchogenic cysts, bronchial atresia, esophageal duplication, neuroblastoma, brain heterotopia.

The differential diagnosis from CDH is not easy. The macrocystic form of CCAM can be confused with CDH left-sided; the intrathoracic stomach may resemble the macrocystic form. Highlighting intestinal peristalsis or emptying the herniated stomach can yield the diagnosis in favor of CDH. In addition, the size of the abdomen is normal, and the abdominal organs are in the normal position in case of CCAM (**Figures 7** and **8**).

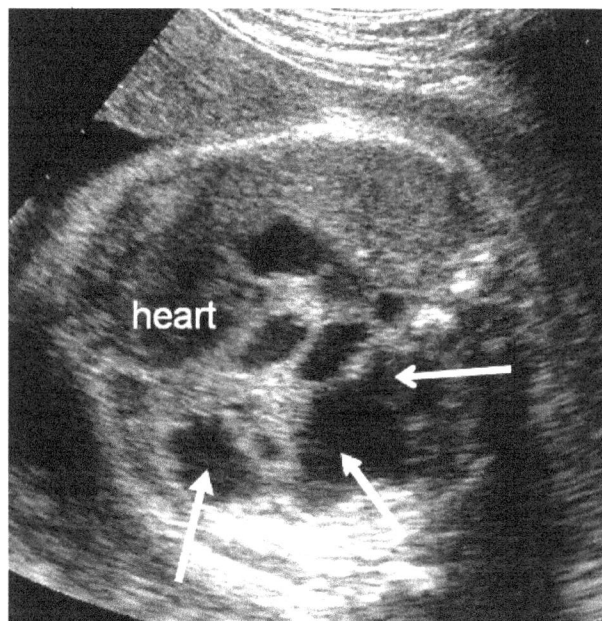

Figure 2. CCAM macrocystic: white arrow—lung cyst.

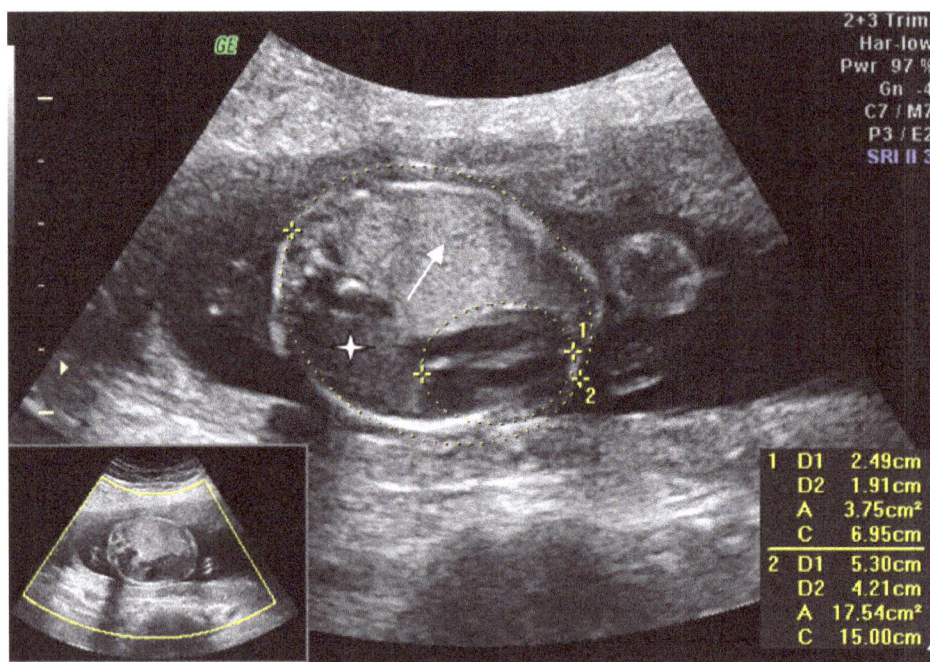

Figure 3. CCAM microcystic: arrow—lung mass, star—normal lung.

Bronchogenic cysts are uniloculated, rarely multicystic, located adjacent to the bronchus, but difficult to distinguish from the macrocystic form of CCAM. Pericardial teratoma may contain large cysts but they are usually associated with the pericardial fluid. The main differential diagnosis of microcystic form of CCAM is with BPS and CDH right

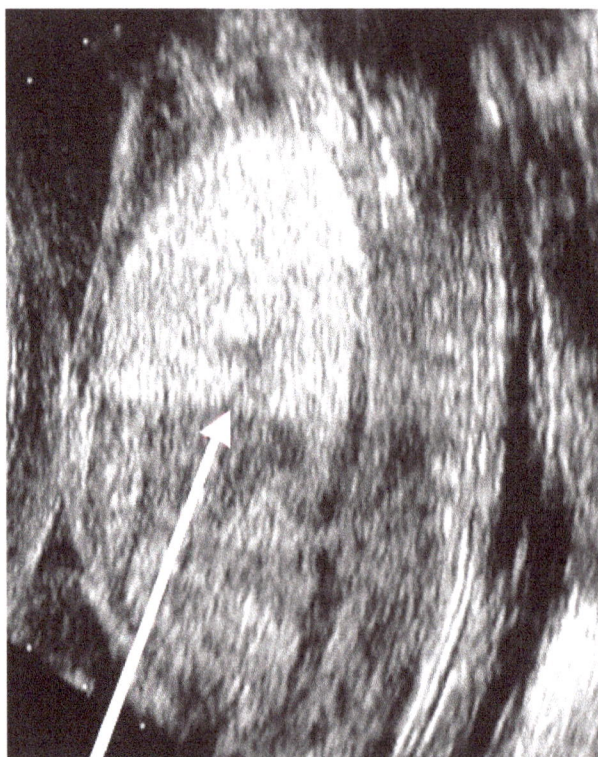

Figure 4. CCAM microcystic: white line—enhancement of diaphragm.

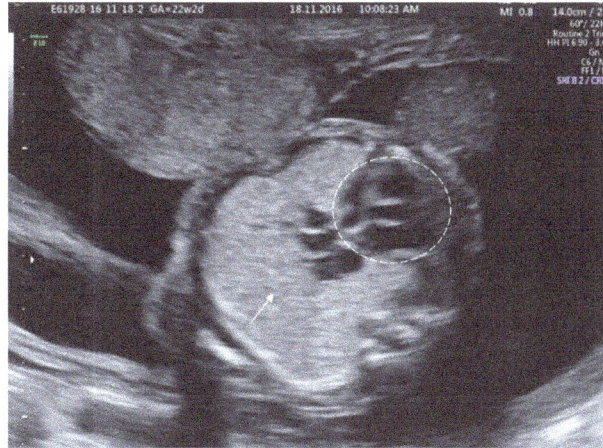

Figure 5. CCAM microcystic: arrow—lung mass, circle—cardiac shift.

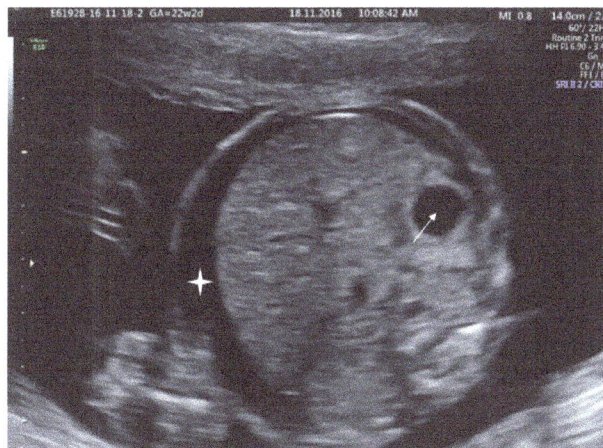

Figure 6. Fetal hydrops: arrow—stomach and star—ascites.

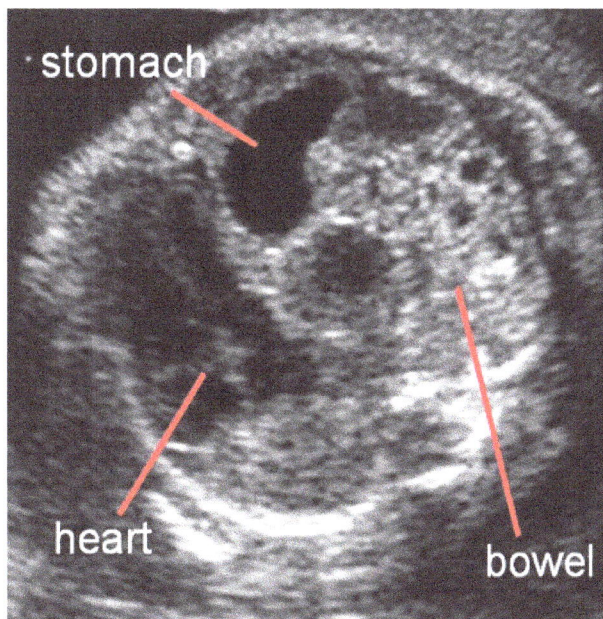

Figure 7. Differential diagnosis CCAM versus CDH left.

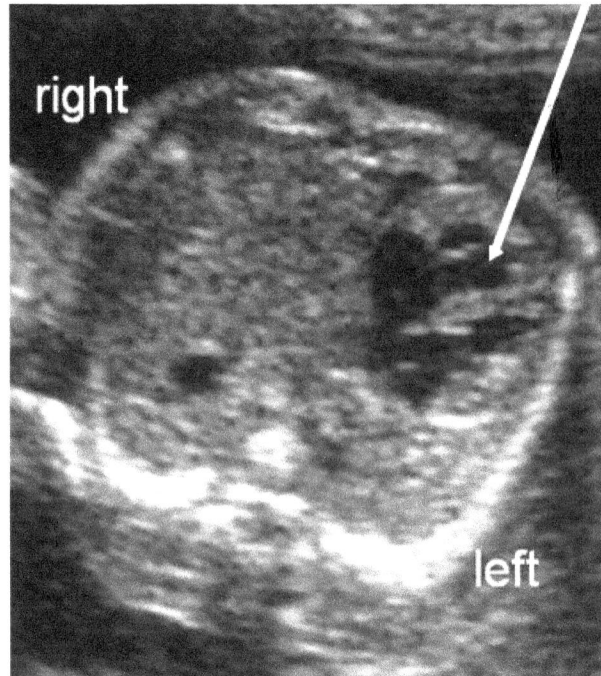

Figure 8. Differential diagnosis CCAM versus CDH right: white line—heart shift.

associated with liver herniation. Basically, the main distinguishing ultrasound element is that in BPS, vascularization originates from the systemic circulation, primarily the direct branch from the descending aorta, which can be easily demonstrated with Doppler color or HD-flow Color Doppler [9, 10]. The differentiation criteria between CCAM and BPS are shown in **Table 1**.

Therefore, the identification of the systemic circulation for a lung tumor mass is pathognomonic for BPS. Recently, Cass described 6 cases of CCAM that also had systemic vasculature and specific histological elements for BPS and CCAM, so these lesions were called hybrid lesions [10]. CDH right with hernia of the liver determines a significant mediastinal shift and secondary pulmonary compression. The highly hyperechogenic aspect of the CCAM microcystic form requires the differentiation from neuroblastoma as well. The association of CCAM with extrapulmonary abnormalities ranges from 0 to 26%, renal agenesis or dysgenesis being the most common associations [11, 12].

	CCAM	BPS
Location	Any lobes	Inferior left
Vascularization	Pulmonary	Systemic
Airway communication	Yes	No
Cysts	Yes	No

Table 1. Differential diagnosis CCAM versus BPS.

2.3. Prognostic

CCAM is not associated with syndromes, the risk of chromosomal anomalies being extremely low. In the absence of hydrops, the long-term outcome of the fetuses with CCAM is good. The incidence of hydrops is 10% in cases of a large cystic mass [12]. Termination of pregnancy before 24-week gestation remains an option for the couple. In cases of prenatal diagnosis of CCAM, the parents should be counseled about the good prognosis even though the CCAM could need a surgical postnatal resection.

The most important factor for prognosis is the presence of hydrops, which is the most important predictor of poor prognosis. If hydrops is present, the chances of survival are very low, perinatal demise being the most frequent outcome, around 100%.

Another prognostic factor has been established with the use of 3D ultrasound, in determining the CAM volume ratio, (CVR) [13]. This parameter is calculated by dividing the volume of CCAM by the HC (head circumference). That is diameter $(L \times AP \times T) \times 0.52$ divided by the HC. If CVR is more than 1.6 the incidence of hydrops is 75%.

2.4. Prenatal management

It is important to emphasize that the mass has an important potential growth between 20 and 26-week gestation, then there is a plateau, and afterwards the mass tends to regress. Thus, since the volume of a mass is not expected to increase after 26 weeks, and if there is no hydrops, then it is unlikely for the hydrops to appear after 26-week gestation. In cases of large masses, it is recommended to plan delivery in a tertiary center because of the risk of lung hypoplasia, cardiovascular decompensation and high mortality. The postnatal risk is high for large masses and low for small-medium masses (**Figure 9**).

Prenatal fetal therapy is indicated in cases that develop hydrops or cardiac failure.

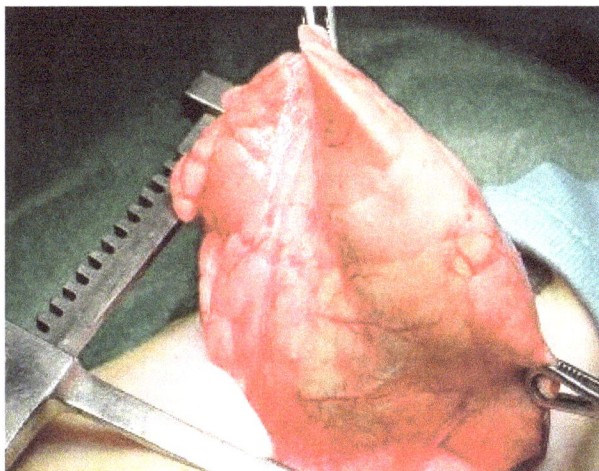

Figure 9. CCAM microcystic intraoperator view.

Karyotyping is not an indication if other anomalies are not present. However, amniocentesis for karyotyping is appropriate if fetal treatment is balanced or when the parents request it [14]. The attitude in CCAM associated with hydrops depends on the CVR value. Thus, if the CVR is less than 1.6 and we do not have a dominant cyst, then weekly fetal monitoring is indicated to identify early signs of hydrops. If we are dealing with a dominant cyst, even if CVR is less than 1.6, the fetus has a major risk of developing hydrops and a thoracoamniotic shunt should be considered at first signs of hydrops appearance. If CVR is above 1.6, the likelihood of developing hydrops is very high and monitoring is required 2 times a week.

The fetal therapy available nowadays is as follows: corticotherapy, in utero fine needle aspiration of macrocysts or thoracoamniotic shunt, laser vascular ablation and, finally, sclerotherapy [15]. A fetus with hydrops below 32-week gestation with a macrocystic lesion of CCAM will benefit from thoracoamniotic shunt. Also, the surgical resection is an option.

Corticosteroid treatment can be followed by the regression of the mass and it is especially indicated in cases of microcystic lesions. If CVR is equal to 1.6, corticosteroid therapy is indicated. Either fine needle aspiration or thoracoamniotic shunt improve the outcome of fetuses with macrocystic CCAM complicated with hydrops/hydrothorax. Microcystic lesions resulting in fetal hydrops of CCAM may need laser ablation of the feeding vessel, to improve survival and with regression of the lesion. The sclerotherapy is also indicated in microcystic cases and it is used Ethanolamine. But it must be emphasized that in most cases fetal CCAM needs only serial fetal surveillance, every 2 or 3 weeks, to confirm regression in size or the remaining at the same size.

3. Bronchopulmonary sequestration

3.1. Definition and incidence

Bronchopulmonary sequestration (BPS) represents a cystic mass of nonfunctioning pulmonary tissue with the blood supply from the systemic vessels and not from the pulmonary arteries.

The incidence reported is 0.5–6.0% of all prenatally diagnosed pulmonary lesions [16].

Pulmonary sequestration can be: intrapulmonary and extrapulmonary. Intrapulmonary sequestration (IPS) represents almost 75% of the cases, but this form is rarely diagnosed in utero. The abnormal lung tissue lies within the normal lung tissue. This variety is produced by the bronchial obstruction.

Extrapulmonary sequestration (EPS) is the most commonly form diagnosed in the prenatal life. The abnormal lung tissue has its own pleural covering, so the abnormal pulmonary tissue is separated from the normal pulmonary tissue and the pathologic tissue drains in the systemic circulation. The extrapulmonary sequestration is considered to be an abnormal pulmonary tissue that has no connection with the bronchial tree. The vascularization is provided by arteries emerging from the aorta.

3.2. Ultrasound diagnosis

The prenatal ultrasound diagnosis of bronchopulmonary sequestration is based on the following elements:

- hyperechoic mass

- a mass with triangular shape, with a paraspinal localization, usually in the base of the left fetal chest.

- small or moderate size

- the large size can cause fetal hydrops

- color Doppler confirm the origin of the tumoral vessels as belonging to systemic vessels

Typically, BPS vascularization, and more specifically EPS, is supplied by a single artery, originating from the aorta (**Figure 10**).

The veins of the BPS drain in the azygos system and hemiazygos. At the opposite end, the venous drainage of the IPS is achieved through the pulmonary veins [17]. The hydrothorax can be associated with BPS, usually ipsilateral, and if it is important, it can cause a mediastinal shift.

Differential diagnosis includes the following: CCAM, bronchial atresia, lobar emphysema, CDH-particularly when the liver or spleen is the only component of herniation, mediastinal teratoma, neuroblastoma, mesoblastic nephroma, segmental thoracic obstruction, and thoracic kidney.

The differential diagnosis between CCAM and BPS, when no systemic feeding vessel is evident, is based on the echogenicity of the mass: the presence of cyst suggests CCAM, while the presence of a hyperechogenic triangular mass suggests BPS (**Figure 11**).

For extrapulmonary BPS, the differential diagnosis includes: mesoblastic nephroma, and neuroblastoma.

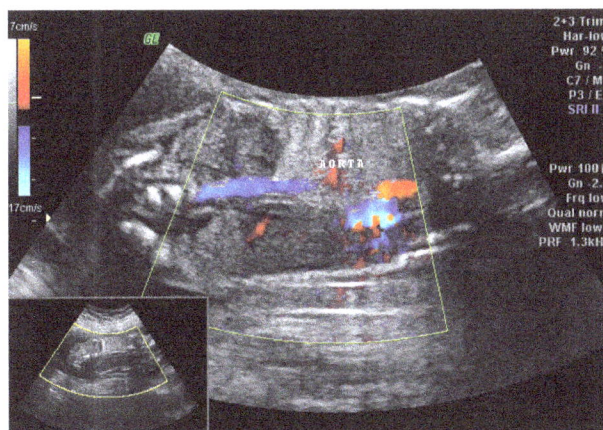

Figure 10. Bronchopulmonary sequestration: systemic vascularization.

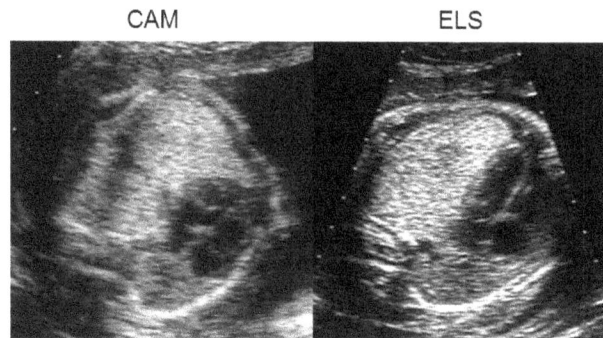

Figure 11. Differential diagnosis CCAM versus BPS.

3.3. Prognosis

The prognosis of BPS is favorable in the absence of other associated abnormalities. In many case series it was found that, similar to CCAM evolution and in BPS cases, there is often present a regression of the lesion [18, 19]. However, in fetuses with BPS associated with fetal hydrops, the prognosis is poor (**Figure 12**).

Fetal hydrops occurs only if a tension hydrothorax develops. The cause of unilateral hydrothorax associated with BPS is not well-defined. The torsion of a vascular pedicle or abnormal pressure gradient between the systemic artery and the pulmonary vein may be the cause [19]. Regardless the etiology, the persistence of the hydrothorax causes pulmonary compression with pulmonary hypoplasia and the impairment of the caval venous drainage due to mediastinal shift.

3.4. Prenatal management

In isolated BPS karyotyping is not mandatory, but it is recommended if any other abnormality is associated. Fetal MRI may be useful for differential diagnosis. The family may choose to terminate the pregnancy if the diagnosis is established before 24 weeks and it is associated with other abnormalities such as: esophageal atresia, neurenteric cyst, CDH, pulmonary hypoplasia, cardiac

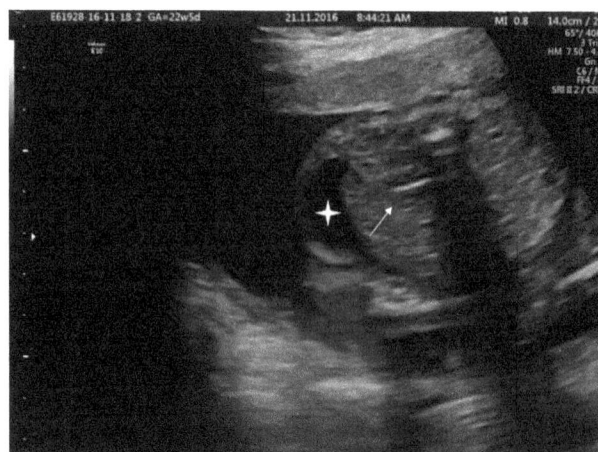

Figure 12. Fetal hydrops and BPS: arrow—BPS mass, star—hydrothorax.

anomalies and bronchogenic cyst. Fetal monitoring is required in the prenatal period, to identify the appearance of the hydrothorax. A fetus with isolated BPS has good chances of survival in the absence of hydrops, polyhydramnios or pleural effusion, because it can regress in 80% of cases. Fetuses over 30-week gestation should be considered for preterm delivery and ex-utero surgical resection. In the presence of hydrops before 30 weeks, placing a thoracoamniotic shunt may be offered. In hydrothorax, installing the thoraco-amniotic shunt may prevent the development of fetal hydrops. The postnatal therapy consists of the endoscopic removal of the pulmonary mass and alternatively the selective embolization of the artery that feeds the tumor [20–22].

In brief, for the two main anomalies CCAM and BPS, we can apply the following therapeutic scheme:

- CCAM/BPS stable as dimensions and stationary as evolution: near-term birth and ex-utero resection

- Regressive CCAM/BPS: term delivery and evaluation

- Progressive CCAM/BPS towards hydrops and mediastinal shift: it depends on the gestational age of the fetus. Thus, if it is less than 32 weeks, then a thoraco-amniotic shunt or resection in utero and cesarean delivery is recommended near term. After 32 weeks' gestational age, the iatrogenic preterm birth and resection ex utero are recommended.

4. Pulmonary hypoplasia and pulmonary agenesis

4.1. Definition and incidence

Congenital pulmonary hypoplasia consists of the lowering of the lung volume in comparison to the lung volume corresponding to the gestational age. The causes of pulmonary hypoplasia are represented by: congenital diaphragmatic hernia (CDH), oligohydramnios, skeletal dysplasia, chest tumors, neuromuscular disorders that obstruct fetal respiratory movements. A rare cause is represented by the obstructive cardiac abnormalities of the right-sided heart, which may be accompanied either by the absence of the development of a single lung or the absence of the development of both lungs. Regardless the mechanism, pulmonary hypoplasia is responsible for the neonatal mortality, of 10–15% [23]. Pulmonary agenesis can be classified into three groups [23, 24]: in group 1, there are bronchial and lung agenesis, in group 2 there is a rudimentary bronchus without bronchial tissue and in group 3 it is a bronchial hypoplasia and a hypoplasia of lung tissue. Pulmonary agenesis is usually unilateral, and occurs at 4 weeks of gestation. The etiology of this anomaly is unknown. The incidence of pulmonary agenesis, either unilateral or bilateral, is very low, 0.0097% or 1 at 10,000 pregnancy [22]. More than half of the fetuses with pulmonary agenesis have other associated abnormalities: gastrointestinal, cardiovascular and genitourinary. Unilateral pulmonary agenesis may be associated with numerous other abnormalities: patent ductus arteriosus (PDA), atrial and ventricular septal defects, anomalous pulmonary venous drainage, tracheoesophageal fistula and duodenal atresia, hemivertebrae with scoliosis, facial abnormalities and limb abnormalities.

4.2. Ultrasound diagnosis

The ultrasound diagnosis is established on the axial section of 4 chambers of the heart. Unilateral pulmonary hypoplasia determines the mediastinal shift to the hemithorax where the lung is absent and the existing lung is highly hyperechogenic. Usually, unilateral pulmonary hypoplasia (especially the right one) is part of the scimitar syndrome, which is an abnormal venous return in the inferior vena cava (both pulmonary veins are absent and replaced with a collecting vein that drains into the inferior vena cava and which at 3D ultrasound resembles a scimitar). In the case of unilateral pulmonary agenesis, the ultrasound aspect is somewhat similar to the one made in case of CDH, by the mediastinal shift, but there is no abdominal viscera noticed inside the rib cage. The color Doppler can be used to highlight the absence of the pulmonary vascular system. Pay attention to differential diagnosis of CDH with pulmonary compression and CCAM, for unilateral lung agenesis advocates the mediastinal shift to the agenesis side and the enlarged hyperechogenic lung herniated in the contralateral chest through the mediastinum.

Bilateral pulmonary hypoplasia is caused by a skeletal dysplasia that is associated with a significant reduction in thoracic volume. Quite rarely, bilateral pulmonary hypoplasia is primary, and it is more commonly secondary to a prolonged oligohydramnios after a long lasting very premature rupture of membrane. The ultrasound diagnosis is also done on the axial section of four chambers view of the heart. The aspect is that the heart fills all the thorax, there is no lung tissue and the rib cage is extremely small. There are nomograms in the literature for thoracic circumference versus gestational age or cardiothoracic ratio.

There is an association of unilateral/bilateral pulmonary agenesis with facial, radial anomalies, genitourinary anomalies, polyhydramnios or oligohydramnios.

The differential diagnosis of unilateral agenesis is done with CDH, CCAM and BPS.

4.3. Prognosis

Bilateral pulmonary hypoplasia is fatal. The risk of chromosomal anomalies is rare, but the risk of association with non-chromosomal syndromes is high. A study comparing eight echographic parameters for the prediction of lethal pulmonary hypoplasia showed that the use of the pulmonary area/abdominal circumference and thoracic circumference/abdominal circumference ratio are the most clinically useful in the prediction of bilateral pulmonary hypoplasia [23]. In the case of unilateral pulmonary agenesis, the duration of neonatal survival is higher for the left one in comparison to right one, probably due to the cardiac and mediastinal shift which is with less distortion of the blood vessels and bronchi. The fetuses with unilateral agenesis have a neonatal risk for repeated bronchopulmonary infections and respiratory distress syndrome. The cause of high neonatal mortality is the pulmonary infection and the association with cardiac abnormalities.

4.4. Prenatal management

In the case of unilateral hypoplasia, no karyotyping is required, but the birth is recommended to occur in a tertiary center because of the risk of orotracheal intubation immediately after the delivery. Bilateral lung agenesis is incompatible with life. In the case of the primary bilateral pulmonary hypoplasia or associated with skeletal dysplasia, the importance of a correct diagnosis is not only for the current pregnancy that will evolve to the exitus of the fetus but also for a future pregnancy because skeletal dysplasia may not occur sporadically but exhibit recessive inheritance. In unilateral pulmonary hypoplasia associated with the scimitar syndrome, neonatal ventilation may be required. Fetal MRI may be useful in distinguishing between the pulmonary agenesis and CCAM [23, 24]. At the same time, the exclusion of associated fetal abnormalities can be done by MRI, in particular: ipsilateral upper extremities, mandible, face, or kidneys. There is no fetal intervention available in pulmonary agenesis.

5. Bronchogenic cysts

5.1. Definition and incidence

It comes from the primitive foregut early in the embryogenesis. It contains the columnar ciliary epithelium and the cartridges. They are usually located intrapulmonary but may also be mediastinal [25], or intrapericardial. They may also be located cervical or infradiaphragmatic. They can basically be located anywhere on the tracheoesophageal tract. It is extremely rare.

5.2. Ultrasound diagnosis

The diagnosis of bronchogenic cysts can be established on the axial section of the four chambers of the heart. It appears as a unilateral, circumscribed, thin wall lesion (**Figure 13**).

They may rarely be multilocular. The bronchogenic mediastinal cyst can compress the trachea or bronchi so that the distal lung becomes dense and expansive, in this way lending the specific echographic aspect for the cystic adenomatoid malformation [26]. The differential diagnosis includes: CCAM, esophageal duplication cyst, pericardial cyst, duplication cyst and lymphangioma. In CCAM, the tissue surrounding the cyst is hyperechogenic.

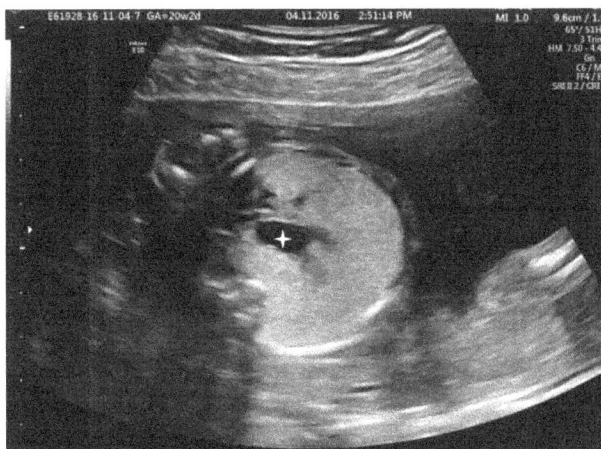

Figure 13. Bronchogenic cyst: star—lung mass.

5.3. Prognosis

One of the few negative prognostic factors is the size of the mass.

5.4. Prenatal management

The presence of bronchogenic cysts does not cause the death of the fetus in utero [25, 26]. It is not recommended to perform karyotyping because the risk of associated chromosomal abnormalities is extremely low. There is, however, the risk of an emergency intubation at birth, so birth is recommended to take place in a tertiary center.

6. Congenital high airway obstruction syndrome (CHAOS—laryngeal atresia)

6.1. Definition and incidence

Congenital high airway obstruction syndrome (CHAOS) occurs due to laryngeal atresia, tracheal atresia, or laryngeal cyst [27]. There are three types of laryngeal atresia: type I-agenesis of glottis, Type II agenesis of larynx, type III-agenesis of both [28]. The laryngeal atresia is difficult to differentiate using ultrasound from tracheal atresia and both are diagnosed based on intrathoracic signs. The exact incidence of this syndrome is unknown, but it is an extremely rare abnormality. The cause of tracheal/laryngeal atresia is not clear, but it appears to be a vascularization deficit during the embryogenic period [29, 30].

6.2. Ultrasound diagnosis

The ultrasound diagnosis is done on the four-chamber axial section. It is noted that both lungs are hyperechogenic, large in size, flattening the diaphragm due to the large volume of the lungs, the heart appears smaller due to the compression exerted by the lungs, the axis of the heart is zero, the dilatation of the tracheobronchial tree can be seen by the accumulation of liquid at its level (**Figure 14**).

On the coronal section, the dilated trachea and bifurcation of this, as well as the diaphragmatic flattening, can be better emphasized. The differential diagnosis of CHAOS does not have what entity to do, because it is a unique anomaly. At most, bilateral CCAM can be considered in the differential diagnosis, but bilateral CCAM is very rare and it does not present a severely increased volume of both lungs.

6.3. Prognosis

This anomaly is fatal. It may be part of the Fraser syndrome [29, 30], which includes: laryngeal atresia, renal agenesis, oligoamnios, microphthalmia, syndactyly, polydactyly. The prognosis is even more severe because the recessive autosomal is transmitted. The risk of chromosomal anomalies is low.

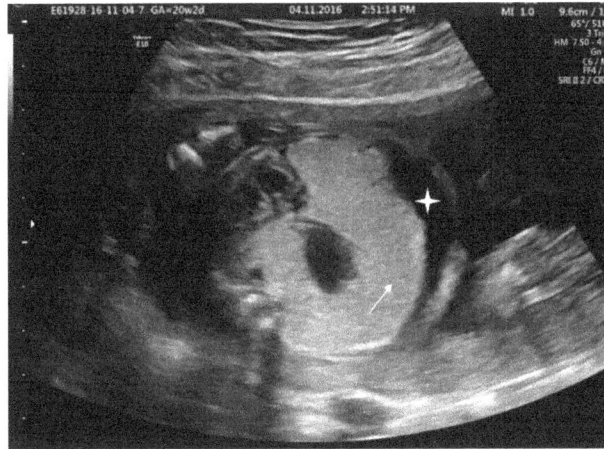

Figure 14. CHAOS: dilatation of tracheobronchial tree.

6.4. Prenatal management

Karyotyping is not indicated because the risk of chromosomal abnormalities is low. The ultrasound should also focus on the exclusion of structural heart or kidney abnormalities. Delivery should take place in a tertiary center. The only option that exists to save a fetus with CHAOS is the EXIT procedure (ex utero intrapartum treatment). So far, only 9 cases have survived through this procedure [29].

7. Fetal hydrothorax

7.1. Definition and incidence

Fetal hydrothorax (FHT) represents the accumulation of fluid in the pleural cavity, between the parietal and the visceral pleura. It can be unilateral or bilateral. It can be isolated or in the context of a generalized hydrops, or associated with other fetal abnormalities.

The incidence is not specified given the variability of the causes, but in the antenatal period, the secondary causes of hydrothorax are more common [31]. The causes that can lead to the occurrence of fetal hydrothorax are multiple: congenital infection (parvovirus, TORCH), iso-immunization, congestive heart failure, Down syndrome, Turner syndrome. Primary FHT is called chylothorax. Secondary FHT usually appears secondary to chromosomal, cardiac, gastrointestinal and infectious abnormalities. FHT generally precedes the installation of fetal hydrops. The appearance of primary FHT is due to a structural defect in the lymphatic system: the obstruction of bronchomediastinal trunks to the venous system, congenital absence of the thoracic duct, congenital hypoplasia of the pulmonary lymphatic vessel [31, 32]. It is a diagnostic of exclusion. In general, primary FHT occurs as a result of the obstruction of secondary lymphatic drainage to a heterogeneous group of developmental defects of the lymphatic system. Unilateral FHT may happen due to a unilateral pathological process such as: congenital diaphragmatic hernia, cystic adenomatoid malformation, pulmonary hypoplasia.

7.2. Ultrasound diagnosis

The diagnosis of fetal hydrothorax is established on the axial image of the four chambers of the heart, as an anechoic area around the pulmonary tissue which limits the mediastinum. Effusions can be unilateral or bilateral (**Figure 15**).

The hydrothorax aspect is that of a peripheral anechoic space in the thorax, compressing the lung tissue. In the case of large bilateral effusions, the aspect is that of the lungs balloting in the rib cage. At the same time, mediastinal shift and the eversion of the diaphragm occur with the displacement of the heart to the contralateral side and they can cause the disruption of the hemodynamic function and the installation of nonimmune hydrops. If the pleural effusion is part of the nonimmune hydrops, then it is also possible to see the edema of the thoracic subcutaneous tissue. It is important to note that FHT associates with the polyhidramnios in over 50% of cases, either due to a mediastinal shift that causes the compression of the esophagus or because of an alteration in the production of amniotic fluid by the compressed lungs.

The differential diagnosis is important because it should be determined whether FHT is primary or secondary. Primary hydrothorax is usually a chylothorax and it is unilateral and is a diagnostic of exclusion. However, the fetus with trisomy 21, Noonan syndrome, and Turner syndrome, may present either unilaterally or bilaterally hydrothorax [31]. For secondary hydrothorax, evidence of specific echographic elements for CDH, CCAM, BPS determines the diagnosis. In the case of the fetuses with hydrops, the presence of fetal anemia should be excluded.

7.3. Prognosis

The most important element of prognosis is whether fetal hydrothorax is associated with non-immune fetal hydrops, because in this situation the fetal mortality is increased. Other negative prognostic factors are FHT associated with cardiac abnormalities or with central nervous system anomalies. The only positive prognostic factor is the presence of FHT without another associated anomaly or other fluid effusion with another location. Isolated small FHT at the fetus without any other abnormalities, without hydrops or abnormal karyotype, has a favorable prognosis, because the fetus usually tolerates well small effusions [31, 32]. What is important to remember is that 10–25% of the cases of chylothorax can regress spontaneously

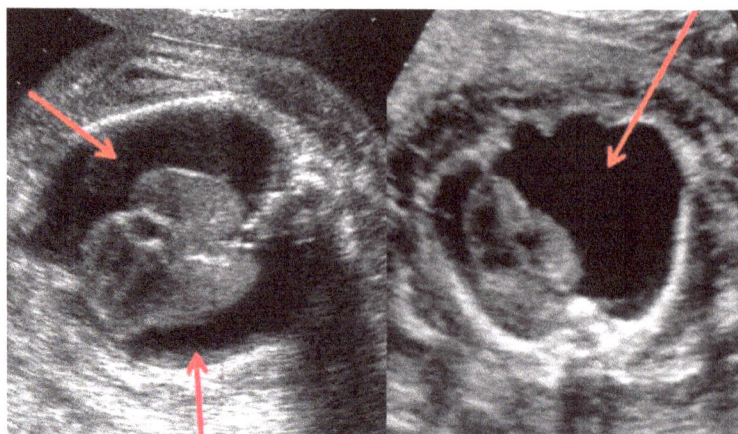

Figure 15. Bilateral hydrothorax: arrow—hydrothorax.

or after only a single drainage [32]. Delivery by vaginal route is an option although there is an increase incidence of the rate of cesarean section [33].

7.4. Prenatal management

It is mandatory to determine the karyotype in FHT due to the increased risk of association with chromosomal anomalies. Even if the fetus tolerates small isolated effusions, a serial echographic surveillance is required because small hydrothorax can progress rapidly to large effusions that may have negative hemodynamic consequences. Therefore, ultrasound monitoring is recommended every 1 or 2 weeks, due to the risk of polyhidramnios and preterm delivery. Birth in a tertiary center is recommended.

If FHT was diagnosed before 24 weeks, the therapeutic interruption of the pregnancy is an option. If the fetus with FHT has more than 32 weeks, then the serial ultrasound at one or 2 weeks distance is recommended, but we can also consider thoraco-amniotic shunt. If the fetus has less than 32 weeks we have three options: thoracocentesis, thoracoamniotic shunt, thoracomaternal cutaneous drainage. The initial step is the thoracocentesis and diagnosis for cell count, culture, or the viral culture. In general, thoracocentesis other than for diagnosis is ineffective because after it is done a re-accumulation of the pleural fluid occurs. The rapidity with which the effusion accumulates after the initial puncture is an indicator of the pleural effusion severity. For this reason, pleural cavity decompression is done through thoracoamniotic shunt. Large FHT is drained through thoracoamniotic shunt especially if hydrops is present. Shunting is especially effective if the fetus has less than 32 weeks of gestation [34]. The failure rate for thoracoamniotic shunt is of 26% [34, 35]. Shunt complications are: blockage, migration, fetal death. If a thoracoamniotic shunt is mounted the incidence of survival increases from 10 to 60%.

8. Fetal mediastinal cysts

8.1. Definition and incidence

Fetal mediastinal cysts are represented by: pericardial cyst, thymic cyst, esophageal duplication cyst, neurenteric cyst. The incidence of these masses is not known because they are rare pathological entities and only case reports are reported. The pericardial cyst is located at the costophrenic right angle level. The pericardial cyst is covered by mesothelium and has fluid content, and is usually asymptomatic. If the size of the cyst is important, then it can be associated with fetal hydrops, or with the change in heart function at birth [17]. If the pericardial cyst size is reduced in size, it can also regress.

The thymic cyst is very rare, representing 4% of postnatal mediastinal cystic masses [17, 35]. Thymic cysts are asymptomatic, but the prenatal diagnosis is possible.

The esophageal duplication cyst exhibits ectopic gastric mucosa, communicating with the gastrointestinal lumen. Sometimes they may not communicate with the gastrointestinal lumen [17, 36]. The communication with the gastrointestinal lumen is located either above the diaphragm or below the diaphragm.

The neurenteric cyst has a connection with the meninges and the spinal cord and it is usually associated with congenital scoliosis or spina bifida.

8.2. Ultrasound diagnosis

The prenatal diagnosis of esophageal duplication cysts is based on the spherical aspect of the cyst, rarely on the tubular aspect, but with a thick, hyperechogenic wall determined by the presence of the gastric mucosa. Usually, the cyst is connected to the esophagus. If the dimensions of the esophageal duplication cyst are large due to the compression effect on the esophagus, the appearance of polyhidramnios may occur [37, 38]. The thymic cyst is formed from remnants of the thymopharangeal duct; they are usually very small and localized to the anterior mediastinum [38]. The ultrasound aspect is of a transonic mass surrounded by the thymic tissue and located in the previous mediastinum.

Pericardial cyst, originating from the pericardium, appears at ultrasound examination as a thin walled, unilocular, fluid-filled transonic mass in the left or the right of the cardiophrenic angle. The cyst wall may communicate with the pericardial space.

Neurenteric cysts are very rare; only eight cases have been diagnosed in the prenatal stage by the ultrasound [37–39]. If the size of the cyst is large, it can exert cardiac compression with the subsequent appearance of the hydrops. It can also exert compressive phenomena on the bronchi, which causes neonatal respiratory distress. Association with anomalies of the membrane can be encountered [40].

The differential diagnosis among the described mediastinal masses is sometimes difficult. Several elements should be considered: pericardial cyst is located in the cardiophrenic angle of the right hemothorax, thymic cysts are located in the anterior mediastinum and are surrounded by thymic tissue, and the enteric duplication cyst is in close contact with the esophagus [41, 42]. For differential diagnosis, we can also use fetal MRI. The origin of the mass can be established sometimes only after perinatal autopsy [43].

8.3. Prognosis

The prognostic thymic cyst is favorable without affecting the condition of the fetus. The pericardial cyst can determine hydrops due to the compression on the heart. However, sometimes even in the case of reduced size, the pericardial cyst can be resorbed. The neurenteric cyst can cause cardiac compression and the appearance of hydrops as secondary effect. The esophageal duplication cyst determines polyhidramnios due to compression on the esophagus. The risk of chromosomal anomalies is absent, so karyotyping is not recommended.

8.4. Prenatal management

The indication of in utero treatment is represented by the presence of hydrops and the presence of compression of the tracheobronchial tree [44]. Puncture with cyst aspiration or the EXIT techniques are the treatment options in such cases.

Acknowledgements

We would like to thank Rahimian Hadi MD, PhD, Regina Maria Hospital, Bucharest, for **Figures 3** and **4**.

Author details

Cringu Ionescu

Address all correspondence to: antoniuginec@yahoo.com

Department of Obstetrics and Gynecology, Clinical Emergency Hospital St Pantelimon, Carol Davila University of Medicine and Pharmacy, Bucharest, Romania

References

[1] Guidelines of the European Respiratory Society and the European Society of Thoracic Surgeons for the management of malignant pleural mesothelioma. The European Respiratory Journal. 2010;**35**:479-495

[2] Stoecker JT, Madewell JER, Drake RM. Congenital cystic adenomatoid malformation of the lung – Classification and morphologic spectrum. Human Pathology. 1977;**8**:155-171

[3] Leninger BJ, Haight C. Congenital cystic adenomatoid malformation of the left lobe lower with compression of remaining lung. Clinical Pediatrics. 1973;**12**:182-186

[4] Langston C. New concepts in the pathology of congenital lung malformations. Seminars in Pediatric Surgery. 2003;**12**:17-37

[5] Laberge JM, Flageole H, Pugash D, et al. Outcome of the prenatally diagnosed congenital cystic malformation: A Canadian experience. Fetal Diagnosis and Therapy. 2001;**16**:178-186

[6] Hernanz Schulman M. Cystic and cystic like lesions of the lung. Radiologic Clinics of North America. 1993;**31**:631-649

[7] Stoecker JT. Congenital airway obstruction malformation: A new name and expanded classification of congenital cystic adenomatoid malformation of the lung. Histopathology. 2002;**41**:144-149

[8] Adzick NS, Harroson MR, Click PL, et al. Fetal cystic adenomatoid malformation prenatal diagnosis and natural history. Journal of Pediatric Surgery. 1985;**20**:483-488

[9] Wilson RD, Hedrick HL, Liechty KW. Cystic adenomatoid malformation of the lung – Review of genetics, prenatal diagnosis and in utero treatment. American Journal of Medical Genetics. Part A. 2006;**140 A**:151-155

[10] Mahle WT, Ryschick J, Tian Z, et al. Echocardiographic evaluation of the fetus with congenital cystic adenomatoid malformations. Ultrasound in Obstetrics & Gynecology. 2000;**16**:620-624

[11] Cass DL, Crombleholme TM, Howello LJ. Cystic lung lesions with systemic arterial blood supply: A hybrid of congenital cystic adenomatoid malformation and broncho-pulmonary sequestration. Journal of Pediatric Surgery. 1997;**32**:986-990

[12] Morin L, Crombleholme TM, Lewis F. Bronchopulmonary sequestration: Prenatal diagnosis with clinicopathologic correlation. Current Opinion in Obstetrics & Gynecology. 1994;**6**:479-481

[13] Cameron HM. Fetal thoracic lesions. Fetal and Maternal Medicine Review. 2003;**14**:23-46

[14] Ionescu C, Calin D, Ples L, Dimitriu M, Bohiltea R, Banacu M. Cystic adenomatoid malformation of the lung associated with trisomy 18. Gineco.eu. Mar 2016;**12**(45):109-112

[15] Crombleholme TM, Coleman B, Hedrick H, et al. Cystic adenomatoid malformation volume ratio predicts outcome in prenatally diagnosed cystic adenomatoid malformation of the lung. Journal of Pediatric Surgery. 2002;**37**:331-338

[16] Dommergues M, Louis-Sylvester C, Mandelbrot, et al. Cystic adenomatoid malformation of the lung: When it is active fetal therapy indicated? American Journal of Obstetrics and Gynecology. 1997;**177**:953-958

[17] Tsao KJ, Albanese CT, Harrison MR. Prenatal therapy for thoracic and mediastinal lesions. World Journal of Surgery. 2003;**27**:77-83

[18] Sauerbei E. Lung sequestration: Duplex Doppler diagnosis at 19 weeks gestation. Journal of Ultrasound in Medicine. 1991;**10**:101-105

[19] Sintzoff SA, Avni EF, Rocmans P, et al. Pulmonary sequestration like anomaly presenting as a spontaneously resolving mass. Pediatric Radiology. 1991;**21**:143-144

[20] Meizner I, Rosenak D. The vanishing fetal intrathoracic mass: Consider an obstructing mucous plug. Ultrasound in Obstetrics & Gynecology. 1995;**5**:275-277

[21] Lee BS, Kim JT, et al. Neonatal pulmonary sequestration: Clinical experience with transumbilical arterial embolization. Pediatric Pulmonology. 2008;**43**:404-413

[22] Sohaey R, Zwiebel W. The fetal thorax: Non cardiac chest anomalies. Seminars in Ultrasound, CT, and MR. 1996;**17**:34-50

[23] Schneider P, Schwalbe E. Die morphologic der missbildungen des menschen und der thiere. Jena: Fischer. 1912;**3**:812-822

[24] Yoshimura S, Masuzaki H, Gotoh H. Ultrasonographic prediction of lethal pulmonary hypoplasia – Comparison of eight different sonographic parameters. American Journal of Obstetrics and Gynecology. 1996;**175**:477-483

[25] Albright EB, Crane JP, Shackelford GD. Prenatal diagnosis of a bronchogenic cyst. Journal of Ultrasound in Medicine. 1988;**7**:91-95

[26] Bagolan P, Bilancioni E, Nahom A. Prenatal diagnosis of a bronchogenic cyst in an unusual site. Ultrasound in Obstetrics & Gynecology. 2000;**151**:66-68

[27] Lim FY, Crombleholme TM, Hedrick HL, et al. Congenital high airway obstruction syndrome: Natural history and management. Journal of Pediatric Surgery. 2003;**38**:940-945

[28] Kalache K, Chaoui R, Tennstedt C, et al. Prenatal diagnosis of laryngeal atresia in cases of CHAOS. Prenatal Diagnosis. 1997;**17**:577-581

[29] Paladini D, Volpe P. Thoracic anomalies. In: Paladini D, Volpe P, editors. Ultrasound of Congenital Fetal Anomalies. CRC Press, Taylor Francis Group; 2014. pp. 253-254

[30] Saadai P, Jelin F, Nijsyndrome EB, et al. Long term outcome after fetal therapy for congenital airway obstruction. Journal of Pediatric Surgery. 2012;**47**:1095-1100

[31] Weber AM, Philipson EH. Fetal pleural effusion: A review and meta-analysis for prognostic indicators. Obstetrics and Gynecology. 1992;**79**:281-286

[32] Moerman P, Vandenberghe K, Devlieger H, et al. Congenital pulmonary lymphangiectasis with chylothorax: A heterogeneous lymphatic vessel abnormality. American Journal of Medical Genetics. 1993;**47**:54-58

[33] Ionescu C, Ples L, Banacu M, Poenaru E, Panaitescu E, Dimitriu M. Present tendencies of elective cesarean delivery in Romania: Geographic, social and economic factors. Journal of the Pakistan Medical Association. Aug 2017;**67**(8):1248-1253

[34] Yaghoobian J, Comrie M. Transitory bilateral isolated fetal pleural effusions. Journal of Ultrasound in Medicine. 1988;**7**:231-232

[35] Paladini D, Chita SD, Allan LD. Prenatal measurement of cardiothoracic ratio in the evaluation of congenital heart disease. Archives of Disease in Childhood. 1990;**65**:20-23

[36] Jung E, Won HS, Lee PR, et al. The progression of mediastinal lymphangiomas in utero. Ultrasound in Obstetrics & Gynecology. 2000;**16**:663-666

[37] Tollefson I, Yoo M, Bland JD. Thymic cysts: Is a correct preoperative diagnosis possible? Report of a case series and review of the literature. European Journal of Pediatrics. 2001;**160**:620-622

[38] Jaggers J, Balsara K. Mediastinal masses in children. Seminars in Thoracic and Cardiovascular Surgery. 2004;**16**:201-208

[39] Gul A, Tekoglu G, Aslan H, et al. Prenatal sonographic features of esophageal and ileal duplication cyst at 18 weeks of gestation. Prenatal Diagnosis. 2004;**24**:969-971

[40] Pleş L, Sima RM, Moisei C, Moga M, Dracea L. Abnormal ultrasound appearance of the amniotic membranes – Diagnostic and significance: A pictorial essay. Medical Ultrasonography. 2017;**19**(2):1-5. ISSN: 2066-864

[41] Bianchi D, Crombleholme TT, D'Alton M, Malone F. Cystic Lesions of the Chest in Fetology Diagnosis and Fetal Patient. 2nd ed. McGraw Hill; 2010. pp. 273-276

[42] Maccaulay KE, Winter TC, Shields L. Neurenteric cyst shown by prenatal sonography. AJR. American Journal of Roentgenology. 1997;**169**:563-565

[43] Şorop-Florea M, Ciurea RN, Ioana M, Stepan AE, Stoica GA, Tănase F, Comănescu MC, Novac MB, Drăgan I, Pătru CL, Drăguşin RC, Zorilă GL, Cărbunaru OM, Oprescu ND, Ceauşu I, Vlădăreanu S, Tudorache Ş, Iliescu DG. The importance of perinatal autopsy. Review of the literature and series of cases. Romanian Journal of Morphology and Embryology. 2017;**58**(2):323-337

[44] Wilkinson K, Albanese CT, Jennings RW. Fetal neurenteric cyst causing hydrops: Case report and literature review. Prenatal Diagnosis. 1999;**19**:118-121

2

Fetal Abdominal Wall Defects

Roxana Cristina Drăguşin, Maria Şorop-Florea,
Ciprian Laurenţiu Pătru, Lucian Zorilă,
Cristian Marinaş, Nicolae Cernea,
Cristian Neamţu and Dominic Gabriel Iliescu

Abstract

Abdominal wall defects (AWDs) represent a group of congenital anomalies that can be diagnosed early during pregnancy even at the time of the first trimester assessment, with direct impact on pre- and postnatal fetal prognosis and management decisions. The most frequent anomalies in this group are gastroschisis and omphalocele. The key method available, that allows the detection of any deviation from the physiologic midgut herniation, is the ultrasound (US) assessment. A precise algorithmic scan approach is imposed not only for an accurate detection of any abdominal wall defect, but also for a proper location of the defect and of the spatial relation to the umbilical cord insertion, fundamentally important in differentiating among various malformations. Other structural or chromosomal anomalies should be excluded. Suitable multidisciplinary counseling should be considered. Unfortunately, in utero surgery, in these cases, has not been yet successful. Postnatal early interventions are usually required in specialized pediatric centers.

Keywords: congenital anomalies, abdominal wall defect, gastroschisis, omphalocele, ultrasound

1. Introduction

Abdominal wall defects (AWDs) define a type of congenital anomalies characterized by the herniation of abdominal organs through an unusual opening surrounding the umbilical cord. The most common two types include omphalocele and gastroschisis. The omphalocele or exomphalos (in Greek, omphalos = umbilicus, kele = hernia, tumors) was firstly described in 1634 by Ambroise Pare, while gastroschisis (in Greek gastro = stomach—the term generally used for abdomen; schisis = fissure, tear or gape) was first described by James Calder, a decade later. Other uncommon AWDS are ectopia cordis (EC), limb–body wall complex, cloacal and bladder exstrophy, urachal cyst, Prune belly syndrome and Cantrell pentalogy [1]. The correct prenatal detection and classification of these fetal malformations are extremely important for subsequent opportunities in parental counseling and pregnancy management. Nowadays, the intensive use of US assessment has allowed an increase in detection rates of AWDs, even from the first trimester nuchal translucency scan.

2. Embryology/pathophysiology and demographics

The embryologic developmental of the ventral body wall is reflected in its malformations. There are two types of defects, respectively, defects in the primaxial component and defects in the abaxial component. The first type of defects is often linked to neural tube-closure defects, whereas the second one manifest as limb–body wall or ventral body wall defects [2, 3]. Several hypotheses with respect to AWDS known as ventral body wall defects have been issued [4]. The embryologic origin of ectopia cordis, gastroschisis and bladder exstrophy is not yet known, but is thought to be more closely linked than that for omphalocele [5, 6]. It is considered that an abnormal closure of the ventral body wall folds during the 4th week of development is the main cause for these entities. In cases of gastroschisis, exposure to a teratogenic factor was suggested to be influential [7]. Some studies suggest that poor socio-economic status and prenatal care, as well as teratogens (e.g. recreational drugs, salicylates, paracetamol and pseudoephedrine) may be important contributors to the development of gastroschisis [8, 9]. A combination of genetic and environmental factors was also thought to be involved in the origin of gastroschisis, and also ectopia cordis and bladder exstrophy [10–12]. Chromosomal abnormalities are diagnosed in 1.2% of infants with gastroschisis [13], whereas approximately half infants (54–57%) with omphalocele present with aneuploidies or gene disorders [14]. However, one risk factor associated with gastroschisis was identified in young maternal age, mothers under 20 years old having the highest risk [10]. The oldest embryologic hypothesis date from 1963, and state the potential teratogenic effect on the folds, which result in gastroschisis [15]. Another theory pleads for the rupture of the amniotic membrane at the base of the umbilical cord [16] or for the disruption of the omphalomesenteric (yolk-sac and vitelline) artery, resulting in infarction and necrosis at the base of the umbilicus [17]. As there is no evidence that for the amniotic rupture almost exclusively on the right side and that the omphalomesenteric artery offers blood supply to the paraumbilical region of the abdominal wall [18], the first and oldest theory may be overlooked [5]. On the other hand, omphalocele is a different entity, with a known etiology, thought to be the failure to return of the loops of bowel after the physiological herniation from the 6th to 10th week post-fertilization, when the fetal midgut extends into the extraembryonic celom, occupying the proximal segment of the umbilical cord [19]. A physiological hernia seldom exceeds 7 mm in diameter or rarely persists after 12 weeks of gestation, when the midgut returns to the abdominal cavity [20]. Other pathogenic theories include failure of complete lateral-body migration and closure of the body wall [15]. Omphalocele is more prevalent in older mothers.

The prevalence of the two most frequent entities of AWDs is reported to be for gastroschisis 3.09 per 10,000 births, with a live birth prevalence of 2.63 per 10,000 and for omphalocele 3.29 and 1.13 per 10,000, respectively [21]. The prevalence of gastroschisis has increased in the last years, whereas that of omphalocele has remained stable [22]. Regarding the prenatal diagnosis of AWDs, both omphalocele and gastroschisis are easily diagnosed at the 11–14 weeks nuchal scan. So, large studies report sensitivity for both congenital anomalies from 90 to 100% [23, 24]. In fact, reports show that 22 and 35% of the chromosomally normal cases of gastroschisis and omphalocele, respectively, were diagnosed before 14 weeks, and 50 and 30% between 14 and 23 weeks. The overall prenatal detection rate was 91.6% for gastroschisis and 83.3% for omphalocele [21].

3. Prenatal diagnosis and classification of fetal abdominal wall defects

3.1. Gastroschisis

Gastroschisis is an AWD characterized by the herniation of the abdominal viscera represented by bowel loops and occasionally parts of other abdominal organs outside the abdominal wall with no covering membrane or sac, to the right of the insertion of the umbilical cord, and rarely to the left side [25, 26]. Even if the condition is not generally associated with other major congenital or chromosomal anomalies, an accurate fetal anatomy assessment is required. The reported rate of the proportion of gastroschisis associated with major defects is about 10% [27], arthrogryposis being present in a minority of these fetuses [28], with a reported mortality rate of 5–10% in all cases of gastroschisis [29]. Others report a higher rate (14%) of additional associated anomalies, the central nervous system and cardiac malformations being the most common anomalies [30]. Gastroschisis is often classified into simple (as an isolated defect) and complex (as associated with bowel-related complications: intestinal atresia, perforation, stenosis or volvulus) [31]. In cases with intestinal complications, there is a relevant risk of increased morbidity, higher rates of complications, as respiratory distress or sepsis and of course an increased length of hospital stays [32]. The key to an accurate diagnosis is fetal US in routine antenatal care, which affects patient management and prognosis. In the past, the detection was higher in the second trimester, between 16 and 22 weeks of gestation, in approximately 60% of cases, with a false positive rate of 5.3% [33]. Misdiagnosis of gastroschisis as omphalocele has serious implications, as gastroschisis is rarely associated with chromosomal anomalies and unnecessary amniocentesis may be needed with additional risks to the procedure [34]. Nowadays, the diagnosis of gastroschisis can be facilitated ultrasonographically as early as the late first trimester, 12–13 weeks of gestation [35]. After correctly identifying a normal umbilical cord insertion using color Doppler, gastroschisis is detected as herniation of the bowel loops with no covering membrane (e.g. **Figure 1a**). In most cases, the defect is on the right side of the umbilical cord with a normal umbilical cord insertion. Beside the location of the defect, it is important to establish the size and content of the defect and if present, the associated anomalies.

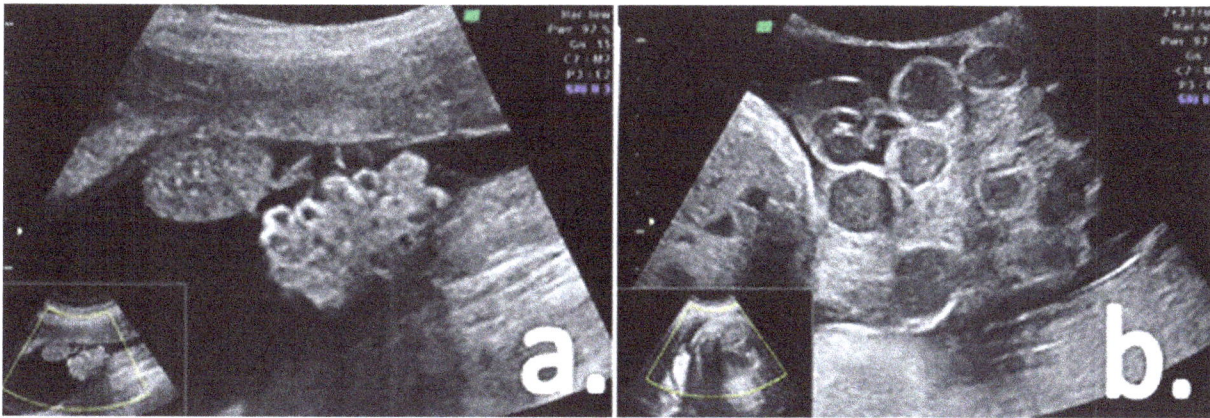

Figure 1. a. Ultrasound image of gastroschisis diagnosed in the second trimester (bowel loops floating in the amniotic fluid with no sac); b. Ultrasound image of gastroschisis diagnosed in the third trimester (thickened, echogenic bowel wall floating in reduced amniotic fluid).

Other ultrasound features may include an abnormal position of the stomach, dilatation of the bowel loops with a thickened and echogenic bowel wall (e.g. **Figure 1b**). Regarding the amniotic fluid, a decreased amount is often reported, rather than an increased amount. Subsequent bowel atresia is a frequent complication in fetuses with gastroschisis, due to inflammation and direct trauma of the amniotic fluid, on the herniated bowel [36]. The significance of certain associated ultrasound features in determining fetal outcome is debated, as prenatal predictors of gastroschisis complications. There is an associated risk of intrauterine death in 5% of cases of gastroschisis [37], as well as an increased incidence of fetal growth restriction or small for gestational age weight fetuses [38]. Antenatal US features of gastroschisis, such as extra- and intra-abdominal bowel dilatation, stomach herniation, stomach dilatation, bowel matting, growth restriction, abnormal umbilical artery (UA) Doppler ultrasounds and abnormal amniotic fluid volume were studied as prognostic factors. However, only extra-abdominal bowel dilatation proved to be a statistically significant marker of complex gastroschisis and associated morbidity [39].The incidence of complex gastroschisis is reported to be 10% [40], with increased risk for complications such as perivisceritis [41], as the amniotic fluid is extremely toxic to the exposed bowel and ischemic injury, because of constriction at the level of the abdominal defect [42]. Regarding the risk of intrauterine demise (IUD), an intense surveillance protocol was proposed and demonstrated to reduce the rate of IUD by 2.2% [43]. The proposed modalities of monitoring included cardiotocography, even daily in the third trimester, and umbilical and middle cerebral artery Doppler [37]. On the other hand, the diagnosis of fetal growth restriction can be difficult, as abdominal circumference measurements are affected by the herniated bowel. Formulas that do not include abdominal circumference can be helpful in fetal weight estimation, but there are still on debate for the moment [44].

3.2. Omphalocele

Omphalocele is another AWDs represented by a midline defect that leads to a herniation into the amniotic cavity through the base of the umbilical cord. The herniated abdominal content is covered by a membrane presented by the peritoneum on the inner side, amnion on the outer side and Wharton's jelly in between [26]. Omphalocele must be differentiated by the physiological midgut herniation that usually disappears before 11–12 weeks of gestation [45]. Omphalocele may be classified in terms of shape, as "conical", that includes hernia of the umbilical cord or "globular", with a large sac having a small diameter base. The size of the defect can be small, up to 5 cm, also called "minor" or more than 5 cm, called "major". The sac may contain bowel loops, small or large intestine, stomach, bladder or ovary or bowel loops and liver [6]. The covering membrane of the omphalocele can be intact, or it can rupture, and the bowel loops can float freely in the amniotic fluid and resemble gastroschisis. The differential diagnosis can include also cord hernia that has a normal insertion into the umbilical ring with intact skin, while in omphalocele the large defect has no muscles or skin. In term of associated anomalies, omphalocele can be syndromic or non-syndromic. About 75% of cases have associated chromosomal and non-chromosomal anomalies [46]. Some authors report a risk for chromosomal abnormalities of 30–40% [34], while other found a lower rate, of only 25% [30]. The most frequent chromosomal abnormalities associated with omphalocele include trisomy 18 (80%), trisomy 13, triploidy and trisomy 21. Other genetic findings described are 45,X, 47,XXY and 47,XXX, partial aneuploidy such as dup (3q), dup (11p), inv. (11), dup (1q), del (1q), dup (4q), dup (5p), dup (6q), del (9p), dup (15q), dup(17q), Pallister-Killian syndrome with mosaic tetrasomy 12p and Miller-Dieker lissencephaly syndrome with deletion of 17p13.3 and uniparental disomy (UPD) such as UPD 11 and UPD 14 [47]. The risk of aneuploidy does not change if the omphalocele contains only bowel or also the liver, but instead correlates with nuchal translucency thickness [14]. Non-chromosomal abnormalities include cardiac defects (50%) (atrial and ventricular septal defects (VSDs) and tetralogy of Fallot (TOF)) and gastrointestinal defects that are present in 40%. Omphalocele is a disorder that characterizes Beckwith-Wiedemann syndrome, together with macroglossia, macrosomia, hypoglycemia, visceromegaly and embryonic tumors [48]. The diagnosis is possible even from the first trimester, after 12 weeks of gestation, during the US genetic assessment (e.g. **Figure 2a** and **b**). Still, no aggressive management should be taken until the second trimester, as in some cases the omphalocele slowly disappears, although no spontaneous resolution have been reported in cases with herniated liver [14, 49]. Omphalocele looks like a smooth central mass, protruding from the anterior abdominal wall covered by membranes (e.g. **Figure 2a** and **b**.). It usually contains small intestine and liver, or other organs such as large intestine, bladder, stomach and spleen. The useful tool to demonstrate umbilical cord is a color Doppler. Polyhydramnios is a specific feature of omphalocele. Ascites can be present as well. Once the diagnosis is established, search for other associated anomalies should be considered. Invasive testing offer is mandatory. Studies have shown that 26–39% of cases are misdiagnosed as isolated omphalocele and actually, associated anomalies are demonstrated postnatally [50, 51]. Regarding the prognosis, it is driven by the presence and nature of the associated anomalies. Also, there is a higher risk for postnatal complications, such as pulmonary hypoplasia with consequently respiratory insufficiency. An omphalocele is considered giant if the defect contains more than 75% of the liver [52]. In cases of a small omphalocele and no associated anomalies, there is a very good prognosis, with a survival around 80–90%. In chromosomal and structural abnormalities associated cases, the mortality rate is around 80–100% [53]. An increased prevalence of deficits in

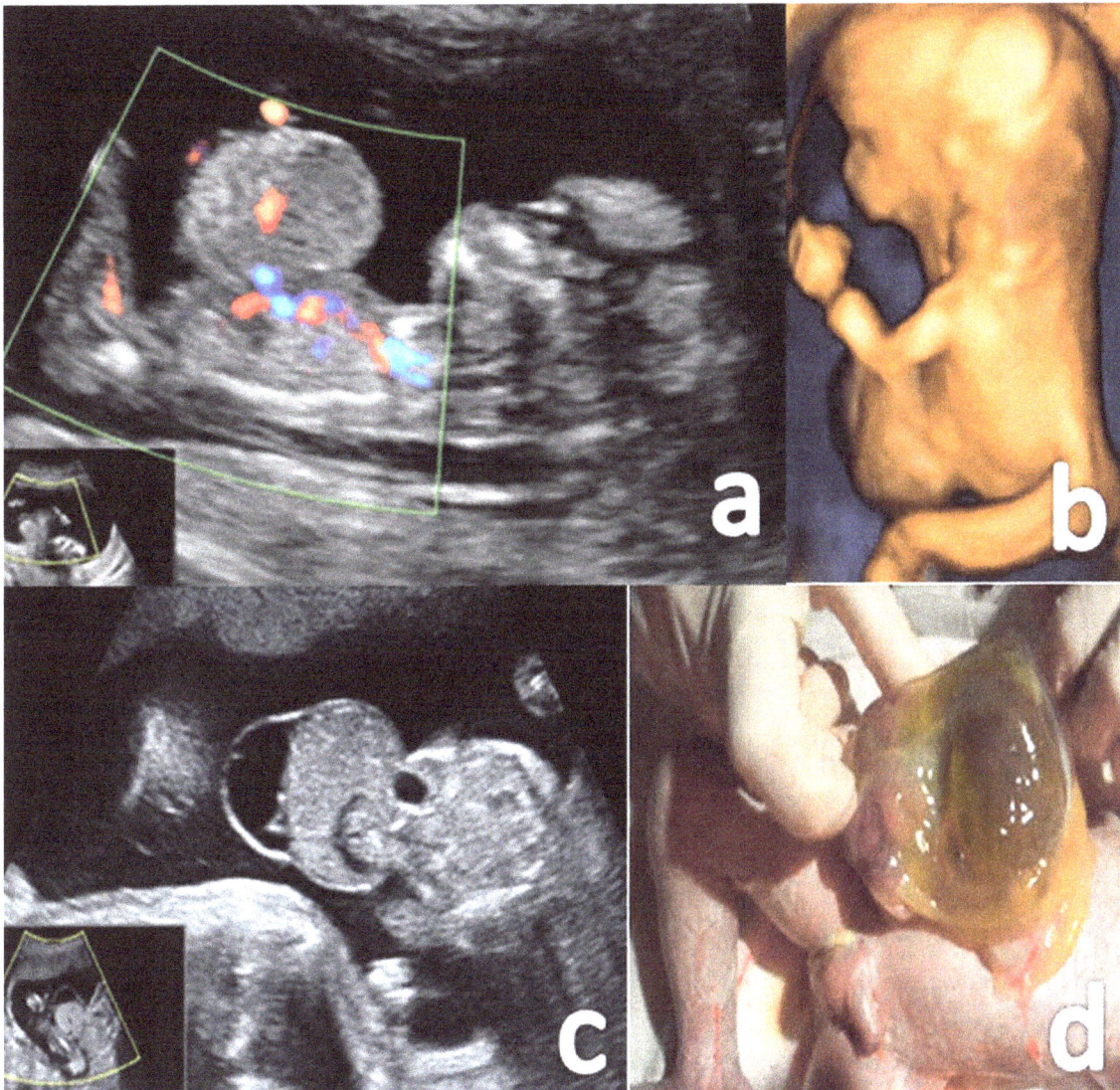

Figure 2. a. Ultrasound image of omphalocele diagnosed in the first trimester (a. Color Doppler image, b. 3D image); c. US image of omphalocele diagnosed in the second trimester; d. Postnatally image of omphalocele.

developmental achievements has been demonstrated in neonates with omphalocele [53]. An accurate prenatal diagnosis includes combining US evaluation with invasive testing. Even if high suspicion of omphalocele in the first trimester, the definitive diagnosis should be established after reevaluating the fetus in the second trimester. Besides karyotyping, also cytogenetic investigations should be offered. Termination of pregnancy is recommended after proper counseling, especially in cases of a large defect and severe associated anomalies.

3.3. Ectopia cordis

Ectopia cordis (EC) is a rare congenital AWD with poor prognosis. The defect is located in the anterior chest wall and abdominal wall, with abnormal placement of the fetal heart outside the thoracic cavity, with associated defect in the parietal pericardium diaphragm, sternum and in most cases cardiac malformation [54] (e.g. **Figure 3a**). The most frequent intracardiac defects include ventricular septal defect (VSD, 100%), atrial septal defect (ASD, 53%), tetralogy of Fallot (TOF, 20%), left ventricular diverticulum (LVD, 20%) and pulmonary hypoplasia [55, 56]. The term of ectopia cordis was described for the first time in 1706, as a generally sporadic malformation [57]. Rarely, it is reported an association with chromosomal abnormalities like trisomy 18, Turner syndrome, 46,XX and 17q+ [58]. The condition affects 5–8/1 million live [59]. EC is classified into different types such as cervical (5%), cervicothoracic and thoracic (65%), thoracoabdominal (20%) and abdominal (10%) [57, 60]. Also, EC can be "partial", if the heart can be visualized pulsating through skin and "complete" when the heart is outside, naked, without the pericardial membrane [55]. The thoracoabdominal EC is one of the five features of pentalogy of Cantrell. The diagnosis of EC is possible using ultrasound assessment as early as the first trimester, even before 11 weeks of gestation [61, 62]. Still the associated abnormalities can be better evaluated in the early second trimester in nearly 90% [63]. Three-dimensional (3D) scan can improve the accuracy in detection of EC in rare cases of minor forms of ectopia cordis [64]. Invasive diagnosis of associated aneuploidy is mandatory in each case of EC [65]. This rare malformation has a poor prognosis, needing intensive care right from delivery, which includes resuscitation and coverage of the exposed heart with saline-soaked gauze pads wrappings, followed by aggressive surgical correction [66]. In most infants, this anomaly is fatal in the first hours or days after birth due to infection, cardiac failure or hypoxemia [67]. Early precise diagnosis of EC is necessary and essential, for a multidisciplinary team to provide optimal parental counseling. The couple must decide whether they opt for termination of pregnancy or for continuing it, despite the poor prognosis. There is no consensus regarding the mode of delivery, and parents should also decide autonomously if they prefer vaginal birth acknowledging the risk for fetal demise during labor. However, the alternative of performing a cesarean section does not change the outcome [63]. Prenatal care and accurate early ultrasound diagnosis is required especially in developing countries, in which the health care system is lacking currently important physical and material resources.

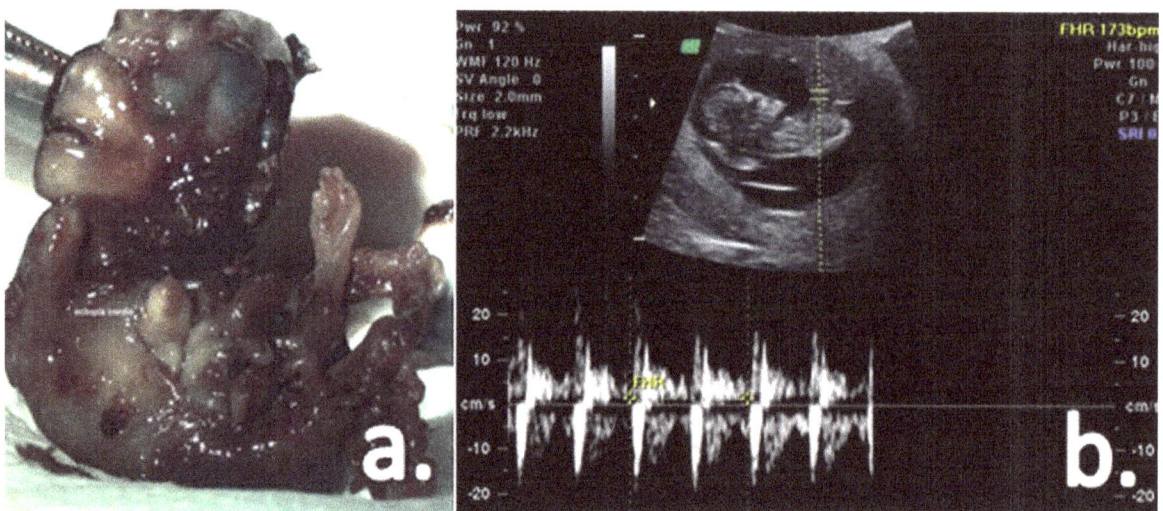

Figure 3. a. Ectopia cordis in a post-abortum fetus; b. Body stalk syndrome (ectopia cordis, fetus attached to the placenta).

3.4. Body stalk syndrome or limb: Body wall complex

Body stalk syndrome (BSS) represents the rarest and most severe AWD. This syndrome was described for the first time in 1987, as an association of three main features: exencephaly, facial clefts or encephalocele, thoraco or abdominoschisis and limb defects [68]. The anomaly is lethal, as there is a herniation of the peritoneal cavity in the extraembryonic coelomic cavity, with the fetus attached to the placenta [69] (e.g. **Figure 3b**). This is due to a large wall defect and due to a short or absent umbilical cord [26]. BSS is also known as the amniotic band syndrome, short umbilical cord syndrome or limb–body wall complex syndrome [70]. Usually, there is no association with chromosomal anomalies; still placental trisomy 16 or maternal uniparental disomy 16 have been reported [71]. The recurrence rate has been demonstrated to be low, and there is no correlation with parental age or fetal gender [68, 72]. The reported prevalence is 0.12 cases per 10,000 births (alive and still births) [73] or even higher 1 in 7500 pregnancies [74]. Two phenotypes have been described, respectively, as placento-cranial and placento-abdominal [75]. The diagnosis of BSS can be established by the end of the first trimester US scan [76] or at 11 weeks' gestation [77]. The US features of BSS show: the fetus is located (in its entirety or partially) outside the amniotic cavity, with an abnormal fetus, that cannot be separated from the placenta, and has lost his anatomic landmarks (**Figure 4a, b**). There can be also thoracoabdominal defects, spinal cord abnormalities, positional limb deformities and abnormalities of umbilical cord and membranes. As the US appearance can be confusing, the examination of the amniotic continuity, content of both the amniotic sac and coelomic cavity and a short umbilical cord helps in differentiating this condition from other AWD [77]. The differential diagnosis includes other polymalformative conditions, such as pentalogy of Cantrell, omphalocele-exostrophy-imperforate anus-spinal defects and isolated gastroschisis [78]. Also, kyphoscoliosis is often seen [74] and oligohydramnios can be present in the second and third trimester, situation in which only MRI can elucidate the anatomic structures [79]. Another finding is the presence of constriction rings, which can entangle the fetus [80]. Also, the fetuses with BSS present an increased nuchal thickness, a short umbilical cord and internal organ malformation, like abnormal mesodermal development [80]. So, the early diagnosis (at 11–13 weeks' gestation) is possible and necessary, as the anomaly is lethal and termination of pregnancy is offered. There is also a risk of spontaneously abortion reported, but in such cases an accurate diagnosis is often impossible. In the special situation represented by a twin pregnancy with a fetus with BSS and another unaffected fetus, the prenatal care should focus only on the healthy twin [80].

3.5. Cloacal and bladder exstrophy

Cloacal exstrophy (CE), even if rare, is a complex anomaly of the urogenital tract and intestinal tract that involves a low AWD with the exstrophy of all the structures that form the cloaca (rectum, bladder and lower genitourinary tract). The main embryologic event that is attributed to CE is represented by the premature rupture of the cloacal membrane before fusion with the urorectal septum. Still, many theories regarding the pathogenesis have been issued such as abnormal overdevelopment of the lower cloaca that prevents mesenchymal tissue migration [81, 82], abnormal fusion of the genital tubercle below the cloacal membrane or

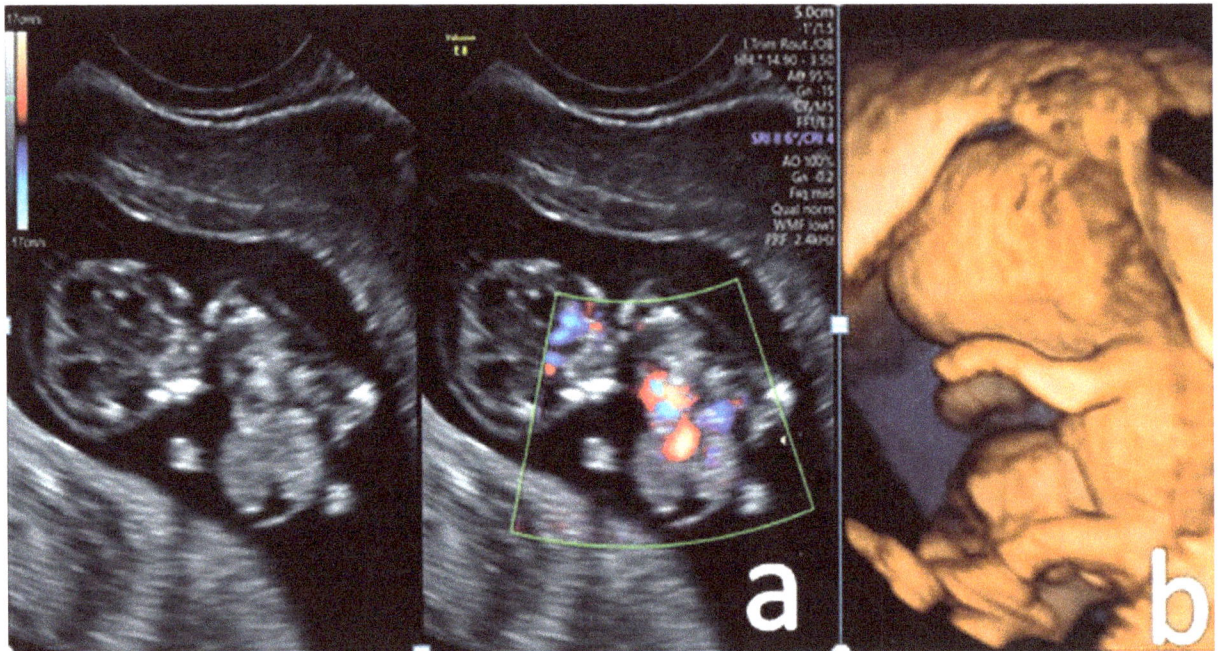

Figure 4. Ultrasound image of a BSS diagnosed in the first trimester: a. Gray scale and color image of the fetus with BSS; b. 3D image of the fetus with BSS.

abnormally caudal position of the body stalk and failure of mesenchymal ingrowth [83]. In the past, the estimated prevalence was reported higher as 1 case in 20,000 births [84], while more current studies describe a rate of 1 case per 200,000–400,000 live births [85]. Female fetuses are more likely to be affected by the anomaly. Prenatal US findings of CE include an absent normal bladder, with a lower abdominal wall defect, with herniated segments of the intestinal tract and a cystic pelvic mass in case of intact cloacal membrane. In fact, the first initial feature is often the omphalocele (in 70–90% of cases), but in a cranial part. Generally, the amniotic fluid index is normal, as the upper urinary tract has no obstruction to flow. Color Doppler examination of both umbilical arteries can help in accurate localization of the bladder [86]. Other associated anomalies may include spinal defects such as sacralization of L5, congenital scoliosis, sacral agenesis [87] and interpedicular widening, or cardiovascular and central nervous system anomalies or single umbilical artery. Also, is reported the association with gastrointestinal malformations such as malrotation (30%), double appendix (30%), absent appendix (21%), short small bowel (19%), small bowel atresia (5%) or abdominal musculature deficiency (1%) [88]. Also, upper urinary tract anomalies can be seen in 60% of cases as pelvic kidney, horseshoe kidney, hypoplastic kidney and solitary kidney, with subsequent hydronephrosis and oligohydramnios [89]. The US diagnosis can also describe "the elephant trunk sign", which is the protrusion of the ileum in the amniotic fluid, resembling the trunk of an elephant [90]. Typically, CE does not associate aneuploidies, but invasive diagnosis can be offered. The survival rates of this type of AWD are approaching 100% these days, because of important operative techniques and perioperative management progress [91]. Still, the reconstructive staged surgical management of patients with CE remains the most challenging for pediatric surgeons and urologists [92]. Early US detection is important, as termination of pregnancy can be offered to the couple before viability, after intense multidisciplinary counseling, especially in cases where a wide range of disorders is associated with CE. If the couple decides to continue with the pregnancy, US assessment can help in correct planning of surgical intervention with minimal damage to the exposed organs.

Bladder exstrophy represents an AWD with a failure of the anterior bladder wall to close normally, due to the lack of muscular or connective tissue [93]. The reported incidence is 0.25–0.5 in 10,000 births, more common in males in the ratio of 2:1 [94]. The main US finding described for prenatal diagnosis is the absence or non-visualization of the bladder, as the bladder is open to the abdominal wall, and urine is released directly into the amniotic fluid. According to the American Institute of Ultrasound in Medicine guidelines, a normal bladder must be demonstrated from the first trimester as a midline fluid-filled structure flanked by the umbilical arteries in color Doppler examination [95]. Other US findings include: lower abdominal protruding mass, formed by the exstrophied bladder, lower umbilical insertion and an umbilical cord cyst and external genitalia malformation, represented by a small penis with anteriorly displaced scrotum. Also, in females, a bifid clitoris and uterine and vaginal anomalies can be identified [93], besides a widening of the iliac crests [96]. The accuracy and sensitivity of the US can be relatively low, as not all signs are always present, and an urachal cyst may mimic the presence of the bladder [97]. Bladder exstrophy should be considered if no urinary bladder is visualized, and there is no oligohydramnios associated or other renal abnormalities. Still, for the differential diagnosis with an empty bladder, the scan of the lower abdomen should be repeated in 15 minutes interval. Also, the exclusion of CE should be made, as the management is more complicated and the prognosis poorer. Prenatal US correct detection of the anomaly helps in parental counseling and recommendation for delivery in the tertiary center, as the prognosis is quite favorable. The postnatal management includes early surgical procedure to close the anterior wall defect within the first 3 days after birth. If the surgical repair is performed later, there is a higher risk of urinary incontinence or uterine prolapsed, infertility and increased risk of bladder adenocarcinoma [86]. Besides the bladder closure, pediatric surgeons must repair also the epispadias simultaneously, or in staged intervention, to offer an acceptable appearance and function of the external genitalia [98].

3.6. Urachal cyst

The urachus is a primitive structure between the umbilical cord and the bladder, in developing fetus. It disappears normally prior to delivery, but in rare cases, parts can persist. The urachal cyst is a sinus considered a congenital urachal remnant abnormalities [99]. It is diagnosed in children, by means of ultrasound and MRI. It usually suspected if there is bleeding in the cyst or infection. The infected urachal cyst can rupture into the peritoneal cavity, leading to peritonitis. The first line treatment is the surgical procedure of complete primary excision with excellent prognosis.

3.7. Omphalocele-exstrophy of bladder-imperforate anus-spinal deformities complex (OIES complex)

OIES complex represents the most severe expression of the abnormal development of the cloaca with the arrest of the urorectal septum in the 7th–8th week of gestation. The reported incidence is rare, of only 0.025–0.04 in 10,000 live births [100, 101]. The diagnosis is accessible early in pregnancy, at the end of the first trimester. The imagistic findings include the presence of omphalocele and bladder exstrophy, associated with anomalies of the spine. The imperforated anus is often found postnatally, even if it can be detected antenatally, but with high suspicion by specialized observer. Other anomalies evaluated with OIES complex are spina bifida, genital anomalies, fistulas, renal anomalies, limb hypoplasia, craniofacial anomalies and single umbilical artery [86]. As the prognosis is poor when multiple structural defects are associated, termination of pregnancy is offered as an option to the couple, after multidisciplinary prenatal counseling. If desire to continue the pregnancy, there is a high risk of preterm delivery, low birth weight or intrauterine death. The proper treatment of OIES complex includes a series of surgeries depending on the severity of the condition [100, 101].

3.8. Prune belly syndrome

The prune belly syndrome is another rare congenital syndrome, characterized by deficient abdominal muscles, urinary tract abnormalities and cryptorchidism in male fetuses. The pathophysiology has not been completely elucidated, as some consider the syndrome as a consequence of severe bladder outlet obstruction and others consider an abdominal muscle deficiency, secondary to a migration defect of the lateral mesoblast between weeks 6 and 7 of pregnancy [102]. The incidence is estimated to be 1 in 35,000 to 1 in 50,000 live births. The antenatal diagnosis is obtained during the second trimester scan, when megacystis is noticed, and an abnormally distended abdomen, in the absence of keyhole sign. However, there are reports in regards to the early US diagnosis [103, 104]. In the most severe form of Prune belly syndrome, a high incidence of oligohydramnios, pulmonary hypoplasia and ultimately still-birth is reported [105]. Often, termination of pregnancy is the couple's option in early pregnancy. The postnatal management may include a single comprehensive surgical approach or a multiple step one, with good long-term results, but with a considerable incidence of iterative surgery and progression of the disease [106].

3.9. Cantrell pentalogy

With an incidence of 5.5 cases per 1 million live births and a male predominance [107], pentalogy of Cantrell is characterized by a midline, supraumbilical AWD, with a defect of the lower sternum, deficiency of the anterior diaphragm, defect in the diaphragmatic pericardium and cardiac anomalies such as septal defects and tetralogy of Fallot [108]. The main event during embryogenesis, thought to be the cause of this rare anomaly, is an abnormal differentiation of the intra-embryonic mesoderm, at approximately 14–18 days after conception [108]. Chromosomal anomalies, such as trisomy 13, 18 and Turner syndrome, are often associated, so the invasive diagnosis is mandatory. Other anomalies observed with pentalogy of Cantrell include craniofacial and vertebral anomalies. US diagnosis of Cantrell's pentalogy is possible early, at 10 weeks' gestation, using 2D and 3D scans [109]. The combination of omphalocele and ectopia cords highly indicates a case of pentalogy of Cantrell [110]. The pentalogy is "complete" if four or all five defects are present, and is "incomplete" when various combination of defects are observed, if a sternal abnormality is present [86]. The AWD may contain stomach, liver,

Abnormality	Covering membrane	Site of defect	Umbilical cord insertion	Additional findings
Omphalocele	Yes	Umbilical insertion	Omphalocele membrane	
Gastroschisis	No	Right of umbilical insertion	Normal insertion	
Umbilical hernia	Yes	No umbilical ring defect	Normal insertion	
Pentalogy of Cantrell	Yes	Above umbilical insertion	Omphalocele membrane	Anterior diaphragmatic hernia, sternal clefting, ectopia cordis, and intracardiac defect.
OEIS complex	Yes	Umbilical insertion	Omphalocele membrane	Bladder exstrophy, imperforate anus, and spina bifida.
Body-stalk anomaly	Herniated organs in extraembryonic coelom	Whole anterior abdominal wall	Cord absent or shortened	Kyphoscoliosis, cranial defects, and limb defects.
Bladder exstrophy	Not applicable	Below umbilical insertion	Low insertion	Non-visualisation of bladder, lower abdominal bulge (exstrophied bladder), small penis with anteriorly displaced scrotum (if male), and widening of the iliac crests.
Cloacal exstrophy	Not applicable	Below umbilical insertion	Low insertion	Renal anomalies, neural tube defect, omphalocele, vertebral anomalies, non-visualisation of the bladder, distended bladder, hydrocolpos, dilated or echogenic bowel, umbilical cord cyst, separated pubic bones, and 'elephant trunk' sign.

OEIS, omphalocele, bladder exstrophy, imperforate anus, spina bifida complex.

Figure 5. Ultrasound findings in fetal abdominal wall defects [26].

bowel or total abdominal contents, evisceration. There is a pleural and pericardial effusion and the fetal heart is completely external or just partially. The prognosis is fatal and the survival is uncommon. Prenatal diagnosis is important as termination of pregnancy is the only option for the couple.

The ultrasound features that best characterize fetal AWDs are presented in **Figure 5** [26].

4. Pregnancy surveillance

In cases with abdominal wall defects, fetal distress was reported in 43% of cases, with an abnormal neurological outcome in 16% of them [111]. There is also the risk of still birth, reported to be 11% in cases of gastroschisis and 20% in cases of omphalocele [112]. Fetuses with gastroschisis often tend to be small for gestational age and to develop oligohydramnios [113, 114]. In such cases, the assessment of fetal weight can be difficult, as measurements of the fetal abdomen are not valid [115]. Placental insufficiency can be indirectly estimated by umbilical artery Doppler velocimetry, cardiotocography and biophysical profile. Still, intrauterine growth restriction and oligohydramnios seem not to worsen the prognosis of fetuses with gastroschisis [116]. Fetal bowel features can be also evaluated, to estimate post-natal bowel complications. A cut-off of 1 cm for bowel diameter was considered a far-seeing marker for bowel damage [117, 118]. Overall, there is not yet a consensus regarding how and when fetal monitoring during pregnancy. Because of the associated risk, recommended attitude is a careful monitoring and a monthly interval control scheme, somewhat arbitrarily chosen. In the third trimester, repeated fetal monitoring is indicated [111]. Hospital admittance was proposed at 35 weeks of gestation, as many patients with fetal AWDs deliver prematurely [112, 115].

5. Mode and time of delivery

Even with recent progress in major medical and surgical specialties, the mode and time of delivery of fetuses with antenatal diagnosed abdominal wall defects remains a controversy. Fetal delivery by elective cesarean section is advocated by some centers [119–125], while others consider a vaginal delivery more suitable in cases with diagnosed fetal abdominal wall defect [126–130]. More so, there is no difference in fetal outcome regarding the mode of delivery [131–135]. In cases of omphalocele, delivery by cesarean section is recommended in cases with a large defect, to prevent the sac rupture and the liver damage during labor [136]. However, some researchers found that features such as the size or liver herniation have no importance in establishing the outcome of vaginal delivery [137]. The gestational age for induced delivery or elective cesarean section is another controversy (preterm versus term delivery). Some authors reported more complications and longer hospitalization in preterm deliveries [138, 139]. Others recommend a preterm delivery to optimize the toxic damage of the amniotic fluid to the herniated bowel in gastroschisis [120, 124, 129, 140]. The most recent study presented good results using a protocol for a preterm elective delivery, between 35 and 36 + 6 gestational age for fetuses with gastroschisis. Preterm delivery is not indicated in cases of omphalocele [26]. Still, most studies agree that in utero transport to a specialized pediatric center, where the defect can be corrected, offers an optimal fetal outcome [126, 141].

6. Postnatal prognosis and management

6.1. Gastroschisis

Postpartum, fetuses with gastroschisis must benefit from intravenous fluid resuscitation and wrapped herniated loops in warm saline as there is an increased risk for water and heat losses by evaporation. Specialized management of gastroschisis includes repositioning of the herniated bowel into the abdominal cavity, with closure of the abdominal wall (primary reduction and repair). In such cases, there is a high risk of respiratory complication. The surgical procedure can be also postponed if the patient is unstable [18], but with subsequent longer time to reach full enteral feeds. In cases of complex gastroschisis, the repair is usually delayed, as anastomosis is impossible immediately after delivery, having an inherent risk of infectious and cholestasis complications [18, 24].

6.2. Omphalocele

In contrast to gastroschisis, there is a low risk of fluid and health losses in neonates with omphalocele, but still a coverage with saline-soaked gauze is required. Postnatal outcome and surgical management depends on the associated anomalies, such as congenital heart disease and pulmonary hypoplasia. Also, fetal gestational age and the size of the defect are relevant [18]. In cases of a small AWD, primary closure is the preferred therapeutic procedure, while in cases of a larger defect, multiple surgeries may be required to repair the considerable defect. Various agents such as povidone-iodine, sulfadiazine, neomycin, silver-impregnated dressings, neomycin, polymyxin and bacitracin ointments have been reported to help with the formation of an eschar of the amnion sac. There are different surgical techniques for the cure of omphalocele that include serial reductions or closing the defect gradually after replacing the sac with a mesh [24].

7. Conclusion

Prenatal ultrasound offers a high accuracy in the diagnosis of fetal abdominal wall defects beginning with the first trimester nuchal scan. Most fetal abdominal wall defects have poor prognosis and termination of pregnancy if often offered at the time of the detection after multidisciplinary counseling. Management of gastroschisis can be challenging, and also is the surgical treatment of complex forms. On the other hand, omphalocele, relatively easy to diagnose and treat, is frequently associated with chromosomal and structural anomalies that worsen the prognosis and the final outcome. The importance of ultrasound diagnosis in early pregnancy must be highlighted. This should be available even in under-developed health systems.

Author details

Roxana Cristina Drăgușin[1]*, Maria Șorop-Florea[1], Ciprian Laurențiu Pătru[1], Lucian Zorilă[1], Cristian Marinaș[2], Nicolae Cernea[1], Cristian Neamțu[3] and Dominic Gabriel Iliescu[1]

*Address all correspondence to: roxy_dimieru@yahoo.com

1 Department of Obstetrics and Gynaecology, University of Medicine and Pharmacy, Craiova, Romania

2 Department of Anatomy, University of Medicine and Pharmacy, Craiova, Romania

3 Department of Physiopathology, University of Medicine and Pharmacy, Craiova, Romania

References

[1] Nyberg DA, Mack LA. Abdominal wall defects. In: Nyberg DA, Mahony BS, Pretorius DH, editors. Diagnostic Ultrasound of Fetal Anomalies: Text and Atlas. St Louis, MO: Mosby Year Book; 1990. pp. 395-432

[2] Hunter AG, Seaver LH, Stevenson RE. Limb-body wall defect. Is there a defensible hypothesis and can it explain all the associated anomalies? American Journal of Medical Genetics. Part A. 2011;**155A**:2045-2059

[3] Iimura T, Denans N, Pourquie O. Establishment of Hox vertebral identities in the embryonic spine precursors. Current Topics in Developmental Biology. 2009;**88**:201-234

[4] Brewer S, Williams T. Finally, a sense of closure? Animal models of human ventral body wall defects. BioEssays. 2004;**26**:1307-1321

[5] Sadler TW. The embryologic origin of ventral body wall defects. Seminars in Pediatric Surgery. 2010 Aug;**19**(3):209-214. DOI: 10.1053/j.sempedsurg.2010.03.006

[6] Evbuomwan I, Lakhoo K. Congenital Anterior Abdminal wall defects: Exomphalos and Gastroschisis. chapter 56, page 348-351. http://www.global-help.org/publications/books/help_pedsurgeryafrica56.pdf

[7] Loane M, Dolk H, Bradbury I. Increasing prevalence of gastroschisis in Europe 1980-2002: A phenomenon restricted to younger mothers? Paediatric and Perinatal Epidemiology. 2007;**21**:363-369

[8] Frolov P, Alali J, Klein MD. Clinical risk factors for gastroschisis and omphalocele in humans: A review of the literature. Pediatric Surgery International. 2010;**26**:1135-1148

[9] Van Dorp DR, Malleis JM, Sullivan BP, et al. Teratogens inducing congenital abdominal wall defects in animal models. Pediatric Surgery International. 2010;**26**:127-139

[10] Rasmussen SA, Frias JL. Non-genetic risk factors for gastroschisis. American Journal of Medical Genetics Part C. 2008;**148C**:199-212

[11] Amato JJ, Douglas WI, Desai U, et al. Ectopia cordis. Chest Surgery Clinics of North America. 2000;**10**:297-316

[12] Martinez-Frias ML, Bermejo E, Rodriguez-Pinilla E, et al. Exstrophy of the cloaca and exstrophy of the bladder: Two different expressions of a primary developmental field defect. American Journal of Medical Genetics. 2001;**99**:261-269

[13] Mastroiacovo P, Lisi A, Castilla EE, et al. Gastroschisis and associated defects: An international study. American Journal of Medical Genetics. Part A. 2007;**143A**:660-671

[14] Khalil A, Arnaoutoglou C, Pacilli M, et al. Outcome of fetal exomphalos diagnosed at 11-14 weeks of gestation. Ultrasound in Obstetrics & Gynecology. 2012;**39**:401-406

[15] Duhamel B. Embryology of exomphalos and allied malformations. Archives of Disease in Childhood. 1963;**38**:142-147

[16] Shaw A. The myth of gastroschisis. Journal of Pediatric Surgery. 1975;**10**:235-244

[17] Hoyme HE, Higginbottom MC, Jones KL. The vascular pathogenesis of gastroschisis: Intrauterine interruption of the omphalomesenteric artery. The Journal of Pediatrics. 1981;**98**:228-231

[18] Hamilton WJ, Mossman HW. Cardio-vascular system. In: Hamilton WJ, Mossman HW, editors. Hamilton, Boyd, and Mossman's Human Embryology. 4th ed. Baltimore, MD: Williams and Wilkins; 1972. pp. 268-271

[19] Sadler TW. Body cavities. In: Sadler TW, ed. Langman's Medical Embryology, 11th ed. Baltimore, MD: Lippincott, Williams, and Wilkins, 2010:155-64

[20] Grigore M1, Iliev G, Gafiteanu D, Cojocaru C, The fetal abdominal wall defects using 2D and 3D ultrasound. Pictorial essay, Med Ultrason. 2012 Dec;**14**(4):341-7

[21] EUROCAT. http://www.eurocat-network.eu [last accessed 08.10.13]

[22] Kirby RS, Marshall J, Tanner JP, et al. Prevalence and correlates of gastroschisis in 15 states, 1995 to 2005. Obstetrics and Gynecology. 2013;**122**:275-281

[23] Syngelaki A, Chelemen T, Dagklis T, et al. Challenges in the diagnosis of fetal non-chromosomal abnormalities at 11-13 weeks. Prenatal Diagnosis. 2011;**31**:90-102

[24] Rossi AC, Prefumo F. Accuracy of ultrasonography at 11-14 weeks of gestation for detection of fetal structural anomalies: A systematic review. Obstetrics and Gynecology. 2013;**122**:1160-1167

[25] Robertson JA, Kimble RM, Stockton K, Sekar R. Antenatal ultrasound features in fetuses with gastroschisis and its prediction in neonatal outcome. The Australian & New Zealand Journal of Obstetrics & Gynaecology. 2017 Feb;**57**(1):52-56. DOI: 10.1111/ajo.12565

[26] Prefumo F, Izzi C. Fetal abdominal wall defects. Best Practice & Research. Clinical Obstetrics & Gynaecology. 2014 Apr;**28**(3):391-402. DOI: 10.1016/j.bpobgyn.2013.10.003

[27] Stoll C, Alembik Y, Dott B, et al. Omphalocele and gastroschisis and associated malformations. American Journal of Medical Genetics. Part A. 2008;**146A**:1280-1285

[28] Ruano R, Picone O, Bernardes L, et al. The association of gastroschisis with other congenital anomalies: How important is it? Prenatal Diagnosis. 2011;**31**:347-350

[29] Grant NH, Dorling J, Thornton JG. Elective preterm birth for fetal gastroschisis. Cochrane Database of Systematic Reviews. 2013:6. Art No.: CD009394. DOI: 10.1002/14651858. CD009394.pub2

[30] Barisic I, Clementi M, Häusler M, et al. Evaluation of prenatal ultrasound diagnosis of fetal abdominal wall defects by 19 European registries. Ultrasound in Obstetrics & Gynecology. 2001;**18**(4):309-316 Crossref, Medline

[31] Molik KA, Gingalewski CA, West KW, et al. Gastroschisis: A plea for risk categorization. Journal of Pediatric Surgery. 2001;**36**:51-55

[32] Arnold MA, Chang DC, Nabaweesi R, et al. Risk stratification of 4344 patients with gastroschisis into simple and complex categories. Journal of Pediatric Surgery. 2007;**42**:1520-1525

[33] Walkiinshaw SA, Renwick M, Hebishch G, Hey EN. How goood is ultrasound in the detection and evaluation of anteriuor abdominal wall defects ? The British Journal of Radiology. 1992 Apr;**65**(772):298-301

[34] Agarwal R. Prenatal diagnosis of anterior abdominal wall defects: Pictorial essay. Gynaecology and Obstetrics. 2005;**15**(3):361-372

[35] Guzman ER. Early prenatal diagnosis of gastroschisis with transvaginal ultrasonography. American Journal of Obstetrics and Gynecology. 1990;**162**(5):1253-1254 Crossref, Medline

[36] Kronfli R, Bradnock TJ, Sabharwal A. Intestinal atresia in association with gastroschisis: A 26-year review. Pediatric Surgery International. 2010;**26**(9):891-894 Crossref, Medline

[37] Fratelli N, Papageorghiou AT, Bhide A, et al. Outcome of antenatally diagnosed abdominal wall defects. Ultrasound in Obstetrics & Gynecology. 2007;**30**:266-270

[38] Nicholas SS, Stamilio DM, Dicke JM, et al. Predicting adverse neonatal outcomes in fetuses with abdominal wall defects using prenatal risk factors. American Journal of Obstetrics and Gynecology. 2009;**201**:383e1-383e6

[39] Robertson JA, Kimble RM, Stockton K, Sekar R. Antenatal ultrasound features in fetuses with gastroschisis and its prediction in neonatal outcome. The Australian & New Zealand Journal of Obstetrics & Gynaecology. 2017 Feb;**57**(1):52-56. DOI: 10.1111/ajo.12565 Epub 2016 Nov 22

[40] Abdullah F, Arnold MA, Nabaweesi R, et al. Gastroschisis in the United States 1988-2003: Analysis and risk categorization of 4344 patients. Journal of Perinatology. 2007;**27**:50-55

[41] Luton D, Guibourdenche J, Vuillard E, et al. Prenatal management of gastroschisis: The place of the amnioexchange procedure. Clinics in Perinatology. 2003;**30**:551-572. viii

[42] Goetzinger KR, Tuuli MG, Longman RE, et al. Sonographic predictors of postnatal bowel atresia in fetal gastroschisis. Ultrasound in Obstetrics & Gynecology; **2013**. http://dx.doi.org/10.1002/uog.12568

[43] Perry H, Healy C, Wellesley D, Hall NJ, Drewett M, Burge DM, Howe DT. Intrauterine death rate in gastroschisis following the introduction of an antenatal surveillance program: Retrospective observational study. The Journal of Obstetrics and Gynaecology Research. 2017 Mar;**43**(3):492-497. DOI: 10.1111/jog.13245

[44] Nicholas S, Tuuli MG, Dicke J, et al. Estimation of fetal weight in fetuses with abdominal wall defects: Comparison of 2 recent sonographic formulas to the Hadlock formula. Journal of Ultrasound in Medicine. 2010;**29**:1069-1074

[45] Byron-Scott R, Haan E, Scott H, Clark K. A population-based study of abdominal wall defects in South Australia and Western Australia. Paediatric and Perinatal Epidemiology. 1998;**12**(2):136

[46] Stoll C, Alembik Y, Dott B, Roth MP. Omphalocele and gastroschisis and associated malformations. American Journal of Medical Genetics. Part A. 2008;**146A**(10):1280-1285

[47] Chen C. Chromosomal abnormalities associated with omphalocele. Taiwanese Journal of Obstetrics & Gynecology. 2007;**46**(1):1-8

[48] Chen CP. Syndromes and disorders associated with omphalocele (I): Beckwith-Wiedemann syndrome. Taiwanese Journal of Obstetrics & Gynecology. 2007;**46**:96-102

[49] Iacovella C, Ghi T, et al. The effect of the contents of exomphalos and nuchal translucency at 11-14 weeks on the likelihood of associated chromosomal abnormality. Prenatal Diagnosis. 2012;**32**:1066-1070

[50] Cohen-Overbeek TE, Tong WH, Hatzmann TR, et al. Omphalocele: Comparison of outcome following prenatal or postnatal diagnosis. Ultrasound in Obstetrics & Gynecology. 2010;**36**:687-692

[51] Porter A, Benson CB, Hawley P, et al. Outcome of fetuses with a prenatal ultrasound diagnosis of isolated omphalocele. Prenatal Diagnosis. 2009;**29**:668-673

[52] Danzer E, Gerdes M, D'Agostino JA, et al. Prospective, interdisciplinary follow-up of children with prenatally diagnosed giant omphalocele: Short-term neurodevelopmental outcome. Journal of Pediatric Surgery. 2010;**45**:718-723

[53] Heider AL et al. Omphalocele: Clinical outcomes in cases with normal karyotypes. American Journal of Obstetrics and Gynecology. 2004;**190**(1):135-141

[54] Goncalo FIMD, Ana PDF, Joaquim MDF. Ectopia cordis: caso clinic. Revista Brasileira de Sa'udeMaterno Infantil. 2014;**14**(3):287-290

[55] Alphonso N, Venugopal PS, Deshpande R, Anderson D. Complete thoracic ectopia cordis. European Journal of Cardiothoracic Surgery. 2003;**23**(3):426-428

[56] Achiron R, Shimmel M, Farber B, Glaser J. Prenatal sonographic diagnosis and perinatal management of ectopia cordis. Ultrasound in Obstetrics and Gynecology. 1991;**1**(6): 431-434

[57] Jimmy S, Keshav B, Rakesh B. Thoracic Ectopia Cordis. BMJ Case Report; 2012

[58] Grethel EJ, Hornberger LK, Farmer DL. Prenatal and postnatal management of a patient with pentalogy of Cantrell and left ventricular aneurysm: A case report and literature review. Fetal Diagnosis andTherapy. 2007;**22**(4):269-273

[59] Apte AV. Thoraco-abdominal ectopia cordis: A rare entity. Case report and review of literature. People's. Journal of Scientific Research. 2008:1

[60] Anderson RH, Shinebourne EA, Macartney FJ. Abnormal positions and relationships of the heart. In: Anderson RH, Shinebourne EA, editors. Paediatric Cardiology. London, UK: Church Livingstone; 1987. pp. 1057-1072

[61] Bick D, Markowitz RI, Horwich A. Trisomy 18 associated with ectopia cordis and occipital meningocele. American Journal of Medical Genetics. 1988;**30**(3):805-810

[62]   Tongsong T, Wanapirak C, Sirivatanapa P, Wongtrangan S. Prenatal sonographic diagnosis of ectopia cordis. Journal of Clinical Ultrasound. 1999;**27**(8):440-445

[63]   Gabriel A, Donnelly J, Kuc A, et al. Ectopia cordis: A rare congenital anomaly. Clinical Anatomy. 2014;**27**(8):1193-1199. DOI: 10.1002/ca.22402

[64]   Chang Y, Yang M-J, Wang P-H, Chen C-Y. Three-dimensional HDlive image of ecto-pia cordis in a twin fetus at 9 gestational weeks. Taiwanese Journal of Obstetrics & Gynecology. 2015;**54**(4):463-464. DOI: 10.1016/j.tjog.2014.07.008

[65]   Sepulveda W, Dezerega V, Gutierrez J. Ectopia cordis in a first-trimester sonographic screening program for aneuploidy. Journal of Ultrasound in Medicine. 2013;**32**(5):865-871. DOI: 10.7863/ultra.32.5.865

[66]   Harrison MR, Filly RA, Stanger P, de Lorimier AA. Prenatal diagnosis and management of omphalocele and ectopia cordis. Journal of Pediatric Surgery. 1982;**17**(1):64-66

[67]   Engum SA. Embryology, sternal clefts, ectopia cordis, and Cantrell's pentalogy. Seminars in Pediatric Surgery. 2008;**17**(3):154-160. DOI: 10.1053/j.sempedsurg.2008.03.004

[68]   Van Allen MI, Curry C, Gallagher L. Limb body wall complex: I. Pathogenesis. American Journal ofMedicalGenetics. 1987;**28**(3):529-548

[69]   Daskalakis G, Pilalis A, Papadopoulos D, Antsaklis A. Body stalk anomaly diagnosed in the 2nd trimester. Fetal Diagnosis and Therapy. 2003;**18**:342-344

[70]   Takeuchi K, Fujita I, Nakajima K, Kitagaki S, Koketsu I. Body stalk anomaly: prenatal diagnosis. International Journal of Gynaecology and Obstetrics. 1995;**51**:49-52

[71]   Chan Y, Silverman N, Jackson L, Wapner R, Wallerstein R. Maternal uniparental disomy of chromosome 16 and body stalk anomaly. American Journal of Medical Genetics. 2000;**94**:284-286

[72]   D'Souza J, Indrajit IK, Menon S. Limb body wall complex. Medical Journal Armed Forces India. 2004;**60**(1):77-80

[73]   Miller ME, Higginbottom M, Smith DW. Short umbilical cord: Its origin and relevance. Pediatrics. 1981;**67**:618-621

[74]   Daskalakis G, Sebire NJ, Jurkovic D, Snijders RJM, Nicolaides KH. Body stalk anomaly at 10-14 weeks of gestation. Ultrasound in Obstetrics and Gynecology. 1997;**10**(6):416-418

[75]   Bhat A, Ilyas M, Dev G. Prenatal sonographic diagnosis of limb-body wall complex: Case series of a rare congenital anomaly. Radiology Case Reports. 2016;**11**(2):116-120. DOI: 10.1016/j.radcr.2016.02.004

[76]   Borade A, Prabhu AS, Prabhu GS, Prabhu SR. Limb-body wall complex. Pediatric Oncall. 2009:6. Art #37

[77]   Panaitescu AM, Ushakov F, Kalaskar A, Pandya PP. Ultrasound features and Manage-ment of Body Stalk Anomaly. Fetal Diagnosis and Therapy. 2016;**40**(4):285-290

[78] Kocherla K, Kumari V, Kocherla PR. Prenatal diagnosis of body stalk complex: A rare entity and review of literature. The Indian Journal of Radiology & Imaging. 2015;**25**(1):67-70. DOI: 10.4103/0971-3026.150162

[79] Higuchi T, Narimatsu Y, Tanaka M. Early second-trimester diagnosis of body stalk anomaly by fetal magnetic resonance imaging. Japanese Journal of Radiology. 2013;**31**(4):289-292

[80] Routhu M, Thakkallapelli S, Mohan P, Ahmed N. Role of ultrasound in body stalk anomaly and amniotic band syndrome. International Journal of Reproductive Medicine. 2016;**2016**:3974139. DOI: 10.1155/2016/3974139

[81] Marshall VF, Muecke EC. Variations in exstrophy of the bladder. The Journal of Urology. 1962;**88**:766-796

[82] Holschneider AM, Hutson JM. Anorectal Malformations in Children: Embryology, Diagnosis, Surgical Treatment, Follow-Up. Berlin, Germany: Springer; 2006

[83] Mildenberger H, Kluth D, Dziuba M. Embryology of bladder exstrophy. Journal of Pediatric Surgery. 1988;**23**(2):166-170

[84] Jeffs RD. Exstrophy, epispadias, and cloacal and urogenital sinus abnormalities. Pediatric Clinics of North America. 1987;**34**:1233-1257

[85] Feldkamp ML, Botto LD, Amar E, et al. Cloacal exstrophy: An epidemiologic study from the international clearinghouse for birth defects surveillance and research. American Journal of Medical Genetics. Part C, Seminars in Medical Genetics. 2011;**157C**(4):333-343

[86] Woodward PJ, Kennedy A, Sohaey R, Byrne JLB, Oh KY, Puchalski MD. Diagnostic Imaging: Obstetrics. Salt Lake City: Amirsys; 2008 7-20i

[87] Loder RT, Dayiogler MM. Association of congenital vertebral malformations with bladder and cloacal exstrophy. Journal of Pediatric Orthopedics. 1990;**12**:38993

[88] Lee EH, Shim JY. New sonographic finding for the prenatal diagnosis of bladder exstrophy: A case report. Ultrasound in Obstetrics & Gynecology. 2003;**21**(5):498-500

[89] Tu W, Chueh J, Kennedy W. Dichorionic Diamniotic twin pregnancy discordant for bladder exstrophy. Advances in Urology. 2009; Article ID 186483, 3 pages

[90] Bischoff A, Calvo-Garcia MA, Baregamian N, et al. Prenatal counseling for cloaca and cloacal exstrophy-challenges faced by pediatric surgeons. Pediatric Surgery International. 2012;**28**(8):781

[91] Vliet Rv, Roelofs LA, Hosman AJ. Clinical outcome of cloacal exstrophy, current status, and a change in surgical management. European Journal of Pediatric Surgery. 2015 Feb;**25**(1):87-93. DOI: 10.1055/s-0034-1387943

[92] Macedo A Jr1, Liguori R, Ortiz V. Cloacal exstrophy: A complex disease. International Braz J Urol. 2013 Nov-Dec;**39**(6):897; discussion 898. DOI: 10.1590/S1677-5538.IBJU. 19-06-2013

[93] Siffel C, Correa A, Amar E, et al. Bladder exstrophy: An epidemiologic study from the international clearinghouse for birth defects surveillance and research, and an overview of the literature. American Journal of Medical Genetics. Part C, Seminars in Medical Genetics. 2011;**157C**(4):321-332

[94] Coulter WJ, Sabbagh MI. Bladder Extrophy and pregnancy. Report of a case. Obstetrics and Gynecology. 1958;**11**:104-107

[95] American Institute of Ultrasound in Medicine. AIUM practice guideline for the performance of obstetric ultrasound examinations. Journal of Ultrasound in Medicine. 2013;**32**:1083-1101

[96] Gearhart JP, Ben-Chaim J, Jeffs RD, et al. Criteria for the prenatal diagnosis of classic bladder exstrophy. Obstetrics and Gynecology. 1995;**85**:961-964

[97] Goyal A, Fishwick J, Hurrell R, et al. Antenatal diagnosis of bladder/cloacal exstrophy: Challenges and possible solutions. Journal of Pediatric Urology. 2012;**8**:140-144

[98] Stec AA, Baradaran N, Schaeffer A, Gearhart JP, Matthews RI. The modern staged repair of classic bladder exstrophy: A detailed postoperative management strategy for primary bladder closure. Journal of Pediatric Urology. 2012;**8**(5):549-555

[99] Hammond G, Yglesias L, Davis JE. The urachus, its anatomy and associated fascia. The Anatomical Record. 1941;**80**:271-274. DOI: 10.1002/ar.1090800302

[100] Olavarria AS, Guillermo Diaz Guerrero L. Answer to case #12. TheFetus.net; 1999. http://www.sonoworld.com/Client/Fetus/case.aspx?id=608&answer=1

[101] Chervenak F. Ultrasound in Obstetrics and Gynecology, Volume 2. Boston: Little Brown and Company; 1993

[102] Tonni G1, Ida V, Alessandro V, Bonasoni MP. Prune-belly syndrome: case series and review of the literature regarding early prenatal diagnosis, epidemiology, genetic factors, treatment, and prognosis. Fetal and Pediatric Pathology. 2013 Feb;**31**(1):13-24. doi: 10.3109/15513815.2012.659411

[103] Kraiem J, Chatti S, Falfoul A. Prune belly syndrome: Early prenatal diagnosis and management. La Tunisie Médicale. 2006 Jul;**84**(7):458-461

[104] Papantoniou N, Papaspyrou I, Mesogitis S, Antsaklis A. Prenatal diagnosis of prune-belly syndrome at 13 weeks of gestation: Case report and review of literature. The Journal of Maternal-Fetal & Neonatal Medicine. 2010 Oct;**23**(10):1263-1267. DOI: 10.3109/14767050903544777

[105] Hoshino T, Ihara Y, Shirane H, Ota T. Prenatal diagnosis of prune belly syndrome at 12 weeks of pregnancy: Case report and review of the literature. Ultrasound in Obstetrics & Gynecology. 01-11-1998

[106] Lopes RI, Tavares A, Srougi M, Dénes FT. 27 years of experience with the comprehensive surgical treatment of prune belly syndrome. Journal of Pediatric Urology. 2015 Oct;**11**(5):276.e1-276.e7. DOI: 10.1016/j.jpurol.2015.05.018

[107] Chandran S, Ari D. Pentalogy of Cantrell: An extremely rare congenital anomaly. Journal of Clinical Neonatology. 2013;**2**(2):95-97

[108] Cantrell JR, Haller JA, Ravitch MMA. Syndrome of congenital defects involving the abdominal wall, sternum, diaphragm, pericardium, and heart. Surgery, Gynecology & Obstetrics. 1958;**107**(5):602-614

[109] Ergenoğlu MA, Akercan F, Sağol S. Prenatal diagnosis of Cantrell pentalogy in first trimester screening: Case report and review of literature. Journal Of The Turkish-German Gynecological Association. 2012;**13**(2):145-148

[110] Desselle C, Sembely C, Perrotin F. Pentalogy of Cantrell: Sonographic assessment. Journal of Clinical Ultrasound. 2007;**35**(4):216-220

[111] Burge DM, Ade-Ajayi N. Adverse outcome after prenatal diagnosis of gastroschisis: The role of fetal monitoring. Journal of Pediatric Surgery. 1997 Mar;**32**(3):441-444

[112] Barisic I, Clementi M, Häusler M, Gjergja R, Kern J, Stoll C. The Euroscan study group. Evaluation of prenatal ultrasound diagnosis of fetal abdominal wall defects by 19 European registries. Ultrasound in Obstetrics & Gynecology. 2001;**18**:309-316

[113] Chen CP, Liu FF, Jan SW, Sheu JC, Huang SH, Lan CC. Prenatal diagnosis and perinatal aspects of abdominal wall defects. American Journal of Perinatology. 1996 Aug;**13**(6):355-361

[114] Blakelock RT, Upadhyay V, Pease PW, Harding JE. Are babies with gastroschisis small for gestational age? Pediatric Surgery International. 1997;**12**:580-582

[115] Salvesen KA1. Fetal abdominal wall defects--easy to diagnose--and then what? Ultrasound in Obstetrics & Gynecology. 2001 Oct;**18**(4):301-304

[116] Johnston R, Haeri S. Oligohydramnios and growth restriction do not portend worse prognosis in gastroschisis pregnancies. The Journal of Maternal-Fetal & Neonatal Medicine. 2016 Dec;**29**(24):4055-4058. DOI: 10.3109/14767058.2016.1154939

[117] Babcook CJ, Hedrick MH, Goldstein RB, Callen PW, Harrison MR, Adzick NS, Filly RA. Gastroschisis: Can sonography of the fetal bowel accurately predict postnatal outcome? Journal of Ultrasound in Medicine. 1994;**13**:701-706

[118] Langer JC, Khanna J, Caco C, Dykes EH, Nicolaides KH. Prenatal diagnosis of gastroschisis: Development of objective sonographical criteria for predicting outcome. Obstetrics and Gynecology. 1993;**81**:53-56

[119] Hadidi A, Subotic U, Goeppl M, Waag KL. Early elective cesarean delivery before 36 weeks vs late spontaneous delivery in infants with gastroschisis. Journal of Pediatric Surgery. 2008;**43**(7):1342-1346. DOI: 10.1016/j.jpedsurg.2007.12.050

[120] Reigstad I, Reigstad H, Kiserud T, Berstad T. Preterm elective caesarean section and early enteral feeding in gastroschisis. Acta paediatrica (Oslo, Norway: 1992). 2011;**100**(1):71-74. DOI: 10.1111/j.1651-2227.2010.01944.x

[121] Glasmeyer P, Mirada A, Sans A. Gastroschisis. Preterm elective cesarean and immediate primary closure: Our experience. Cirugia pediatrica: organo oficial de la Sociedad Espanola de. Cir Pediatr. 2012;**25**(1):12-1.5

[122] Sakala EP, Erhard LN, White JJ. Elective cesarean section improves outcomes of neonates with gastroschisis. American Journal of Obstetrics and Gynecology. 1993;**169**:1050-1053

[123] Dunn JC, Fonkalsrud EW, Atkinson JB. The influence of gestational age and mode of delivery on infants with gastroschisis. Journal of Pediatric Surgery. 1999;**34**:1393-1395

[124] Mesas Burgos C, Svenningsson A, Vejde JH, Granholm T, Conner P. Outcomes in infants with prenatally diagnosed gastroschisis and planned preterm delivery. Pediatric Surgery International. 2015 Nov;**31**(11):1047-1053. DOI: 10.1007/s00383-015-3795-8 Epub 2015 Sep 23

[125] Tawil KA, Gillam GL. Gastroschisis: 13 years' experience at RCH Melbourne. Journal of Paediatrics and Child Health. 1995;**31**(6):553

[126] Quirk JG Jr, Hassad SJ, Wagner C. Outcomes of newborns with gastroschisis: The effects of mode of delivery, site of delivery, and interval from birth to surgery. American Journal of Obstetrics and Gynecology. 1996;**174**:1134-1138

[127] Abdel-Latif ME, Bolisetty S, Abeywardana S, Lui K. Mode of delivery and neonatal survival of infants with gastroschisis in Australia and New Zealand. Journal of Pediatric Surgery. 2008;**43**(9):1685-1690. DOI: 10.1016/j.jpedsurg.2008.03.053

[128] How HY, Khoury J, Siddiqi TA. Is vaginal delivery preferable to elective cesarean delivery in fetuses with a known ventral wall defect? American Journal of Obstetrics and Gynecology. 2000;**182**(6):1527-1534. DOI: 10.1067

[129] Baud D, Langer JC, Kelly EN, Ryan G. Expectant management compared with elective delivery at 37 weeks for gastroschisis. Obstetrics and Gynecology. 2013;**121**(5):990-998. DOI: 10.1097/ AOG

[130] Puligandla PS, Janvier A, Flageole H, Bouchard S, Laberge JM. Routine cesarean delivery does not improve the outcome of infants with gastroschisis. Journal of Pediatric Surgery. 2004;**39**(5):742-745

[131] Salihu HM, Emusu D, Aliyu ZY, Pierre-Louis BJ, Druschel CM, Kirby RS. Mode of delivery and neonatal survival of infants with isolated gastroschisis. Obstetrics and Gynecology. 2004;**104**(4):678-683. DOI: 10.1097/01.aog.0000139513.93115.81

[132] Sipes SL, Weiner CP, Sipes DR 2nd, Grant SS, Williamson RA. Gastroschisis and omphalocele: Does either antenatal diagnosis or route of delivery make a difference in perinatal outcome? Obstetrics and Gynecology. 1990;**76**:195-199

[133] Kitchanan S, Patole SK, Muller R, Whitehall JS. Neonatal outcome of gastroschisis and exomphalos: A 10-year review. Journal of Pediatrics & Child Health. 2000;**36**:428-430

[134] Rinehart BK, Perry KG Jr, Roberts WE. Modern obstetric management and outcome of infants with gastroschisis. Obstetrics and Gynecology. 1999;**94**:112-116

[135] Christison-Lagay ER, Kelleher CM, Langer JC. Neonatal abdominal wall defects. Seminars in Fetal & Neonatal Medicine. 2011;**16**:164-172

[136] Kleinrouweler CE, Kuijper CF, van Zalen-Sprock MM, et al. Characteristics and outcome and the omphalocele circumference/abdominal circumference ratio in prenatally diagnosed fetal omphalocele. Fetal Diagnosis and Therapy. 2011;**30**:60-69

[137] Nasr A, Wayne C, Bass J, Ryan G, Langer JC. Effect of delivery approach on outcomes in fetuses with gastroschisis. Journal of Pediatric Surgery. 2013;**48**(11):2251-2255. DOI: 10.1016/j.jpedsurg.2013.07.004

[138] Soares H, Correia-Pinto J, Guimaraes H. Gastroschisis: Preterm or term delivery? Clinics (São Paulo, Brazil). 2010;**65**(2):139-142. DOI: 10.1590/s1807- 59322010000200004

[139] Serra A, Fitze G, Kamin G, Dinger J, Konig IR, Roesner D. Preliminary report on elective preterm delivery at 34 weeks and primary abdominal closure for the management of gastroschisis. European Journal of Pediatric Surgery. 2008;**18**(1):32-37. DOI: 10.1055/s- 2007-965744

[140] Nasr A, Langer JC. Influence of location of delivery on outcome in neonates with gastroschisis. Journal of Pediatric Surgery. 2012;**47**(11):2022-2025. DOI: 10.1016/j. jpedsurg.2012.07.037

[141] Islam S. Advances in surgery for abdominal wall defects: Gastroschisis and omphalocele. Clinics in Perinatology. 2012;**39**:375-386

3

The Antenatal Detection of Fetal Limb Anomalies

Iuliana Ceausu, Dominic Iliescu, Cristian Poalelungi,
Cristian Posea, Nicolae Bacalbasa,
Dragos Dobritoiu and Liana Ples

Abstract

The etiology of fetal limb abnormalities is very complex, involving different risk factors: chromosomal abnormalities, gene disorders, intrauterine factors, maternal diseases, or exposure to different risk factors. The prevalence of fetal limb anomalies is reported to be approximately 6 in 10,000 live births, and the impairments of the upper limbs seem to present a higher incidence in comparison to the inferior limbs, more often are affected unilaterally and on the right side in comparison to the left side, some being isolate or may associate other anomalies, as a part of an underlying syndrome. According to the current guidelines, the assessment of the fetal limbs should be performed in the late first and early second trimester. Three-dimensional ultrasound provides a better understanding of the fetal anomaly for the parents and helps a better counseling, and it is used to confirm the anomalies detected by the conventional ultrasound. In cases of treatable anomalies, a multidisciplinary approach involving an obstetrician, geneticist, neonatologist, pediatrician, and pediatric orthopedic surgeon is essential to improve the postnatal outcome. Ultrasound examination and genetic counseling for the parents has an important benefit since some conditions present a genetic inheritance, and the recurrence rate in further pregnancies is very high.

Keywords: fetal limbs, malformations, fetal syndrome, ultrasonography, 3D ultrasound, matero-fetal medicine

1. Current recommendations

The evaluation of musculoskeletal system and limbs is a part of the routine fetal ultrasound (US) examination, especially during the first- and second-trimester (ST) screening.

Its assessment is significantly more difficult in the third trimester, as the fetal dimensions and movements frequently alter the visualization of some segments, situated far from the transducer or behind other fetal bony structures.

In the last decades, the 11–13 weeks +6 days of US genetic scan has become an important tool for fetal anatomy assessment. It includes almost all segments of the fetal body and also the upper and lower extremities. The second-trimester anomaly scan remained the standard morphologic evaluation, an audit for the early scan, and a baseline for future US evaluations and interpretation of the fetal development. Still, between the guidelines issued by the major societies, there is a wide variation of the parameters proposed as a minimum for limb evaluation (**Table 1**).

Systematic and careful examination of the extremities is important, at any time. Congenital anomalies may affect one or more limbs and may affect any segment.

Usually, these limb anomalies are isolated, but detection of any of them should be followed by a detailed examination of the rest of the fetal anatomy. In many cases with aneuploidy and genetic syndromes, limb defects are present.

Limb segments included in the protocol recommendations	ISUOG [1]	NHS (UK) [2]	ACOG, AIUM, ACR, SRU [3–5]
Upper and lower limb presence	x	x	x
Femur diaphysis length (measurement)	x	x	x
Metacarpal and metatarsal bones/presence of the hands and feet	x	x	—
Digit count	—	—	—
Fetal movement	x	—	—

ISUOG: International Society of Ultrasound in Obstetrics and Gynecology; NHS, UK: National Health Service in the United Kingdom; ACOG: American College of Obstetricians and Gynecologists; AIUM: American Institute of Ultrasound in Medicine; ACR: American College of Radiology; SRU: Society of Radiologists in Ultrasound.

Table 1. Recommendation for fetal limb evaluation on prenatal ultrasound.

2. Development

The fetal skeleton starts to develop early during gestation. The appendicular and axial skeletons undergo a programmed pattern of endochondral ossification during which a cartilage template is replaced by the bone. In contrast, the calvarium and portions of the clavicle and pubis ossify via membranous ossification, whereby mesenchymal cells differentiate directly into osteoblasts [6].

Limb buds begin to develop during the fourth to fifth gestational week (GW) as clusters of mesenchymal cells covered by the ectoderm, but before the end of the seventh GW, the anatomy of the embryonic pole is difficult to observe. The upper limb development precedes the lower limbs in bud appearance, differentiation, individualization, movements, and final size. The process starts from proximal to distal, with the humerus and femur first, then ulna and radius, tibia and fibula, metacarpal and metatarsal bones, and lastly phalanges [7]. Then, the mandible, maxilla, and clavicles ossification centers appear at 8 weeks of gestation; appendicular skeleton, ilium, and scapula by 12 weeks; and metacarpals and metatarsals by 12–16 GW [6].

3. First-trimester assessment

During the so-called nuchal 'or genetic scan, a morphologic evaluation is recommended. Nuchal translucency (NT) assessment is more sensitive at an earlier gestation, 11–12 weeks of gestational age, but the optimal moment of the first-trimester anomaly scan is reported after 12 GW [8–11]. Regardless of scan timing, the fetus needs to be assessed in all planes: longitudinal, axial, and coronal. The examination may be performed transabdominal, and if necessary transvaginal, and a combination of the two approaches might give the best results [12]. In our experience, the completion of the basic protocol regarding the assessment of the fetal skeleton rarely requires an increased gestational age or the transvaginal approach, but we should keep in mind that the imaging of the fingers and feet was reported consistently and is achieved only after 12 GW [13]. Still, there was an important and constant technological progress in ultrasound capabilities since the respective researches that enables the operators to use modern systems and high-resolution probes for an earlier and a better visualization of fetal anatomy and especially the echogenic structures.

The exam should detect both upper limbs, which are often found in front of the fetal thorax or face, in semiflexed position. The lower limbs are generally flexed at the hip at this gestation. The fingers are relatively easy to assess in the first trimester as number and position, including the thumb, because they frequently lie in the same ultrasound plane. Feet can also be identified, but the number of toes may be difficult to assess because of their small size. The tendency of the ankles to have an inward position may result in an overdiagnosis of clubfoot in the first trimester. The proximal long bones—femur and humerus—can be seen and measured at the first-trimester scan, although their dimensions are not part of the routine biometry at this developmental stage.

The performance of the routine first-trimester anomaly scan was reported satisfactory in a recent study [14], where all the examinations were performed transabdominal and the vast majority of limb abnormalities detected prenatally were identified in the first trimester (82%). In the respective group, 77.8% of the total limb abnormalities were diagnosed prenatally and 63.9% on the first-trimester scan.

These encouraging results followed a previous large screening study regarding the results of routine fetal anomaly evaluation at the time of genetic scan [15], where only one third of the skeletal abnormalities were diagnosed (34.12%). In the respective group, all cases of body stalk anomaly were diagnosed, but none of those with unilateral or bilateral talipes, club or claw hand, and digital defects. The correct diagnosis was made in the majority of cases of a missing hand or foot (77.8%), or polydactyly (60%), and half of the lethal skeletal dysplasia (50%) and isolated shortening of one of the long bones (50%). The only case of ectrodactyly was missed, and arthrogryposis was not suspected during the first-trimester scan.

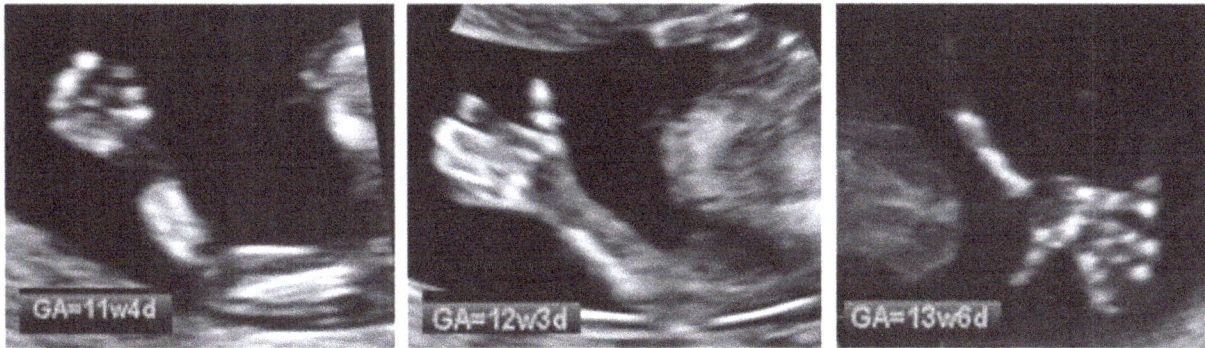

Figure 1. Normal aspects of fetal hand in the late first trimester.

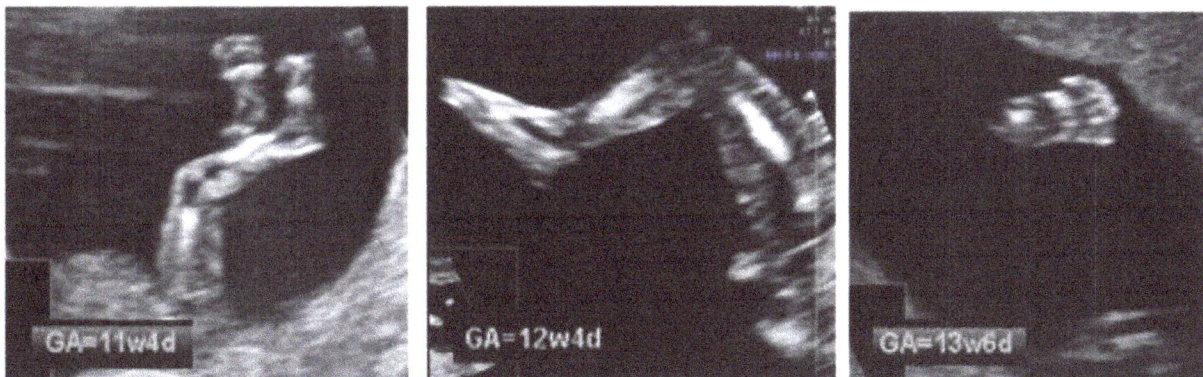

Figure 2. Normal aspects of fetal foot in the late first trimester.

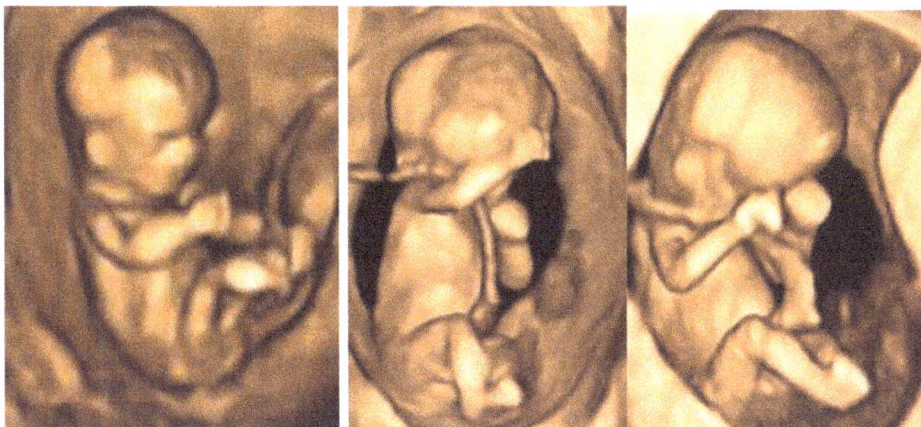

Figure 3. The whole fetus, imaged by 3D static ultrasound (surface rendering mode). The harmonious development and relationship between limbs' segments are easy to asses.

It was suggested that a systemic sequential approach scanning from proximal to distal until the entire limb is observed, and the strict operational training and audit and the use of high-resolution ultrasound machines may improve the early diagnosis of limb defects [14].

As for the most frequent limb anomalies diagnosed early in pregnancy, not only transverse limb reduction defects [14] but also radial aplasia and club hand [16] were proposed in different studies.

An abnormal nuchal translucency may accompany major skeletal abnormalities [17] and sometimes may be the only early sign in conditions with discrete if any early features [18–20]. Narrowing of the thorax with secondary mediastinal compression and abnormal cutaneous collagen deposition were discussed as possible causes (**Figures 1–3**).

4. Second-trimester assessment

Most of the authors agree that the fetal anatomy may readily be assessed at 20–24 WG, because:

- The pregnant uterus is completely lifted up in the maternal abdomen.

- The fetus may present favorable positions and axis for scan.

- The fetus is also enough developed to be seen, leading to good results if scanning for anomalies.

Some important studies underlined a statistically significant difference being able to perform a complete fetal morphology scan if US is performed at 18 to 19 + 6 (in 76% of cases) versus 20 to 22 + 6 weeks of gestation (in 90% of cases) [21–24]. However, with the improved technological capabilities of the ultrasound equipment, the gestational age for confidently assessment is constantly lowering. On the other hand, due to absorption of sound phenomenon, the visualization of the skeleton is easier than for other fetal systems (e.g., the cardiovascular system). Also, the skeletal system is already completely developed, unlike other structures (e.g., central nervous system components, as the corpus callosum or vermis). Therefore, the fetal skeletal evaluation may be proposed and successfully performed in the routine early second-trimester scan (**Figures 4–7**).

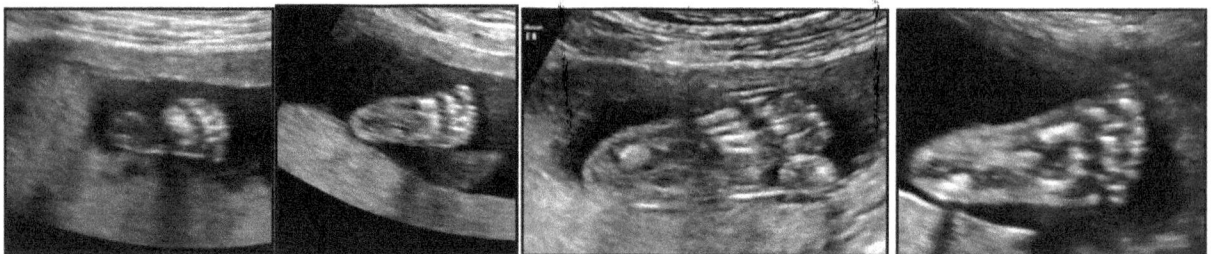

Figure 4. 2D conventional US images of normal feet at 17 weeks of amenorrhea (WA) and at 23 WA. The normal position of the toe is readily observed. In many cases, numbering the digits is possible.

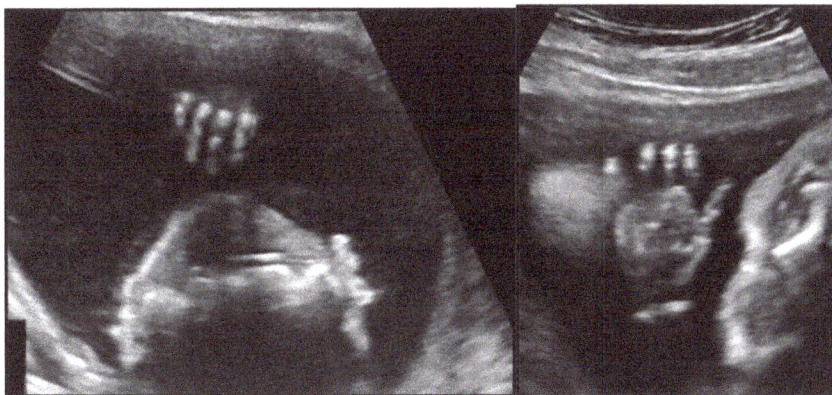

Figure 5. 2D conventional US images of normal fetal hands in midtrimester. Similarly, numbering the fingers is possible and, in certain cases, even the phalanges. As seen, in most cases, the thumb lies in a different plane than the other four fingers. Due to hand anatomy, thumb visualization may not be simultaneous than the other fingers. Yet, confirming the presence of the opposable finger is considered important, due to the prehension function of the hand.

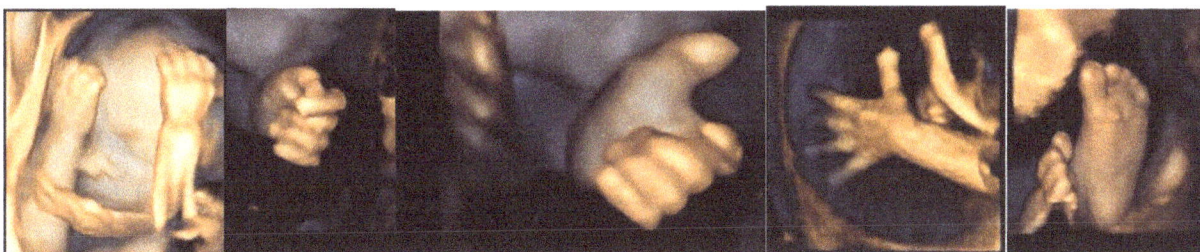

Figure 6. Hands and foot, imaged by 3D static ultrasound (surface rendering mode). Using this technique, the demonstration of the extremities is easier, despite the different spatial arrangement of the thumb.

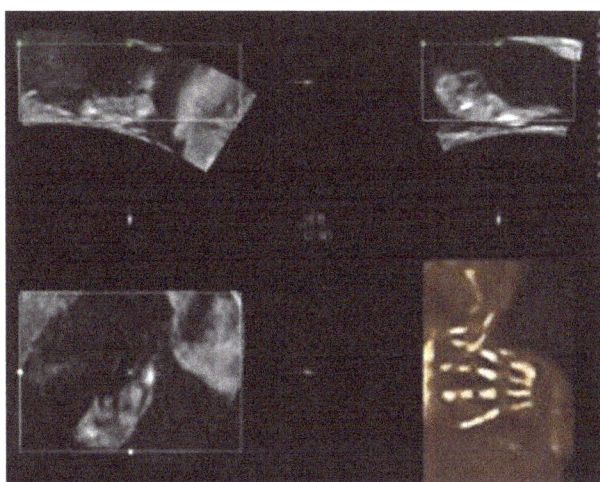

Figure 7. Hand imaged by 3D static ultrasound (skeletal mode). The technique makes the confirmation of the normal number of phalanges of each finger easier.

5. Third-trimester assessment

Later in the second trimester and in the third trimester, despite the increase in the size of the fetus, morphological examination of the limbs is more difficult because:

- the fetal position is maintained for longer periods, due to the reduced mobility;

- the limb's segments have a complete flexion, and the proximal limb's position is maintained toward the fetal axis;

- the amniotic fluid volume decreases, especially at term; and

- the bone ossification increases, impairing the visualization of the underlying structures.

In certain cases, in the late second and third trimester, the secondary anatomy changes due to functional disturbances (some forms of skeletal dysplasia, fetal tumors, segmental deformations secondary to compression in oligohydramnios, multiple pregnancies, or other pathologies) become evident. Thus, even in cases with a normal morphological examination in the second trimester, the examination of the upper and lower members should be attempted in the third trimester. The commendation is stronger if such conditions are suspected.

In the third trimester, the evaluation of the fetal well-being includes the limbs and hand movements, as part of the Manning classical biophysical profile.

6. Literature

Historically, the sensitivity of prenatal ultrasound for detection of musculoskeletal and limb anomalies has been low. In 1991, Levi published a series of 16,072 pregnant women with prenatal ultrasound and found a 45.32% sensitivity for detection of any type of anomaly, with a 23.26% sensitivity for detection of limb and skeletal anomalies [25]. In 1992, Stoll found a 15% sensitivity for isolated anomalies and 48% sensitivity for multiple anomalies for the second-trimester prenatal ultrasounds [26]. The most meaningful result of these early studies is the high specificity of scanning in terms of skeletal abnormalities [25, 26]. This is important, because conditions with high false-positive rates can mislead parents and clinicians in their decisions and recommendations.

Detection of major anomalies has improved over time as a result of improvements in technology and skills, although detection of limb anomalies remained low. The Eurofetus study, in 1999, showed an overall sensitivity for detection of any anomaly to be 61%, with identification of musculoskeletal anomalies much lower and similar to the findings of Levi et al. at 18% [27].

It seems that detection of proximal limb reduction defects is better (23–50%) than detection of hand or finger limb reduction defects (0–8%) [28]. The 2005 EUROCAT study of 4366 fetuses with different anomalies reported a prenatal detection rate for both upper and lower limb reduction defects of 34% [29]. In a more recent study, a higher prenatal detection rate was found for limb reduction defects with associated malformations (49%), if compared to isolated limb reduction defects (25%) [30]. Pajkrt et al. also found a high detection rate for fetuses with short or absent radii and/or ulnae associated with aneuploidy or genetic syndromes (70%) [31]. In another large study, Gray et al. found that 31% of upper extremity anomalies were detected prenatally; however, only 18% were correctly diagnosed [32]. The missed malformations were also located distally (hand and fingers).

The difficulties in detection of upper extremity anomalies may be related to the current guidelines. They mandate only a cursory examination of the upper and lower limbs during the standard second-trimester (ST) examination. This may contribute to the high false-negative rate [33].

7. Technique

The standard examination includes measurements of fetal biometry, in order to estimate the gestational age and fetal weight. It includes the biparietal diameter (BPD), the head circumference (HC), the abdominal circumference (AC), and the femur length (FL) [34]. The measurements of the humerus length (HL) and the transcerebellar diameter (TCD) are optional in many settings. Yet, the fetal biometry may be completed with other segment measurements, as Jeanty proposed over three decades ago [35]. Benefits of such an approach are investigated recently [36]. For almost all fetal structures, nomograms were created, in order to accurately estimate the gestational age.

For limbs examination is recommended to start the sweep proximally. The long bones must be measured in their entirety ("end to end") in a parallel plane to the probe. The examination aims to confirm the normal mineralization and the absence of fractures. The "shortening" diagnosis is allowed only if a previous scan certifies gestational age (preferably, a first-trimester scan).

The forearm and lower leg contain two long bones. In routine examination their presence and normality should be confirmed. If differences between them are suspected or in the presence of other anomalies, all measurements and comparison with the standard data for the gestational age should be done. At the elbow, the ulna is located medially to the radius and has a much higher extremity in relation with humerus. At the wrist, its position depends on the degree of rotation of the forearm.

The image of the foot is obtained in a transverse section to show the heel, the sole, and toes. The position of the big toe with respect to the other toes can be evaluated readily. The length of the foot is not a part of the routine examination, but is important in assessment of skeletal dysplasias and in cases of short femur. If the dimensions of foot remain in normal range for the gestational age and the femur is short, the femur/foot length ratio will be significantly decreased (0.9). In fetuses with constitutionally short femur, this ratio will remain normal.

The ideal window for visualizing the fetal hands is at the late first and early second trimester, when the fingers tend to be extended and abducted. US examinations will be less accurate later in pregnancy, due to fetal position and flexed digits [37]. By some authors, the use of three-dimensional (3D) and 4D US, as well as fetal MRI, improves detection of hand anomalies [32, 37–42]. However, the technique is not currently recommended for routine use by The American College of Obstetricians and Gynecologists [3, 33].

8. Types of limb abnormalities

The most common types of limb anomalies include abnormal number of digits (the higher frequency having polydactyly), abnormal hand/foot position, limb reduction defects, and arthrogryposis. It seems that unilateral limb defects are rarer.

Abnormal hand position is defined as clenched hands or overlapping digits. Arthrogryposis is defined as fetal joint contractures and rigidity.

Counting the fingers is not part of routine scan. Polydactyly is more common in some ethnic groups, such as African Americans. It may occur isolated or may affect both hands and feet.

In amniotic band syndrome, fingers can be missing. This is due to the arrest in development and not as a primary defect in the blastulation process.

In some rare syndromes such as ectrodactyly-ectodermal dysplasia-cleft syndrome (EEC syndrome), missing fingers occur in association with complex malformations. EEC syndrome is a rare form of ectodermal dysplasia. It is an autosomal dominant disorder, inherited as a genetic trait. EEC includes also vesicoureteral reflux, recurrent urinary tract infections, obstruction of the nasolacrimal duct, decreased pigmentation of the hair and skin, missing or abnormal teeth, enamel hypoplasia, absent punctae in the lower eyelids, and photophobia. Occasional, cognitive impairment, kidney anomalies, and conductive hearing loss may appear.

In the development of fetal limbs the free movement itself has a very important role. This is favored by the proximity of fluid in the uterine cavity. The limbs should move freely within each joint. Normal movement assures the normal positions of the hip, knee, elbow, ankle, and wrist joints.

Apparition of abnormal angulation of the ankle joint (ankle clubbing, talipes equinovarus) is frequent, with a prevalence of 1 in 100 live births. The best image is to get a coronal section of the ankle, in which the extended ankle straight along is seen, in a normal spatial relationship with the lower leg. In ankle clubbing, the ankle deviates medially. In the third trimester, especially when the amniotic fluid decreases, a slight subjective angulation of the ankle is common. The key feature for ruling out a true clubbing is the normal shape of the foot. Unilateral ankle clubbing is usually an isolated defect. Bilateral clubbing should be investigated for chromosomal anomalies and genetic syndromes.

The wrist is very flexible and the position of the fingers is also variable. Thus, the examination can find them in a wide variety of positions. In late second trimester and third trimester, the resting position is fisting. The hand can be stimulated to open, showing all four fingers and the thumb. Due to the anatomy of the hand, the thumb is visible in a different plane from the rest of the fingers. Due to this particular context, the diagnosis of abnormal hand position is more difficult than in distal limb.

9. Rationale of screening

All limb anomalies, other than isolated polydactyly, have an increased risk for associated nonskeletal malformations, aneuploidy, stillbirth, neonatal neurodevelopmental delay, and pregnancy termination [43]. This information influences the guiding of evaluation and management, the counseling of parents, and the delivery planning.

The abnormal number of fingers or abnormal position of fingers (Campylodactyly or clinodactyly) is associated with an increased risk of an underlying fetal syndrome.

An image of "sandal gap" anomaly has a weak association with trisomy 21.

The shortening of the humerus seems to have a slightly better predictive value than shortening of the femur in screening for aneuploidies, especially for trisomy 21.

In skeletal dysplasias, the shortening or fracture of long bones is a criterion for diagnosis. The site and the type of shortening are important in establishing an accurate diagnosis (**Table 2**).

Limbs segments	Proximal	Midsegments	Distal segments
Term*	(Humerus/femur)	(Radius and ulna/tibia and Fibula)	(Hand and foot)
Normal (N)**	N	N	N
Rhizomelia	Short	N	N
Mesomelia	N	Short	N
Acromelia	N	N	Short
Micromelia	Short	Short	Short

*The term does not include the malformation, fractures, or absence of the bones.

**Normal measurements is related to an accurate gestational age, ideally established in the first trimester of pregnancy.

Table 2. Terminology in long bone abnormalities.

The upper limb anomalies (and especially radial hypoplasia or aplasia) are phenotypical features of a number of syndromes.

The primary advantage of prenatal diagnosis of upper extremity anomalies is the opportunity for more refined prenatal counseling [44]. Parents are given the chance to discuss their child's diagnosis with a variety of specialists and to receive genetic counseling. For treatable anomalies, a team may be assembled to prepare for postnatal care. Some families will consider pregnancy termination for major untreatable anomalies, and several studies have shown higher rates of pregnancy termination after early prenatal diagnosis of major untreatable anomalies [25, 28, 29, 45].

10. Personal experience

We selected from our archive several suggestive cases of limb abnormalities (**Figures 8–19**):

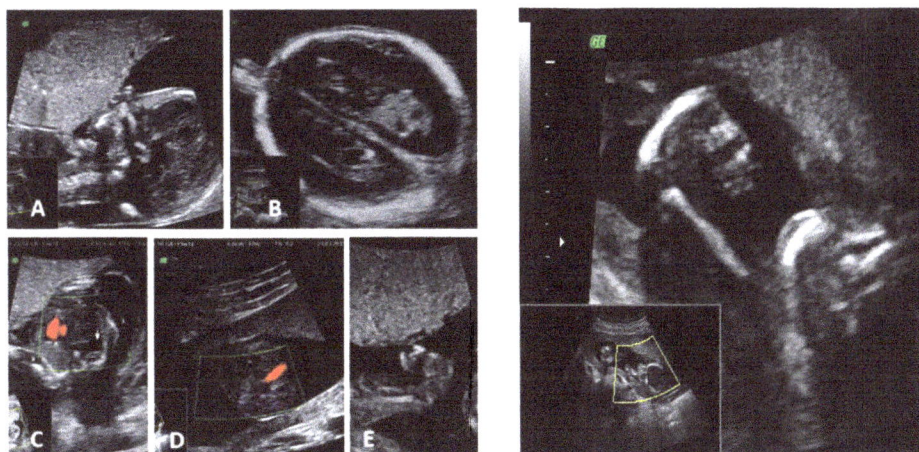

Figure 8. Trisomy 18, diagnosed in early pregnancy. The left image composite shows (A) the abnormal facial profile, the nuchal edema, and the absent nasal bone; (B) multiple choroid plexus cysts; (C) axial plane of the fetal thorax with dextroposition of the fetal heart and presence of the stomach in the thorax, both suggesting diaphragmatic hernia; (D) single umbilical artery crossing lateral to the fetal bladder; and (E) skeletal abnormality and persistent malposition of the fetal arm. In the right-hand image—a detail: the radial aplasia, very characteristic for the syndrome.

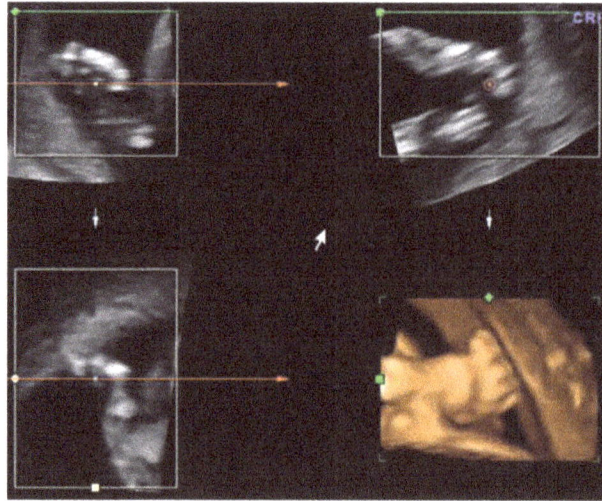

Figure 9. 3D ultrasound images (surface rendering mode), applied in a case of polydactyly. The case was scanned in the first trimester, and the volume was acquired by means of transvaginal scan.

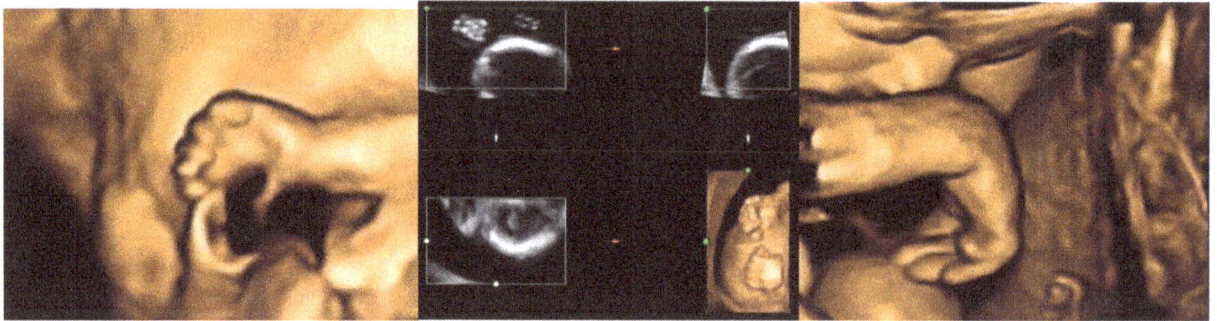

Figure 10. 3D ultrasound images (surface rendering mode), applied in cases of polydactyly in the second trimester; the volume datasets were acquired by means of transabdominal scan. The images were used in the parental counseling process.

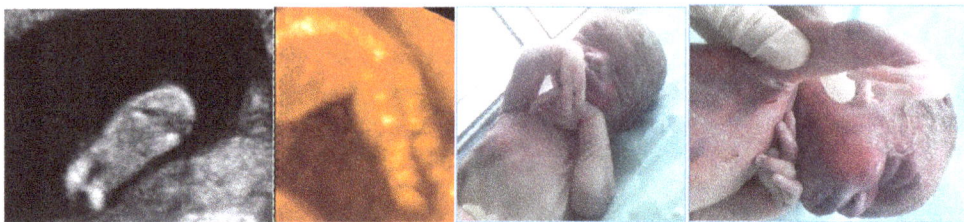

Figure 11. Ectrodactyly: conventional 2D ultrasound, 3D ultrasound skeletal mode, and pathological specimen correlated.

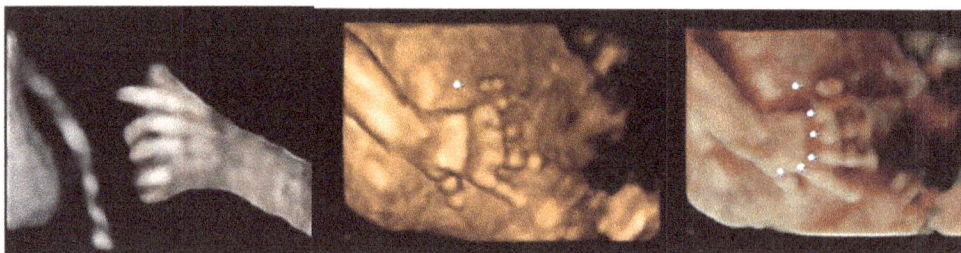

Figure 12. Unilateral postaxial polydactyly type I. Different techniques for acquiring the 3D volume datasets: surface rendering, skeletal mode, and HD life. The case evolved with spontaneous amputation in utero (reproduced with permission of authors) [39].

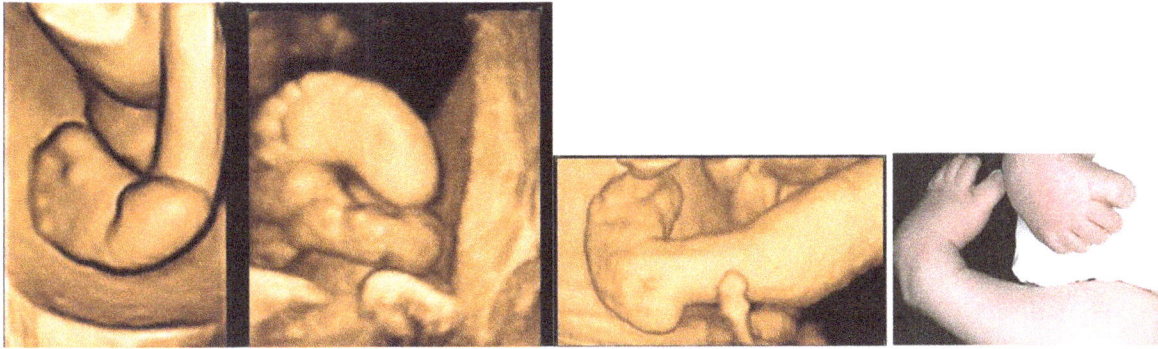

Figure 13. Different cases of clubfoot.

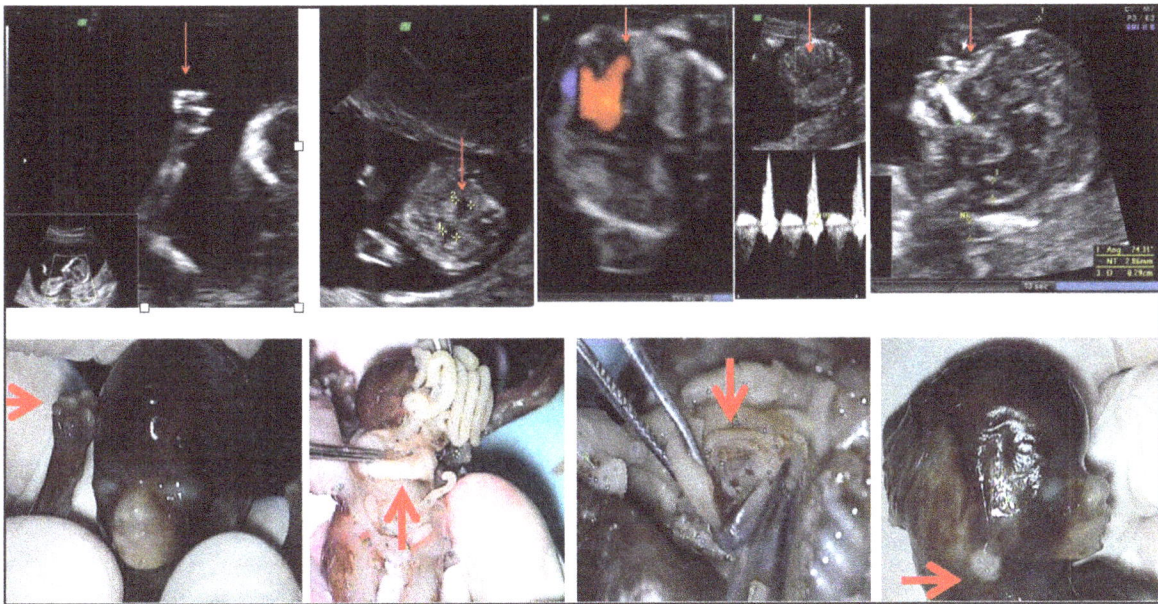

Figure 14. A paucisymptomatic case of trisomy 18, diagnosed in the late first trimester. The upper row demonstrated the ultrasound features: club hand, bilateral pyelectasis, atrioventricular defect, abnormal spectral Doppler at the tricuspid valve interrogation, and unremarkable profile. All these features were compared with the pathological specimen details. The added information were horseshoe kidneys and low set years.

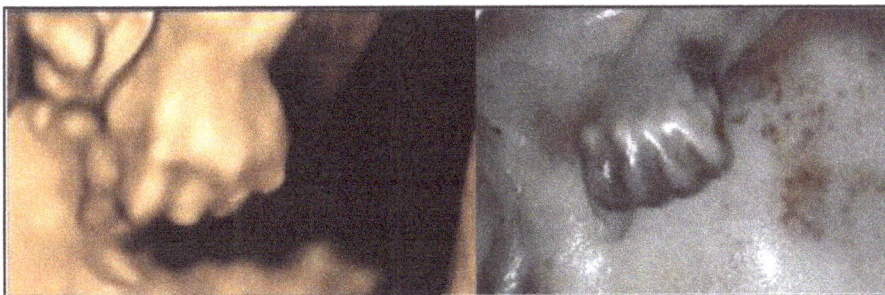

Figure 15. Persistent abnormal hand position. The ultrasound and pathologic data are displayed (the thumb overlapping finger 2). In this case trisomy 13 was diagnosed. The fetus had multiple-associated congenital malformations.

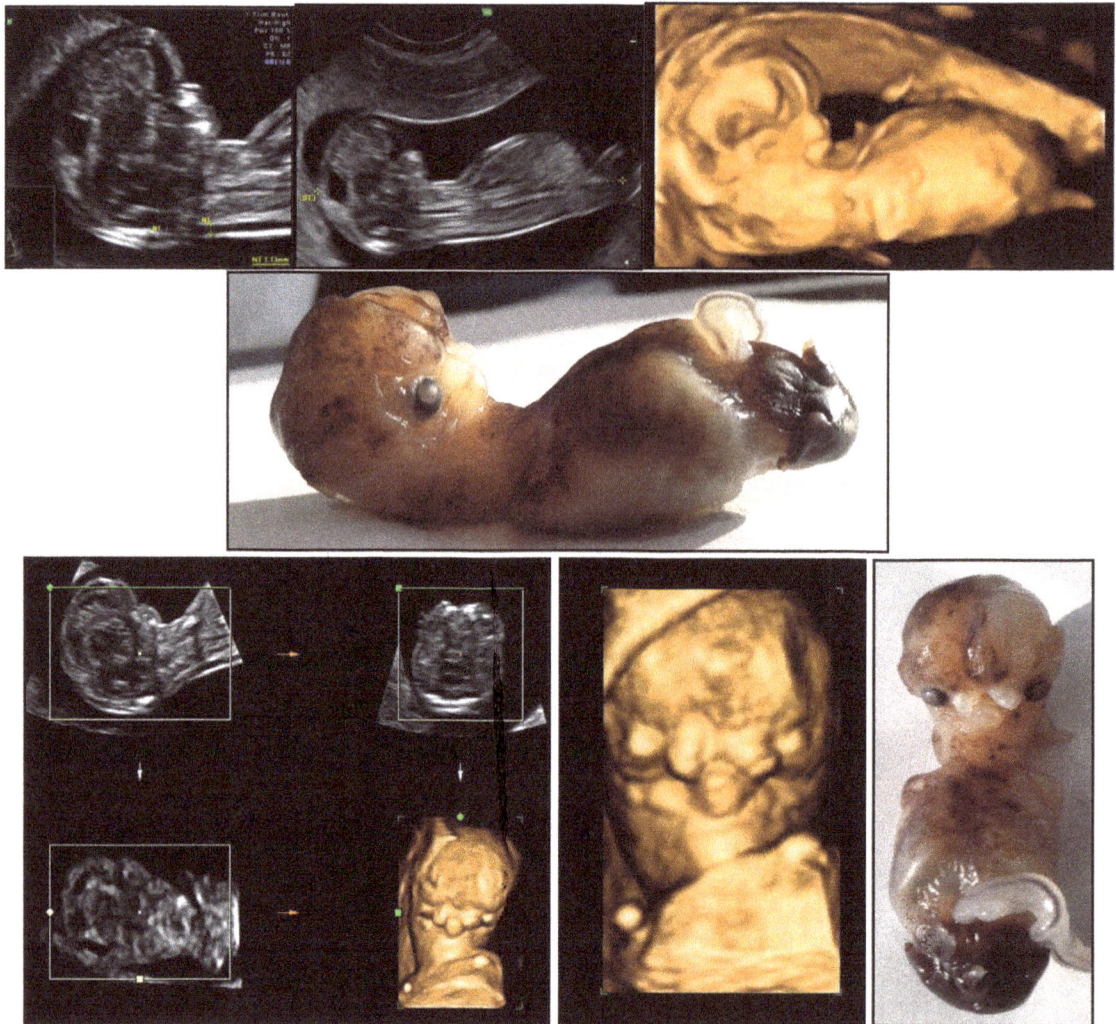

Figure 16. A rare case of complex severe facial malformation, in association with tetraamelia. The 2D conventional ultrasound, the 3D static surface rendering mode, and the pathologic data are correlated.

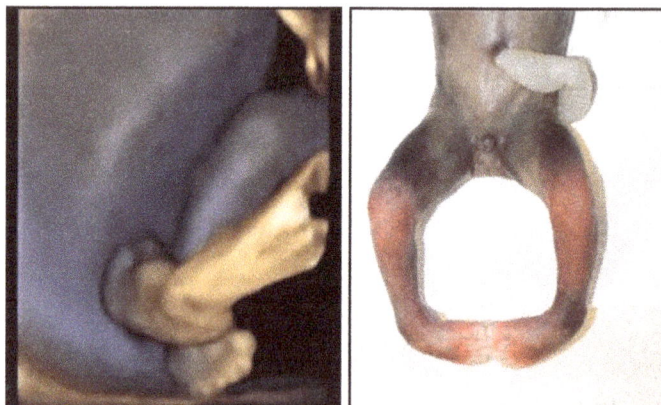

Figure 17. Bilateral clubfoot (genu varum), seen prenatally and post abortion.

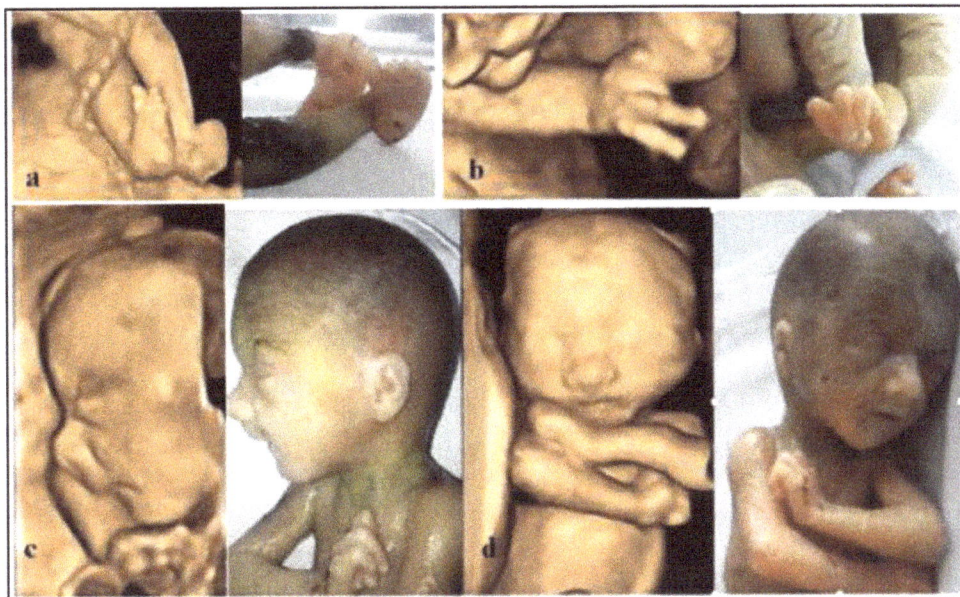

Figure 18. A case of fetal akinesia deformation sequence. The fetus had a complete normal 12 weeks of scan. The mother self-presented for decreased active fetal movements. The matching details obtained by means of volumetric ultrasound and pathology can be observed: Abnormal feet position[a], campylodactyly [b], ulnar deviation of the hands [c], multiple joints contracture (arthrogryposis) [b, c, d], short neck, facial anomalies, hypertelorism, telecanthus, posterior angulation of the ears, and small mouth [c, d].

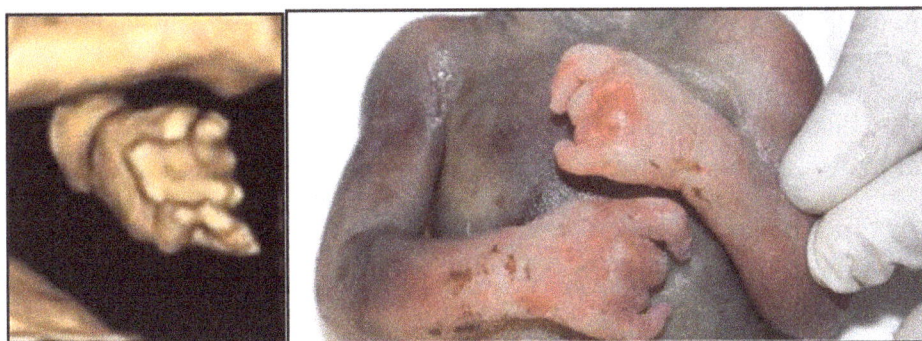

Figure 19. Abnormal position of the hand, with camptodactyly and overlapping fingers.

Author details

Iuliana Ceausu[1]*, Dominic Iliescu[2], Cristian Poalelungi[1], Cristian Posea[1], Nicolae Bacalbasa[1], Dragos Dobritoiu[1] and Liana Ples[3]

*Address all correspondence to: iulianaceausu2004@yahoo.com

1 Department of Obstetrics–Gynecology, University of Medicine and Pharmacy "Carol Davila," "Dr. I. Cantacuzino" Hospital, Bucharest, Romania

2 Department of Obstetrics–Gynecology, University of Medicine and Pharmacy, Craiova, Romania

3 Department of Obstetrics–Gynecology, University of Medicine and Pharmacy "Carol Davila," "Sf. Ioan" Emergency Hospital, Bucharest, Romania

References

[1] Salomon LJ, Alfirevic Z, Berghella V, et al. Practice guidelines for performance of the routine mid-trimester fetal ultrasound scan (ISUOG). Ultrasound in Obstetrics & Gynecology. 2011;**37**:116-126

[2] NHS Fetal Anomaly Screening Programme Handbook. June 2015. Available from: https://www.gov.uk/government/uploads/system/uploads/attachment_data/file/456654/FASP_programme_handbook_August_2015.pdf

[3] American College of Obstetricians and Gynecologists. Ultrasonography in pregnancy. Obstetrics and Gynecology. 2009;**113**:451-461. ACOG Practice Bulletin No. 101

[4] American Institute of Ultrasound in Medicine. AIUM practice guideline for the performance of obstetric ultrasound examinations. Journal of Ultrasound in Medicine. 2010;**29**:157-166

[5] http://www.acr.org/guidelines https://www.acr.org/-/media/ACR/Files/Practice-Parameters/us-ob.pdf

[6] Eames BF, de la Fuente L, Helms JA. Molecular ontogeny of the skeleton. Birth Defects Research. Part C, Embryo Today. 2003;**69**:93-101

[7] Schoenwolf GC, Larsen WJ. Larsen's Human Embryology. 4th ed. Philadelphia, PA: Elsevier Churchill Livingstone; 2009

[8] Souka AP, Pilalis A, Kavalakis Y, et al. Assessment of fetal anatomy at the 11-14-week ultrasound examination. Ultrasound in Obstetrics & Gynecology. 2004;**24**(7):730-734

[9] Iliescu D, Tudorache S, Comanescu A, Antsaklis P, Cotarcea S, Novac L, Cernea N, Antsaklis A. Improved detection rate of structural abnormalities in the first trimester using an extended examination protocol. Ultrasound in Obstetrics & Gynecology. 2013;**42**(3):300-309

[10] Becker R, Albig M, Gasiorek-Wiens A, Entezami M, Knoll U, Wegner RD. The potential of first trimester anomaly scan and first trimester fetal echocardiography as screening procedures in a medium risk population. The Journal of Obstetrics and Gynecology of India. 2005;**55**(3):228-230

[11] Iliescu D, Cara M, Tudorache S, Antsaklis P, Ceausu I, Paulescu D, Novac L, Cernea N, Antsaklis A. Challenges in sonographic detection of fetal major structural abnormalities at the first trimester anomaly scan. Donald School Journal of Ultrasound in Obstetrics and Gynecology. 2015;**9**(3):239-259

[12] Nicolaides KH. Screening for fetal aneuploidy at 11 to 13 weeks. Prenatal Diagnosis. 2011;**31**:7-15

[13] Timor-Tritsch IE, Monteagudo A, Peisner DB. High-frequency transvaginal sonographic examination for the potential malformation assessment of the 9-week to 14-week fetus. Journal of Clinical Ultrasound. 1992;**20**(4):231-238

[14] Liao YM, Li SL, Luo GY, Wen HX, Ouyang SY, Chen CY, Yao Y, Bi JR, Tian XX. Routine screening for fetal limb abnormalities in the first trimester. Prenatal Diagnosis. 2016; **36**(2):117-126

[15] Syngelaki A, Chelemen T, Dagklis T, Allan L, Nicolaides KH. Challenges in the diagnosis of fetal non-chromosomal abnormalities at 11-13 weeks. Prenatal Diagnosis. 2011; **31**(1):90-102

[16] Rice KJ, Ballas J, Lai E, et al. Diagnosis of fetal limb abnormalities before 15 weeks: Cause for concern. Journal of Ultrasound in Medicine. 2011;**30**(7):1009-1019

[17] Ngo C, Viot G, Aubry MC, et al. First-trimester ultrasound diagnosis of skeletal dysplasia associated with increased nuchal translucency thickness. Ultrasound in Obstetrics & Gynecology. 2007;**30**(2):221-226

[18] De Biasio P, Ichim IB, Scarso E, et al. Thanatophoric dysplasia type I presenting with increased nuchal translucency in the first trimester. Prenatal Diagnosis. 2005;**25**(5):426-428

[19] Vimercati A, Panzarino M, Totaro I, Chincoli A, Selvaggi L. Increased nuchal translucency and short femur length as possible early signs of osteogenesis imperfecta type III. Journal of Prenatal Medicine. 2013;**7**(1):5-8

[20] Viora E, Sciarrone A, Bastonero S, et al. Increased nuchal translucency in the first trimester as a sign of osteogenesis imperfecta. American Journal of Medical Genetics. 2002; **109**(4):336-337

[21] Romero R. Routine obstetric ultrasound. Ultrasound in Obstetrics & Gynecology. 1993; **3**:303-307

[22] Schwarzler P, Senat MV, Holden D, et al. Feasibility of the second-trimester fetal ultrasound examination in an unselected population at 18, 20 or 22 weeks of pregnancy: A randomized trial. Ultrasound in Obstetrics & Gynecology. 1999;**14**:92-97

[23] Vintzileos AM, Ananth CV, Smulian JC, et al. Routine second-trimester ultrasonography in the United States: A cost-benefit analysis. American Journal of Obstetrics and Gynecology. 2000;**182**:655-660

[24] Timor-Tritsch IE. As technology evolves, so should its application: shortcomings of the "18-week anatomy scan.". Journal of Ultrasound in Medicine. 2006;**25**:423-428

[25] Levi S, Hyjazi Y, Schaapst JP, et al. Sensitivity and specificity of routine antenatal screening for congenital anomalies by ultrasound: The Belgian Multicentric Study. Ultrasound in Obstetrics & Gynecology. 1991;**1**(2):102-110

[26] Stoll C, Alembik Y, Dott B, Roth MP, Finck S. Evaluation of prenatal diagnosis by a registry of congenital anomalies. Prenatal Diagnosis. 1992;**12**(4):263-270

[27] Grandjean H, Larroque D, Levi S. The performance of routine ultrasonographic screening of pregnancies in the Eurofetus Study. American Journal of Obstetrics and Gynecology. 1999;**181**(2):446-454

[28] Stoll C, Wiesel A, Queisser-Luft A, et al. Evaluation of the prenatal diagnosis of limb reduction deficiencies. EUROSCAN Study Group. Prenatal Diagnosis. 2000;**20**(10):811-818

[29] Garne E, Loane M, Dolk H, et al. Prenatal diagnosis of severe structural congenital malformations in Europe. Ultrasound in Obstetrics & Gynecology. 2005;**25**(1):6-11

[30] Stoll C, Alembik Y, Dott B, Roth MP. Associated malformations in patients with limb reduction deficiencies. European Journal of Medical Genetics. 2010;**53**(5):286-290

[31] Pajkrt E, Cicero S, Griffin DR, van Maarle MC, Chitty LS. Fetal forearm anomalies: Prenatal diagnosis, associations and management strategy. Prenatal Diagnosis. 2012;**32**(11):1084-1093

[32] Gray BL, Calfee RP, Dicke JM, Steffen J, Goldfarb CA. The utility of prenatal ultrasound as a screening tool for upper extremity congenital anomalies. Journal of Hand Surgery. 2013;**38**(11):2106-2111

[33] Reddy UM, Abuhamad AZ, Levine D, Saade GR. Fetal Imaging Workshop Invited P. Fetal imaging: Executive summary of a Joint Eunice Kennedy Shriver National Institute of Child Health and Human Development, Society for Maternal-Fetal Medicine, American Institute of Ultrasound in Medicine, American College of Obstetricians and Gynecologists, American College of Radiology, Society for Pediatric Radiology, and Society of Radiologists in Ultrasound Fetal Imaging Workshop. American Journal of Obstetrics and Gynecology. 2014;**210**(5):387-397

[34] Hadlock FP, Harrist RB, Deter RJ, et al. Fetal femur length as a predictor of menstrual age: Sonographically mea-sured. AJR. American Journal of Roentgenology. 1982;**138**:875-878

[35] Jeanty P, Rodesch F, Delbeke D, et al. Estimation of gestational age form measurements of fetal long bones. Journal of Ultrasound in Medicine. 1984;**3**:75-79

[36] Villar J, Giuliani F, Bhutta ZA, et al. Postnatal growth standards for preterm babies: The preterm postnatal follow-up study of the INTERGROWTH-21stst project: A multicentre population study. The Lancet Global Health. 2015;**3**:e681-e691

[37] Bae DS, Barnewolt CE, Jennings RW. Prenatal diagnosis and treatment of congenital differences of the hand and upper limb. The Journal of Bone and Joint Surgery. American Volume. 2009;**91**(Suppl. 4):31-39

[38] Kennelly MM, Moran P. A clinical algorithm of prenatal diagnosis of radial ray defects with two and three dimensional ultrasound. Prenatal Diagnosis. 2007;**27**(8):730-737

[39] Tudorache S, Dragusin RC, Florea M, Patru CL, Novac M, Iliescu DG. Reversional unilateral postaxial polydactyly type I in fetal life: A case report. Obstetrica și Ginecologia. 2016;**4**

[40] Langner I, Stahnke T, Stachs O, Lindner T, Kühn JP, Kim S, Wree A, Langner S. MR microscopy of the human fetal upper extremity—A proof-of-principle study. BMC Developmental Biology. 2016;**16**(1). https://doi.org/10.1186/s12861-016-0123-z

[41] Palacios-Marqués A, Oliver C, Martín-Bayón T, Martinez-Escoriza JC. Prenatal diagnosis
      of caudal dysplasia sequence associated with undiagnosed type I diabetes. BML Case
      Reports. 2013;**2013**. pii: bcr2013009043 10.1136/bcr-2013-009043

[42] Nemec SF, Kasprian G, Brugger PC, Bettelheim D, Amann G, Nemec U, Rotmensch S,
      Graham JM Jr, Rimoin DL, Lachman RS, Prayer D. Abnormalities of the upper extremi-
      ties on fetal magnetic resonance imaging. Ultrasound in Obstetrics & Gynecology.
      2011;**38**(5):559-567

[43] Dicke JM, Piper SL, Goldfarb CA. The utility of ultrasound for the detection of fetal
      limb abnormalities—A 20-year single-center experience. Prenatal Diagnosis. 2015;**35**(4):
      348-353

[44] Rypens F, Dubois J, Garel L, et al. Obstetric US: Watch the fetal hands. Radiographics.
      2006;**26**(3):811-829; discussion 830-811

[45] Crane JP, LeFevre ML, Winborn RC, et al. A randomized trial of prenatal ultrasono-
      graphic screening: Impact on the detection, management, and outcome of anomalous
      fetuses. The RADIUS Study Group. American Journal of Obstetrics and Gynecology.
      1994;**171**(2):392-399

4

The Neonate with Minor Dysmorphisms

Simona Vlădăreanu, Mihaela Boț, Costin Berceanu,
Claudia Mehedințu and Simona Popescu

Abstract

Congenital anomalies are present in at least 10% of all neonatal intensive care unit admissions, of whom many have an underlying genetic condition. About 50–60% of human congenital anomalies are of unknown etiology, and approximately one- third are caused by genetic factors. A smaller percentage of birth defects are the result of chromosomal aberrations and gene mutations. Around 1 in 40 or 2.5% of all newborns have a malformation at birth. This may be an isolated malformation or may occur together with other malformations and/or dysmorphic features as part of a malformation syndrome. Around 4000 malformation syndromes have now been delineated. Many are associated with medical problems and making a specific syndrome diagnosis can influence immediate medical management. However, the infant with dysmorphism often does not have a major malformation, and may simply have an appearance that is unusual compared with the general population and of unaffected close relatives. The chapter intends to provide semnificative data concerning the approach and management of a dysmorphic neonate, mainly when there are minor anomalies and will offer all those relevant data and try to establish a protocol guide for the approach of the dimorphic neonate.

Keywords: congenital, anomalies, neonate, dysmorphic, syndrome

1. Introduction

Dysmorphology is the branch of clinical genetics that attempts to interpret the human growth patterns and structural defects.

Often, the neonatologist has the opportunity to be the first to identify a congenital anomaly in the neonates. Thus, the presence of a neonatal dysmorphic syndrome (be it major or minor) must be shared with the parents, something that may certainly cause feelings of anxiety.

Addressing the diagnosis of a dysmorphic newborn is similar to the diagnosis of systemic diseases – it relies on analyzing the family history and on performing a meticulous examination of signs and expressions, in an effort to identify a syndrome [1].

The steps to be taken after identifying a neonatal dysmorphism are to confirm the diagnosis through cytogenetic testing via molecular techniques (in order to confirm/exclude a genetic etiology), followed by family counseling by the neonatologist-geneticist team.

After many years spent 'looking after little patients', we hereby discuss a number of anomalies and abnormal physical characteristics, isolated or associated, together with the genetic syndromes in which they can be included.

Since the neonatologists are the first to evaluate the neonates, they must be familiar with various major and minor dysmorphisms. The diagnosis of a syndrome depends on good clinical skills, knowledge of phenotypic features of various syndromes and the experience of the examiner.

Dysmorphism [1] is a morphological anomaly of a structure, a deviation from the norm, and can be classified as major or minor. Major abnormalities may be surgical, medical or cosmetic, and they may be markers for other malformations too. Minor anomalies do not have significant surgical or cosmetic importance, though many genetic syndromes can be recognized based on basis of minor anomalies.

2. Mechanisms of occurrence

Anomalies may occur through three mechanisms [2], each having different implications for the diagnosis:

- *The malformative mechanism* causes structural defects, resulting from an inherently abnormal development process, a primary error in morphogenesis. Malformations include congenital heart, lips, and palate abnormalities. These types of malformations are most commonly associated with a genetic disease or a genetic predisposition.

  ○ The malformation sequence results from a single primary malformation, as is the case with lumbar neural tube defects.

  ○ Malformative syndrome results from several different biological errors during morphogenesis.

- *The deforming mechanism* is an anomaly resulting from the action of prenatal mechanical forces on normal fetal structures. The femur, the fingers (that become overlapped) and the head (that grows into an unusual shape) can be affected. Deformations are rarely genetic, and the recurrence risk is usually low.

- *The disruptive mechanism* causes structural defects resulting from the destruction or interruption of normal intrinsic tissue, such as limbs reduction in amniotic band sequence or certain types of intestinal atresia due to vascular insufficiency [3]. The anomalies are rarely caused by a genetic condition and unlikely to occur in a future pregnancy.

Other terms used to describe the congenital anomalies are:

- Dysplasia, which is an abnormal cellular organization within a tissue, causing structural abnormalities (for example changes in bone structure and cartilage in skeletal dysplasia).

- Association, which is a group of abnormalities that occurs more frequently than expected, but which do not have a predictable pattern or a unique etiology.

3. Incidence

The incidence of congenital abnormalities is approximately 10% of total admissions in neonatal intensive care units (NICUs). Many of them have underlying genetic syndromes. Worldwide, around 7.9 million children (6% of births worldwide) are born with congenital anomalies [4] annually.

Minor anomalies, the subject of this chapter, appear to be isolated more frequently. About 15% of neonates are diagnosed with one minor anomaly (**Table 1**). About 71% of them are found in head, neck and hands. Among neonates diagnosed with an isolated minor anomaly, 3% have a major associated abnormality.

Affected segment	Minor anomaly diagnosed
Head and throat	• Asymmetric crying facies
	• Aplasia cutis congenital
	• Mild micrognathia
	• Flat nasal bridge
	• Upturned nose
	• Large fontanel
Eyes	• Brushfield spots
	• Inner epicanthal folds
	• Telecanthus and hypertelorism
	• Slanting of palpebral fissures
Ear	• Lack of helical fold
	• Posteriorly rotated pinna
	• Preauricular with or without auricular skin tags
	• Auricular (preauricular) pit or sinus
	• Small pinna
	• Folding of helix
	• Darwinian tubercle
	• Crushed (crinkled) ear
	• Asymmetric ear sizes
	• Low-set ears

Affected segment	Minor anomaly diagnosed
Skin	• Dimpling over bones
	• Capillary hemangioma (face, posterior neck)
	• Mongolian spots (African Americans, Asians)
	• Sacral dimple
	• Pigmented nevi
	• Redundant skin
	• Cutis marmorata
	• Café au lait spot
Hand	• Simian creases
	• Bridged upper palmar creases
	• Clinodactyly of the fifth finger
	• Hyperextensibility of thumbs
	• Single flexion crease of fifth digit (hypoplasia of middle phalanx)
	• Partial cutaneous syndactyly
	• Polydactyly
	• Short, broad thumb
	• Narrow, hyperconvex nails
	• Hypoplastic nails
	• Camptodactyly
	• Shortened fourth digit
Leg	• Partial syndactyly of second and third toes
	• Asymmetric toe length
	• Clinodactyly of second toe
	• Overlapping toes
	• Nail hypoplasia
	• Wide gap between hallux and second toe
	• Deep plantar crease between hallux and second toe
Others	• Mild calcaneovalgus
	• Hydrocele
	• Shawl scrotum
	• Hypospadias
	• Hypoplasia of labia majora

Table 1. Minor anomalies seen in various systems.

0.8% of neonates have two minor anomalies associated, and 11% of them have a major associated abnormality.

The presence of three or more minor abnormalities is rare (about 0.5%), and in most cases (90%), neonates also associate a major malformation.

4. Classification

4.1. Minor head and throat anomalies

4.1.1. Asymmetric crying facies

Asymmetric crying facies (ACF) is a minor abnormality, characterized by lowering the corner of the mouth on the unaffected side when crying or sketching a grimace. This is caused by the congenital absence of the anguli oris depressant muscle. The ACF neonates show both nasolabial folds with normal, symmetrical depth and do have the normal ability to lift their forehead and close both eyes. This anomaly must be distinguished from facial nerve paralysis, which is less common [5]. In 20–70% of cases, ACF is associated with other congenital abnormalities, the most common being head/neck, cardiovascular, musculoskeletal, genitourinary and gastrointestinal.

Once this anomaly has been identified, genetic testing is recommended (FISH test or chromosomal microarray comparative genomic hybridization) because ACF is especially associated with 22q11 deletion syndrome (also known as velocardiofacial or DiGeorge syndrome). In this syndrome, the facial dysmorphism coexist with structural heart anomalies, long fingers/limbs, thymus aplasia/hypoplasia and kidney abnormalities. The postnatal follow-up protocol recommends close monitoring of growth and development, evaluation of thyroid and parathyroid function, immunological, hearing and ophthalmic evaluation, echocardiography, renal ultrasonography and the treatment of possibly associated anomalies [6].

4.1.2. Aplasia cutis congenita

Aplasia cutis congenita (ACC) is the congenital absence of the skin, and may occur on any part of the body. It affects the scalp in 70–80% of the cases (**Figure 1**), either as solitary lesions or associated with skull and dura mater defects [2, 7]. Aplasia cutis congenita is a rare anomaly in neonates. Over 500 cases have been reported since the first description, by Cordon in 1767. Due to the unreported cases, their real incidence is unknown. An estimate of the incidence is about 3 out of 10,000 births [8].

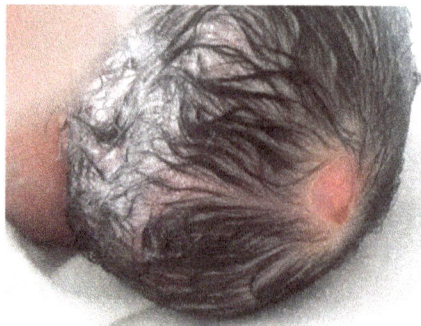

Figure 1. Aplasia cutis congenita.

The pathophysiological mechanism of aplasia cutis congenita is unclear; some theories suggest the involvement of factors such as obstetrical trauma, intrauterine infections with varicella zoster or herpes virus, as well as teratogenic agents, such as cocaine and methimazole [7, 9].

When this anomaly is confirmed, a series of additional investigations are required to determine if there are also other associated malformations that describe a genetic syndrome.

Adams-Oliver's syndrome includes (alongside ACC and limb defects) cutis marmorata telangiectatica congenita, central nervous system abnormalities and cardiovascular abnormalities. To diagnose this genetic syndrome, cerebral and spine (MRI) imaging, limb radiographs, echocardiography and genetic tests with genes ARHGAP31, DOCK6, RBPJ, EOGT [7, 10] sequencing are required. Adams-Oliver Syndrome can be transmitted either autosomal dominant or autosomal recessive. ACC has also been associated with trisomy 13 [11].

ACC may evolve with complications (local infection, meningitis, bleeding and superior sagittal sinus thrombosis). The mortality rate lies between 20 and 50% and depends on the size of the lesion and its association with other malformations.

4.1.2.1. Management

Small sized ACC, located laterally to the median line, is usually a unique congenital anomaly and does not require further evaluation. In sizeable defects, located on the median line, with a membranous appearance that raises the suspicion of a simultaneously damage of the skull and dura mater, cerebral and spinal MRI are recommended. A subjacent neural tube defect must be confirmed or excluded. Treatment for ACC is usually conservative [7].

4.1.2.2. Prognosis

The outcome is usually very good, small defects evolving toward healing within a few weeks through progressive epithelization and atrophic, hairless scarring [8]. In rare cases, hemorrhage and local infections may appear. Large defects of the scalp can be surgically repaired using autologous or biological grafts.

If aplasia cutis congenita is associated with other anomalies, the outcome depends on their severity.

Deep and small defects of the scalp and skull close spontaneously during the first year of life. Larger-sized defects require surgical correction.

Scalp defects that interest the skull and dura mater can be complicated by sagittal sinus thrombosis and are associated with a mortality rate greater than 50%.

4.1.3. Mild micrognathia

Micrognathia is a rather frequent clinical craniofacial abnormality, caused by congenital mandibular hypoplasia (**Figure 2**). It is usually associated with a deficient gonial angle, ascending ramus, and mandibular corpus.

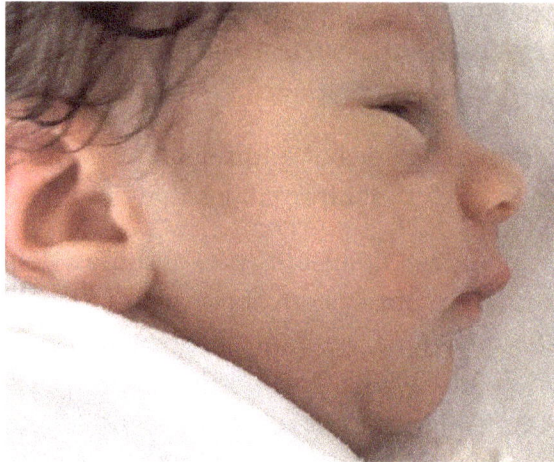

Figure 2. Mild micrognathia associated with retrognathia.

It can appear as a minor and isolated abnormality, or may be severe, as part of a genetic syndrome, frequently causing postnatal complications.

Congenital mandibular hypoplasia occurs either through intrauterine deformation or malformative mechanisms, as a result of a primary intrinsic growth disorder [12, 13].

The mandible is formed from the neural crest, beginning with the onset of the 4th week of gestation, the cells migrating to the upcoming region of the head and neck and with the initiation of the formation of the gill arches. From the first branching arch, two prominences develop, the mandibular and the maxillary one. The mandibular protrusion will form the mandible, and the jaw will form the jaw bone, the zygomatic bone and the squamous part of the temporal bone.

It is likely that congenital mandibular hypoplasia results from poor or insufficient development of the neural crest, or by means of altered migration process to the first branch of the gill, during the 4th week of gestation.

The diagnosis of micrognathia in neonates requires a careful clinical evaluation, to identify other associated craniofacial abnormalities, such as cleft palate or the coexistence of other congenital anomalies. The maxillary, the zygomatic bone, the temporal bone, the cranial vault and the cervical spine represent the other anatomical regions that can be affected.

In the clear majority of cases that include, among the first clinical signs – micrognathia, the diagnosis of genetic syndromes can be suspected on clinical examination. Subsequently, the case requires confirmation by genetic testing, as in deletion syndrome 22q11 cases.

Approximately 60 syndromes associated with micrognathia have been described, such as [12]:

Aneuploidic syndromic

- Trisomy 9
- Trisomy 13
- Trisomy 18

Non Aneuploidic syndromic

- Fryns syndrome

- Goldenhar syndrome (hemifacial microsomia)

- Hydrolethalus syndrome

- Lethal multiple pterygium syndrome

- Nager syndrome

- Pena Shokeir syndrome

- Pierre Robin sequence

- Seckel syndrome

- Smith Lemli Opitz syndrome

- Stickler syndrome

- TAR syndrome

- Treacher Collins syndrome (mandibulofacial dysostosis)

Micrognathia can result in a malocclusion (poor bite), where the teeth and jaws do not line up properly, or in more severe cases, in difficulties in breathing or swallowing. Underdeveloped mandibles can also cause severe psychological and functional impact in the growing of the child, and may be associated with life-threatening complications such as obstructive sleep apnea [12].

4.2. Minor eye anomalies

Although there is a wide variety of ocular morphology (in terms of gender, ethnicity and age), a careful analysis of some dysmorphological entities and objective measurements during the clinical examination can help diagnose some features outside of the normal standards, which may help identifying a syndrome.

4.2.1. Brushfield spots

Brushfield spots are white, yellow-colored spots on the anterior surface of the iris or small white-gray areas around the pupil.

Brushfield spots are observed in 20% of normal neonates, regardless of the color of their eyes. 85% of people with blue eyes show these spots (**Figure 3**).

They are also very common (80%) in the iris of children with trisomy 21. In children with Down syndrome and brown eyes, these spots are visible in 15–17% of cases only, being masked by normal pigmented cells. In cases with black eyes, they cannot be identified.

Brushfield spots should be differentiated from normal stromal condensation called "Kunkmann Wolffian bodies", which are light-colored, located peripherally in the iris and are not considered to be ocular dysmorphisms.

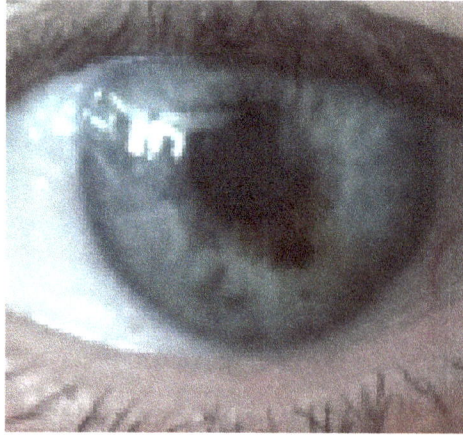

Figure 3. Brushfield spot.

4.2.2. Inner epicanthal fold

Epicanthal fold represents the oblique or vertical skin fold [14], which starts from the upper eyelid to the lower eyelid, covering the inner corner of the eye and it is most frequently bilateral (**Figure 4**). This feature is also named plica palpebronasalis or the historically Mongolian fold.

These skin folds appear through the excessive development of the skin across the nasal bridge. This excess skin presents a certain tension determined by the ectopic orbicularis oculi muscle fibers and connective tissue [15], leading to residual horizontal skin over the nasal bridge.

One of the main facial features that is often closely associated with the epicanthic fold is the elevation of the nasal bridge [16].

Factors influencing this facial trait are: geographical ancestry, age and certain pathological conditions such as blepharophimosis, palpebral ptosis.

The epicanthic fold may be an isolated congenital anomaly, or it may be a manifestation of other syndromes [17, 18]. Approximately 60% of people with Down syndrome have this fold, named "the Mongoloid fold" by John Langdon Down. In Zellweger's syndrome, epicanthic folds are present and prominent [19]. Other pathological conditions that highlight this epicanthic fold are the fetal alcohol syndrome, phenylketonuria, Turner syndrome and Smith-Lemli-Opitz syndrome.

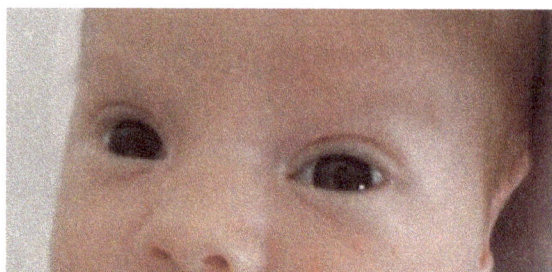

Figure 4. Inner epicanthal fold.

Four types of epicanthic folds [20] have been identified:

1. Epicanthus tarsalis: the fold is most prominent along the upper eyelid - the normal anatomical variant of the Asian eyelid

2. Epicanthus inversus: the fold is most prominent along lower eyelid - associated with blepharophimosis syndrome

3. Epicanthus palpebralis: involves both upper and lower eyelids

4. Epicanthus superciliaris: the fold originates from the brow and follows down to the lacrimal sac

The evolution of epicanthic folds is favorable: a mild degree of epicanthus disappears most frequently with further development of the nose and massive facial bone [20, 21].

Surgical correction is only occasionally required. One of the surgical indications is in the case of epicanthus inversus, which does not resolve on its own with further growth and development of the face [15].

4.2.3. Telecanthus and hypertelorism

Telecanthus is the increased distance between the medial canthi of both eyes, with normal interpupillary distance. This condition is different to hypertelorism, which refers to an increased distance between the orbits [22].

Telecanthus may appear secondary to obstetrical traumas such as naso-orbito-ethmoidal fractures, and it may be an ethnic marker. It could also represent the expression of sinus or orbital tumors, or it may be associated with syndromes such as:

*   Sinus polyps – Kartagener syndrome

*   Down syndrome

*   Turner syndrome

*   Klinefelter syndrome

*   Fetal alcohol syndrome

*   Cri du chat syndrome

*   Dubowitz syndrome

*   Noonan syndrome

*   SHORT syndrome

Hypertelorism is a clinical sign in a wide range of affections and syndromes such as:

*   Edwards syndrome

*   1q21.1 duplication syndrome

- Basal cell nevus syndrome

- DiGeorge syndrome

- Loeys-Dietz syndrome

- Apert syndrome

- Neurofibromatosis

- Leopard syndrome

- Crouzon syndrome

- Wolf-Hirschhorn syndrome

- Andersen-Tawil syndrome

- Waardenburg syndrome

- Cri du chat syndrome

Since hypertelorism is a facial dysmorphism associated with a large and diverse number of congenital disorders and syndromes, the mechanism of hypertelorism is heterogeneous.

A number of theories have attempted to pinpoint this anomaly, such as: the early ossification of the lower wings of the sphenoid, the increasing width of the ethmoid sinuses, the formation and abnormal development of the skull, which can be seen in syndromes such as Apert and Crouzon [22].

4.2.4. Slanting of palpebral fissures

In the normal eye, the eyelids are generally positioned so that the lateral canthus is about 1 mm higher than the medial canthus. The palpebral slant is the direction of the slant of a line that goes from the outer corner of the eye to the inner corner.

The upper or lower slant of the palpebral fissure can be a genetic or ethnic feature (Asian population), but there are a number of conditions and syndromes manifested through this anomaly, isolated or in association with others, such as the Treacher Collins syndrome, Franceschetti (oculo-mandibulo-facial) syndrome, Down syndrome, fetal alcohol syndrome or other genetic disorders.

The identification of an abnormal slant of the palpebral fissure requires a thorough medical examination with an analysis of family history, a physical exam to detect other associated disorders/abnormalities and paraclinical investigations (karyotype), enzyme assays and metabolic studies [23].

4.3. Minor ear anomalies

The incidence of ear malformations is approximately 1 in 3800 newborns [24] and accounts for 50% of all ENT (Ear, Nose, and Throat) malformations. The most common malformations are unilateral and localized in the outer and middle ear.

Auricular malformations in newborns may be genetic (associated with syndromes or not, with family history, spontaneous mutations) or intrauterine (acquired by deformation mechanisms).

External ear malformations may involve the orientation, position, size, and external configuration of the pinna. The absence of the external ear can be identified (anotia).

4.3.1. Preauricular and auricular ear tags and pits

Auricular and preauricular ear tags and pits (**Figures 5** and **6**) are frequent findings on routine neonatal physical examinations, occurring at a frequency of 1 in 12,500 births [25]. The incidence of spontaneous formation of external ear pits in the non-syndromic population ranges between 0.3 and 1.3%, it equally affects both sexes and it has no race predilection. The incidence of unilateral preauricular sinus is 1.3% and that of bilateral preauricular sinus is 0.3%. The rate of genetic transmission of bilateral preauricular sinus was higher in children with a parent with this condition, compared to the cases of unilateral preauricular sinus.

The ear begins to develop in the 6th week of gestation, from the first and second branchial arches. A series of 6 mesenchymal proliferations is formed, known as hillocks of His, which subsequently fuse to form the definitive auricle. The first three hillocks are derived from the first branchial arch and form the tragus, crus of the helix and helix, and the other three hillocks are derived from the second arch and form the antihelix, scapha, and the lobule.

Auricular fistulas may be caused by faulty or incomplete fusion of the hillocks or by localized folding of the ectoderm. Genetic tests suggest that preauricular fistula appears due to an abnormality in chromosome 8q11.1-q13.3 [25].

Preauricular tags may be caused by supernumerary development of the first 3 hillocks of the first branchial arch.

Auricular fistulas are small, pigmented, benign congenital formations [26], located in the tegument and auricular and periauricular soft tissues, anywhere along a line drawn from the tragus to the angle of the mouth. They were first described by Van Heusinger in 1864.

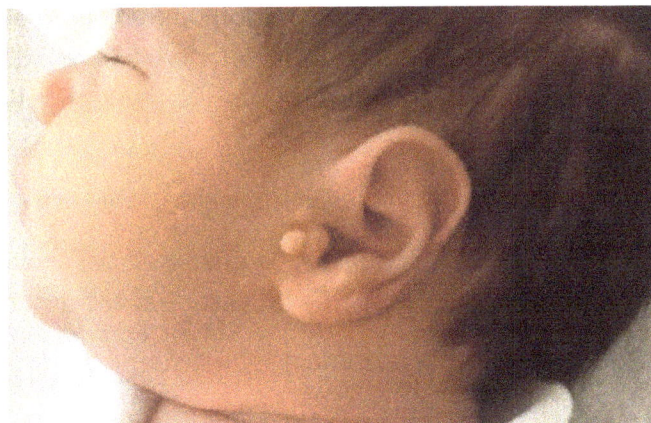

Figure 5. Preauricular tag.

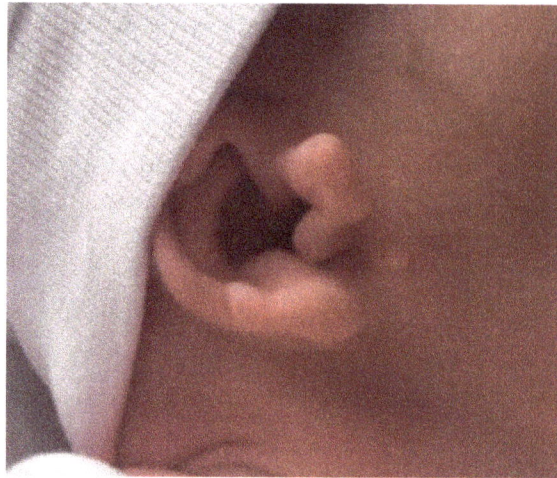

Figure 6. Preauricular tag.

Auricular fistulas are small pits/openings, located anywhere at the anterior margin of the auricle, from crus of the helix to helix, and are lined by squamous epithelium.

These auricular abnormalities can be found in isolation or as part of a genetic syndrome. All newborns will need a hearing assessment later because outer ear abnormalities can be associated with additional abnormalities such as shape abnormalities (helical ear pits), asymmetry, posterior angulation, small size, absent tragus, and narrow external auditory meatus [26], middle or inner ear malformations, and with progressive hearing loss.

These patients should be examined for any other malformations in an attempt to include the anomaly in a genetic syndrome such as [2, 26–29]:

- **Craniofacial microsomia**: association of auricular nodules with other external ear abnormalities, progressive hearing loss, palatoschisis, maxillary and/ or mandibular hypoplasia and renal abnormalities. These children require audiological assessment and renal ultrasonography, and from the point of view of genetic diagnosis, karyotype testing.

- **Branchio-oto renal syndrome (BOR)**: the association of auricular fistulae with other outer ear abnormalities, renal abnormalities and Brachial cleft fistulae. These children require auditory and renal echography, and from the point of view of genetic diagnosis, EYA1, SIX5, SIX1 sequencing is required.

- **Beckwith-Wiedemann syndrome**: auricular fistulae associated with ear lobe asymmetry

- **Oculo-auriculo-vertebral dysplasia (Goldhar Syndrome)**: associates auricular nodules, upper eyelid coloboma, outer ear deformities and vertebral abnormalities

- **Chromosome arm 11q duplication syndrome**: Preauricular tags or pits

- **Chromosome arm 4p deletion syndrome**: Preauricular dimples or skin tags

- **Chromosome arm 5p deletion syndrome**: Preauricular tags

De novo appearance of these auricular abnormalities associated with those on the face and neck may be related to the use of propylthiouracil in early pregnancy to treat maternal hyperthyroidism [30].

When auricular fistulae and nodules are isolated, no further evaluation is required for these children [2].

Most cases with typical location of auricular and preauricular fistulas are asymptomatic and do not require surgery. They can retain epithelial and sebum debris, and can evolve to subcutaneous cysts or infection. This may in turn lead to cellulitis or abscess, and may require aspiration of the collection if the antibiotic therapy is not responding. In cases of recurrent cyst infection, surgical excision of the cyst and the fistula tract is indicated. A preauricular fistulae may vary in length, may have a sinuous tract or may be extensively branched. If there are auricular fistulas and subcutaneous cysts, they adhere to the auricular perichondritis. Thus, complete elimination of the fistula or cyst should also include a portion of the auricular perichondritis at the base of the lesion [26]. Auricular and preauricular nodules can be excised for esthetic reasons.

4.3.2. Microtia

Microtia is a congenital anomaly characterized by the underdevelopment of the outer ear, while anotia is the complete absence of the ear. Because microtia and anotia have the same origin, they can be described as microtia-anotia [31].

Microtia can be unilateral or bilateral and its frequency is of approximately 1–3 to every 10,000 births [32]. In the case of unilateral microtia, the right ear is most frequently affected [31].

Etiologically, the administration of the teratogenic agent called isotretinoin (Accutane®) during pregnancy may lead to these congenital auricular abnormalities (anotia/microtia).

The pathogenesis of microtia is heterogeneous, and there have been indications of unique genetic mutations or its presence as a family trait [33].

Microtia has a broad spectrum of phenotypic aspects, from the uncomplicated hereditary one, (which is transmitted as a dominant feature, and it is most often harmless), to severe, complicated forms of hearing loss. From a clinical point of view, four grades of microtia have been described:

- **Grade I:** A less than complete development of the external ear with identifiable structures and a small but present external ear canal

- **Grade II:** A partially developed ear (usually the top portion is underdeveloped) with a stenotic external ear canal producing a conductive hearing loss

- **Grade III**: the most common form of microtia: Absence of the external ear with a small peanut-like vestige structure and an absence of the external ear canal and ear drum.

- **Grade IV:** Absence of the total ear or anotia.

Isolated microtia is relatively common, but it can be found in newborns in association with other facial dysmorphisms, such as hemifacial microsomia, Goldenhar syndrome or Treacher

Collins syndrome [34], jaw deformities, vertebral anomalies [35], heart defects, limb abnormalities, renal abnormalities and holoprosencephaly [32, 36].

Auricular atresia is the underdevelopment of the middle ear and auditory canal, and it occurs relatively frequently in conjunction with microtia, since newborns with microtia have no external opening to the ear canal, although the cochlea and the other internal ear structures are usually present. The degree of microtia usually correlates to the grade of underdevelopment of the middle ear [37, 38].

The assessment of newborns and infants with microtia-anotia should include a thorough clinical examination for the detection of associated structural defects, pediatric audiological test, multi-disciplinary consultation with the genetic specialist, pediatric otolaryngologist, and pediatric plastic surgeon.

4.3.2.1. Management

A minor anomaly does not require surgical correction. When the auricle is very deformed or absent (grades III and IV), reconstruction is often required for esthetic reasons. Most reconstructive interventions are recommended after the age of 6–10 years old, when the ear pavilion has 80% of the size of an adult ear.

The management of a microtia case associated with an auditory meatus defect is performed by long term periodic audiological monitoring, especially if there is an atresia of the auditory meatus, with the possible placement of an amplification device, especially in the case of the bilateral forms [39].

The surgical procedure for restoring the pinna is complex and is performed in several stages, with esthetic results that vary greatly, as the outer ear structure is difficult to duplicate [40]. A plastic surgical alternative is the use of a synthetic prosthetic pinna or a pinna obtained via the three-dimensional printing technology, but the research is still underway [41].

4.3.3. Macrotia

Macrotia refers to an oversized or enlarged but well-developed auricle without any other malformations of the ear (**Figure 7**). The most exaggerated portion of the ear is the scaphoid fossa. The condition is usually bilateral and symmetric.

Generally, it has an autosomal dominant pattern of transmission and an unknown pathogenesis [42].

Macrotia is commonly associated with the following syndromes:

- Marfan Syndrome: large auricle with dropped, floppy cartilage

- Fragile X-syndrome: macrotia with floppy cartilage, associated with mild or profound X-linked retardation [43].

- Cerebro-oculo-facial-skeletal syndrome (COFS): macrotia associated with neurogenic arthrogryposis, microcephaly, micro-ophthalmia.

- Variant of De Lange type 2 syndrome [44]: characterized by macrotia associated with severe microcephaly, mild mental retardation, muscular hypotonia and dysmorphic faces (flat profile, mild ptosis, short nose with a large tip and anteverted nares, narrow mouth, retrognathism).

4.3.3.1. Management

Otoplasty can improve the shape, position and proportion of the ear. It is a reconstructive surgery procedure that attempts to harmonize the ratio between ear and face.

4.4. Minor skin anomalies

4.4.1. Capillary hemangioma

It is a congenital vascular abnormality which consists of an agglomeration of neo-formation capillary vessels, manifested in the form of variable reddish-purple patches (**Figures 8** and **9**). These patches are mainly located on the face, neck and lips, but they can appear on any area of the body. They are diagnosed by clinical inspection.

Capillary hemangiomas occur only in the layers of the skin, and they do not develop in depth. They generally appear within a few weeks after birth, but they may appear in infants too and most frequently disappear spontaneously in 1–2 years. A special form of this anomaly is the 'birthmark', the clinical form that appears on the nape or covers a portion of the face and has a violet color [45, 46].

4.4.1.1. Management

Capillary hemangiomas are prone to irritation and ulceration. Each lesion must be evaluated individually, and the practitioner may opt to treat it selecting an alternative therapeutic route.

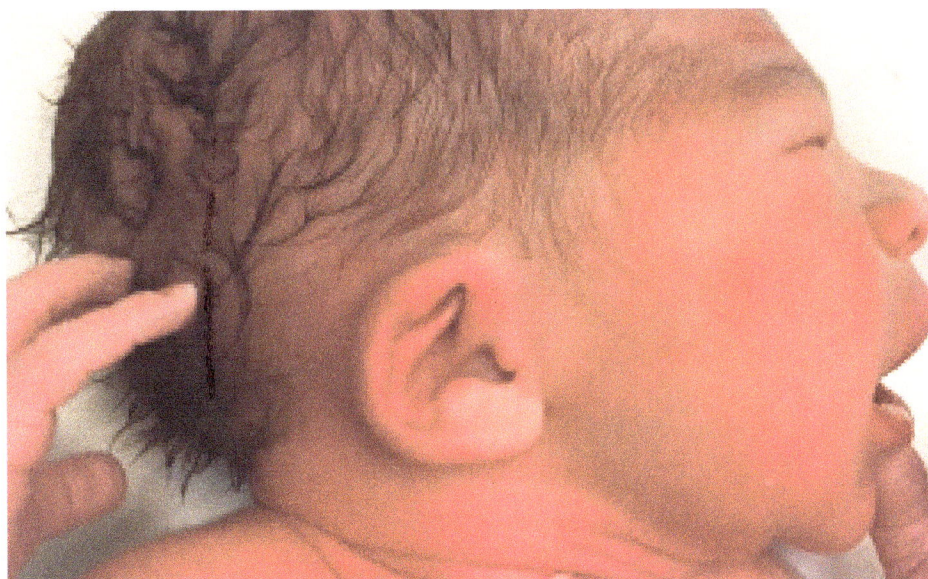

Figure 7. Bilateral macrotia with abnormal shape of the auricle.

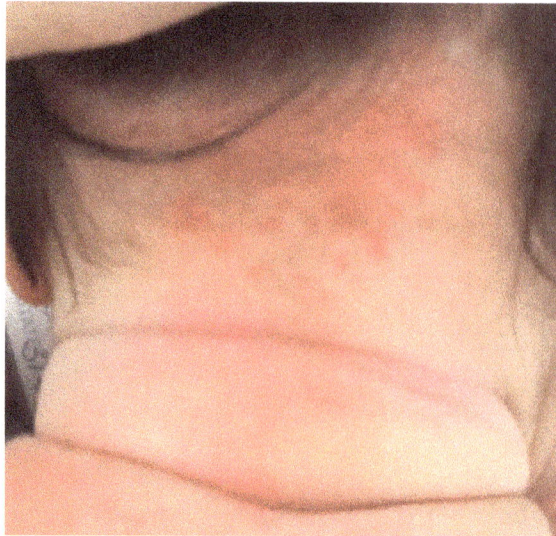

Figure 8. Capilary hemangioma – Posterior neck.

The treatment can be surgical and dermatological-medical and may consist of the surgical excision of hemangiomas, laser pulses, cryosurgery and systemic administration of glucocorticoids. Oral propranolol may be administered in order to reduce the size of hemangiomas may be a therapeutic option [47].

4.4.2. Mongolian spots (Africans, Americans, Asians)

Mongolian Spots, also known as Mongolian Blue Spots or congenital dermal melanocytosis, represent a congenital condition characterized by the presence of smooth spots, irregular-shaped with wavy borders, dark blue to brown, with a normal skin texture [48]. They may be present from birth or may appear within the first few weeks of life during the neonatal period.

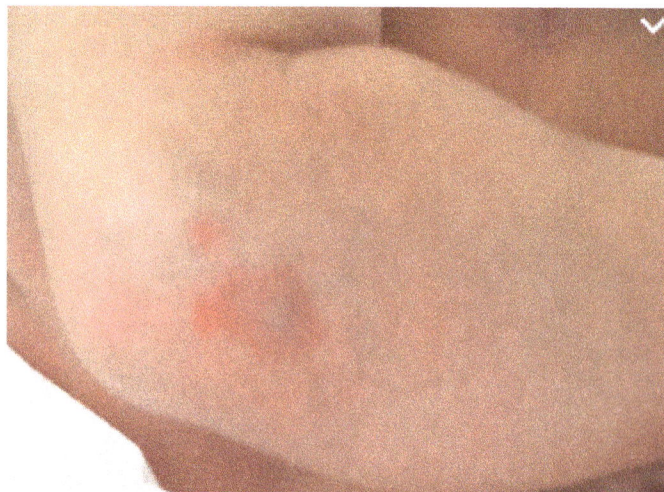

Figure 9. Capilary hemangioma – Forearm.

Mongoloid Spots represent an agglomeration of dermal melanocytes and is not a clinical sign associated with a disease or syndrome.

Depending on the location of melanocytes on the surface of the skin, the coloration of the Mongoloid Spots change. If they are superficially located, the color of the spots is brown, and the deeper they are, the color tends more and more to have a blue shade [48, 49].

Mongoloid Spots are most commonly diagnosed at birth due to specific coloration and localization, and no additional investigation methods are required. They are found with a frequency of 90% in the black population and the Native Americans, in about 80% of Asian infants, 70% of Hispanic individuals and in a reduced proportion of 5–10% of Caucasian children [48, 49]. Incidence is lower in preterm infants compared to full-term infants, and in terms of gender distribution, the incidence is higher in boys.

Most spots are located on the buttocks, lumbosacral (**Figure 10**), deltoid and dorsal region, on the limbs and in rare cases on the face or on the occipital region. There may be single or multiple spots, ranging in size from 1 to 2 cm to tens of cm [50].

4.4.2.1. Management

No treatment is recommended, as Mongoloid spots generally disappear spontaneously at the age of 1–4 years, most frequently in the first year of life. If they do not disappear until puberty, they remain permanent, a situation that occurs in approximately 5% of cases [51].

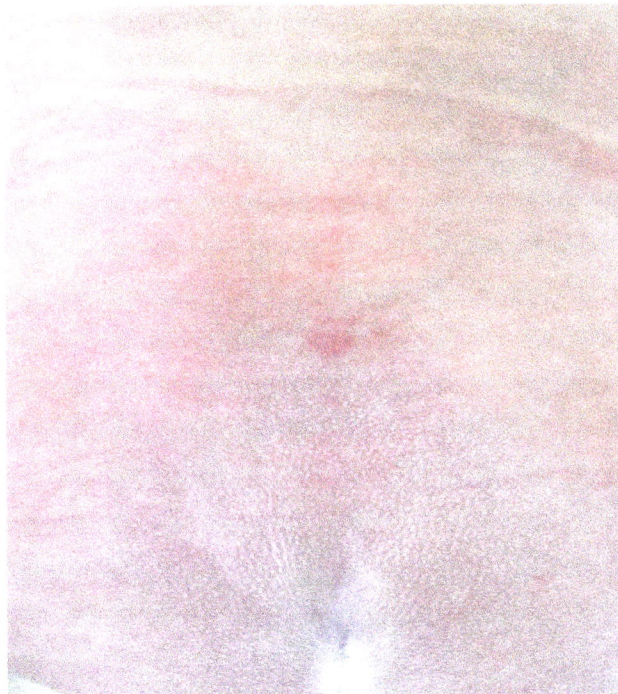

Figure 10. Mongoloid spot – Lumbosacral region.

4.4.3. Cutis marmorata telangiectatica congenita

Cutis marmorata telangiectatica congenita is a rare congenital vascular disorder that manifests itself by affecting the blood vessels of the skin by alternating a vascular network with a vasodilation and vasoconstriction process which gives the skin a marbled appearance. It is accentuated by cold temperatures, but it does not disappear when exposed to warmer temperatures [52].

It should not be confused with Cutis Marmorata, which is a normal, adaptive, physiological response of the newborn to exposure to low temperatures. This disorder is due to a neurological and vascular immature system, it varies between the constriction and dilation of blood vessels, and it occurs most frequently in the hands and feet.

Very few cases of cutis marmorata telangiectatica congenita have been reported worldwide - less than 100 cases [53], but in reality it is more common than that. Mild forms are not that rare, but they are not reported [54].

The pathophysiological mechanisms are still unclear, with most cases occurring sporadically, although rare cases were reported in some families. Studies indicate the primary involvement of capillaries, venules and veins, and possibly arterioles and lymphatic vessels.

The hypothetical mechanisms that have been proposed are environmental factors, peripheral neural dysfunctions, failure of the development of mesodermic vessels in an early embryonic stage and autosomal dominant inheritance with incomplete penetrance [52, 55].

Diagnosis: skin manifestations may be associated with the asymmetry of extremities, macrocephaly, glaucoma, cutaneous atrophy, chronic skin ulcerations, neurological anomalies, vascular anomalies (nevus flammeus, Sturge–Weber syndrome, Klippel-Trénauna syndrome, Adams Oliver syndrome), psychomotor and /or mental retardation [56].

Management: in general, there is no treatment for this condition, but the associated anomalies can be treated. In the case of limb asymmetry, without motor dysfunction, there is the possibility of inserting an "elevation" device for the shorter leg during early childhood. Laser therapy has not been successful in the treatment of this vascular skin disorder, possibly due to many dilated capillaries and veins in the deep layers of the skin.

Prognosis: the prognosis is favorable in most cases, when patients experience an isolated cutaneous abnormality. In most cases, the marbled appearance regresses spontaneously during the first year of life due to the normal maturation process, with the thickening of the epidermis and dermis. In fewer cases, lesions can continue for up to 10 years or throughout the patient's life.

4.4.4. Pigmentary nevi

Pigmentary nevi, also known as melanocytic nevi, are benign neoplasms present from birth - congenital melanocytic nevi may develop throughout life.

Pigmentary nevi appear with a high frequency as uniform, beige, brown or skin-color formations, sometimes protruding, circular or oval, with regular, smooth, well-defined margins, of 6 mm in diameter [57, 58].

Histopathologically, they are cellular (melanocyte) benign clusters that change very little in life, have a slow growth, and never invade the surrounding tissues. The number of nevi is influenced both genetically - the family history is very important - and from the sun exposure of the infant [59].

Congenital pigmentary nevi over 20 cm in diameter have an increased risk of malignancy.

Pigmentary nevi are commonly diagnosed clinically or using the dermatoscope.

The management of pigmentary nevi depends on the type of nevus and the degree of uncertainty of the diagnosis. Benign ones require nothing else than monitoring after the neonatal period [60, 61], while those with special characteristics - asymmetry, uneven, irregular margins, color variations, diameter > 6 mm - very rare cases, require biopsy with histopathology, immunohistochemistry and electron microscopy [57, 62].

4.5. Minor hand anomalies

4.5.1. Camptodactyly

Camptodactyly is the irreversible flexion of one or both interphalangeal joints at the level of one or more fingers, being most frequently a congenital condition.

It can be diagnosed antenatally [63–65] "in utero" or postnatally, being a clinically obvious deformity, which subsequently requires imaging investigations. An abnormal insertion of lumbrical and flexor digitorum tendons of the hand is often noted.

Camptodactyly may occur sporadically, de novo or by autosomal dominant inheritance.

It may be an isolated clinical manifestation or clinical expression in syndromes such as Trisomy 18 and 13, Freeman Sheldon Syndrome, Pena Shokeir Syndrome, CACP Syndrome (Camptodactyly, Arthropathy, Coxa vara, Pericarditis), arthrogryposis [63, 65–67].

4.5.2. Clinodactyly

Clinodactyly is a congenital malformation consisting of the lateral deflection of the fingers by affecting the first interphalangeal joint, which interests any finger, especially the pollex and the auricular fingers (the fifth finger), (**Figure 11**).

Clinodactyly is a descriptive term, which refers to a radial angulation at a common interphalangeal joint in radio-ulnar or palmar planes, and can often be a normal anatomical variant.

The incidence varies, ranging between 1 and 18%, as it is most frequently under-reported.

Clinodactyly may be a very common isolated clinical manifestation in the context of a family history [68] - with autosomal recessive inheritance, but it may also occur in several syndromes, in association with other locomotor abnormalities or in other organs and systems.

Clinodactyly is seen in over 60% of children with Down syndrome [63], Klinefelter syndrome, trisomy 18, Turner syndrome, Cornelia de Lange Syndrome, Feingold Syndrome, Roberts Syndrome, Russell-Silver Syndrome or Fanconi Syndrome. It may also be a clinical manifestation associated with other abnormalities such as macrodystrophia lipomatosa and brachydactyly type A3.

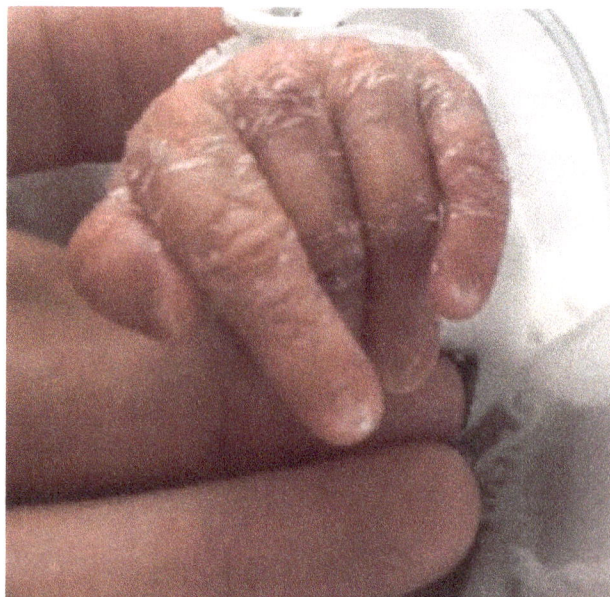

Figure 11. Clinodactily of the fifth finger.

Considering the presence of this sign in multiple chromosomal anomalies, some authors consider it a "soft sign", if detected in an antenatal ultrasound scan.

If the clinodactyly is isolated, it has an excellent prognosis.

Usually, the treatment is not necessary. If necessary - because of emotional stress due to esthetic reasons or the impairment of the fine hand movements - the treatment is surgical [69]. For surgery, preoperative radiographs of the pollex are performed, establishing the size of the graft and the degree of angulation necessary to restore the normal function of the distal phalange.

4.5.3. Polydactyly

It is one of the most common congenital abnormalities of upper limbs, seen in all ethnicities, and it refers to the presence of additional fingers, being usually bilateral [70]. Most often, polydactyly affects the upper and lower limbs synchronously. Supernumerary fingers do not usually have adequate muscle connections [71, 72].

The classification of this condition is based on the location of the additional fingers, the polydactyly being:

• Postaxial (duplicated finger V),

• Mesoaxial/central (duplication of fingers II, III, IV),

• Preaxial (duplicated thumb),

• Mixed.

Polydactyly may appear isolated, de novo, sometimes autosomal dominant inherited or may be associated with syndromes [73, 74] such as Bardet-Biedl Syndrome, Carpenter Syndrome, Elis-Van Creveld Syndrome, Fanconi Syndrome, Greig Syndrome, Holt-Oram Syndrome, Meckel-Gruber

Syndrome, Pallister-Hall Syndrome, Smith-Lemil-Opitz Syndrome, Trisomy 13, Trisomy 18, Short Rib Polydactyly Syndrome Type I (Saldino-Noonan Type) (Majewski type), Trisomy 21, Townes-Brocks Syndrome.

Usually, polydactyly is diagnosed antenatally, but if it is postnatally discovered, it requires paraclinical investigations in order to be included in one of the genetic syndromes, except for cases of family history. The investigations are performed using imaging techniques (MRI, CT scan, ultrasound examination), followed by genetic consultation in case of association with other malformations. The most commonly associated malformations are syndactyly, hypoplasia or aplasia of long bones, hydrocephalus, microcephaly, spina bifida, ventricular septal defect, atrial septal defect, esophageal atresia, duodenal atresia, anal imperfection, abdominal wall defects, renal agenesis, polycystic kidney disease, hydronephrosis, diaphragmatic hernia, anophthalmia, cheilopalatoschisis.

In the case of isolated polydactyly, no treatment is required. If this anomaly affects the mobility and gross/fine movements of the fingers/hands, the treatment is always surgical.

4.6. Minor foot anomalies

4.6.1. Partial syndactyly of the second and third toe

Syndactyly is one of the most common congenital limb malformations involving the fusion of two or more fingers due to the failure of separation process during the development of limbs in the first trimester. In the lower limbs, the most common location is between the second and the third finger [75].

It is a heterogeneous clinical phenotype, as it may be: unilateral or bilateral, symmetrical or asymmetrical, partial or complete, cutaneous or bony, involving only the phalanges and/ or metatarsal bone, or may extend to tarsal bones or even the calf bones.

Partial syndactyly of the second and third toe may appear as a clinically isolated phenotype (the most common is zygodactyly) [75] or may be associated with syndromes such as:

- Pfeiffer syndrome [76–79] - type V acrocephalopolysyndactyly has as its etiology a dominant autosomal genetic defect in which mutations occur in the FGFR1 gene (fibroblast growth factor receptor 1) and in the FGFR2 gene (fibroblast growth factor receptor 2). In this syndrome, the partial syndactyly of the second and third toe is accompanied by other malformations such as craniosynostosis, facial hypoplasia, hypertelorism, brachydactyly.

- Carpenter syndrome - type II acrocephalopolysyndactyly is an autosomal recessive genetic disorder in which mutations occur in RAB23, a hydrolysis involved in transmembrane regulation [80]. Carpenter syndrome associates, besides partial syndactyly and polydactyly, with auricular, cardiac and genital abnormalities.

- Smith-Lemli-Opitz syndrome is an autosomal recessive genetic disorder of cholesterol biosynthesis [81]. This syndrome associates with syndactyly and microcephaly, micrognathia, genital malformations, auricular malformations, autism spectrum disorders.

Partial syndactyly of the second and third toe does not affect the motor function, and therefore does not require correction.

4.6.2. Dysplastic nails

Insufficient development of nails [82] may occur in isolation or in many genetic malformations such as:

- Simpson-Golabi-Behmel Syndrome (Bulldog Syndrome). The most common etiology of this syndrome is the mutations in the GPC3 gene to chromosome X [83]. Nail hypoplasia is accompanied by other clinical manifestations such as macrosomia, hypertelorism, polydactyly, macrostomia, macroglossia.

- Fetal Alcohol Syndrome [84]. Prenatal exposure to alcohol causes numerous fetal malformations, including nail dysplasia accompanied by: microcephaly, facial hirsutism, short palpebral fissures.

- Fryns Syndrome. This syndrome is a genetic disorder inherited in an autosomal recessive manner, in which dysplastic nails occur along with other minor and major malformations such as diaphragmatic hernia, hirsutism, distal phalangeal hypoplasia, Dandy-Walker malformation, agenesis of corpus callosum.

4.6.3. Phalanx anomalies: digital deformities

The small bones and soft tissues of the feet can be affected by systemic disorders, and frequently, the findings are quite unique and virtually help diagnose some genetic or metabolic disorders [85]. Sometimes the changes in the structural bones of the feet, metacarpals and metatarsals, or the phalangeal units are so astonishing that they ensure the diagnosis of peculiar and rare syndromes.

There are many disorders – some genetic, some neoplastic, some inflammatory – which sometimes produce extraordinary changes in the patient's feet. In some cases, phalanx abnormalities occur as a result of the sucking of the finger by the fetus, causing elongation and hypertrophy (**Figures 12** and **13**).

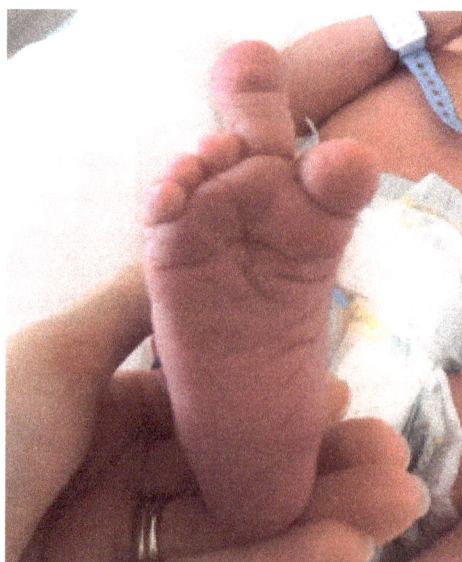

Figure 12. Phalanx anomalies.

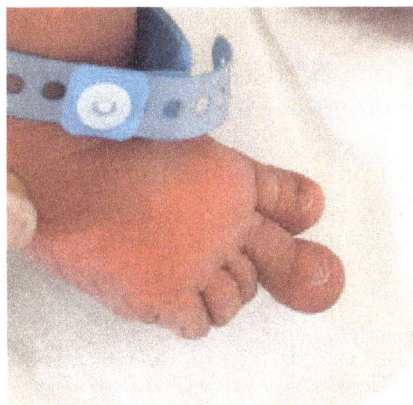

Figure 13. Phalanx anomalies.

A small listing includes synovial chondromatosis, fibrous dysplasia, tumoral calcinosis, Maffucci syndrome, Ollier's disease, hereditary multiple osteocartilaginous exostosis, type 1 neurofibromatosis, pigmented villonodular synovitis, hyperparathyroidism, or gout.

Author details

Simona Vlădăreanu[1]*, Mihaela Boț[1], Costin Berceanu[2], Claudia Mehedințu[1] and Simona Popescu[1]

*Address all correspondence to: simconst69@gmail.com

1 University of Medicine and Pharmacy "Carol Davila", Bucharest, Romania

2 University of Medicine and Pharmacy of Craiova, Romania

References

[1] Tewari VV, Mehta R, Tewari K. Dysmorphic neonate: An approach diagnostic in the current era. Pediatric Dimensions. ISSN: 2397-950X

[2] Jones LK, Adam MP. Evaluation and diagnosis of the dysmorphic infant. Clinics in Perinatology. 2015 Jun;**42**(2):243-248. DOI: 10.1016/j.clp.2002.002

[3] Adam M, Hudgins L. The importance of minor anomalies in the evaluation of the newborn. NeoReviews. 2003;**4**:e99-e104

[4] Lobo I, Zhaurova K. Birth defects: Causes and statistics. Nature Education. 2008;**1**(1):18

[5] Shapira M, Borochowitz ZU. Asymmetric crying facies. NeoReviews. 2009;**10**:e502-e509

[6] Cancrini C, Puliafito P, Digilio MC, et al. Clinical features and follow-up in patients with 22q11.2 deletion syndrome. The Journal of Pediatrics. 2014;**164**:1475-1480

[7] Tollefson MM. Aplasia cutis congenita. NeoReviews. 2012;**13**:e285-e292

[8] Wan J. Aplasia Cutis Congenita. Medscape. Updated: May 12, 2017

[9] Yoshihara A, Noh J, Yamaguchi T, et al. Treatment of graves' disease with antithyroid drugs in the first trimester of pregnancy and the prevalence of congenital malformation. The Journal of Clinical Endocrinology and Metabolism. 2012;**97**:2396-2403

[10] Cohen I, Silberstein E, Perez Y, et al. Autosomal recessive Adams-Oliver syndrome caused by homozygous mutation in EOGT, encoding an EGF domain-specific O-GlcNAc transferase. European Journal of Human Genetics. 2014;**22**:374-378

[11] Carey J. Trisomy 18 and 13 syndromes. In: Cassidy S, Allanson J, editors. Management of Genetic Syndromes. 3rd. New York: John Wiley & Sons; 2010. pp. 807-823

[12] Kumar P, Burton B. Congenital Malformation. Evidence-Based Evaluation and Management. McGrowHill Medical 2008. 0-07-159356-X. Chapter 14. Micrognathia. Pg 101-104

[13] Sperber GH. Craniofacial Development. London: BC Decker Inc; 2001. pp. 127-138

[14] Bowling B. Congenital malformations: Epicanthic folds. In: Kanski's Clinical Ophthalmology: A Systematic Approach. 8th ed. S.l.: Elsevier; 2016. p. 57

[15] Li G, Wu Z, Tan J, Ding W, Luo M. Correcting Epicanthal folds by using asymmetric Z-plasty with a two curve design. Journal of Plastic, Reconstructive & Aesthetic Surgery. 2016;**69**(3):438-440. Web. 20 Apr. 2017

[16] Montagu A. Growing Young. N.Y: McGraw Hill; 1989. p. 40

[17] Hammer. In: McPhee SJ, Gary D, editors. "Pathophysiology of Selected Genetic Diseases". Pathophysiology of Disease: An Introduction to Clinical Medicine. 6th ed. New York: McGraw-Hill Medical; 2010. Chapter 2. ISBN: 978-0-07-162167-0

[18] Pham V. Common Otolaryngological Congenital Abnormalities. UTMB, Dept. of Otolaryngology; 2010

[19] Kalyanasundaram S. Peroxisomal disorder-unusual presentation as failure to thrive in early infancy. Indian Journal of Pediatrics. 2010;**77**:1151-1152

[20] Foster JA et al. Basic and Clinical Science Course: Section 7. American Academy of Ophthalmology; 2016-2017

[21] Goldberger E. Epicanthus and its variants among Caucasians. Archives of Ophthalmology. 1936;**16**(3):506-515. Web. 20 Apr. 2017

[22] Bentz LM, by Renato Ocampo, John A. Persing. Pediatric Plastic Surgery, Hypertelorism

[23] Dollfus H, Verloes A. Developmental anomalies of the lids. In: Hoyt CS, Taylor D, editors. Pediatric Ophthalmology and Strabismus. 4th ed. Elsevier Saunders; 2013:chap 18

[24] Bartel-Friedrich S, Wulke C. Clasification and diagnosis of ear malformation. GMS Current Topics in Otorhinolaryngology - Head and Neck Surgery. 2007;**6**: Doc05. Published online 2008 Mar 14

[25] Zou F, Peng Y, Wang X, et al. A locus for congenital preauricular fistula maps to chromosome 8q11.1-q13.3. Journal of Human Genetics. 2003;**48**(3):155-158

[26] Ostrower ST, Bent JP. Preauricular Cysts, Pits, and Fissures. Otolaringology and Facial Plastic Surgery. Medscape; Updated: Feb 07, 2017

[27] Heike CL, Hing AV, Aspinall CA, et al. Clinical care in craniofacial microsomia: A review of current management recommendations and opportunities to advance research. American Journal of Medical Genetics. Part C, Seminars in Medical Genetics. 2013;**163C**:271-282

[28] Kugelman A, Tubi A, Bader D, et al. Pre-auricular tags and pits in the newborn. The Journal of Pediatrics. 2002;**141**:388-391

[29] Wang RY, Earl DL, Ruder RO, et al. Syndromic ear anomalies and renal ultrasounds. Pediatrics. 2001;**108**:e32-e32

[30] Andersen SL, Olsen J, Wu CS, et al. Severity of birth defects after propylthiouracil exposure in early pregnancy. Thyroid. 2014 Jun 25

[31] De la Cruz A, Kesser BW (1999). "Management of the unilateral atretic ear". In Pensak M. Controversies in Otolaryngology—Head and Neck Surgery. New York: Thieme Medical Publishers. pp. 381-385

[32] Harris J, Källén B, Robert E. The epidemiology of anotia and microtia. Journal of Medical Genetics. 1996;**33**(10):809

[33] Luquetti DV, Heike CL, Hing AV, Cunningham ML, Cox TC. Microtia: Epidemiology & genetics. American Journal of Medical Genetics. Part A. 2012 Jan;**158A**(1):124-139

[34] Katsanis SH, Cutting GR (July 2004). "Treacher Collins Syndrome". GeneReviews

[35] Brent B. Auricular repair with autogenous rib cartilage grafts: Two decades of experience with 600 cases. Plastic and Reconstructive Surgery. 1992;**90**(3):355-374

[36] Llano-Rivas I, González-del Angel A, del Castillo V, et al. Microtia: A clinical and genetic study at the National Institute of pediatrics in Mexico City. Archives of Medical Research. 1999;**30**:120

[37] Kountakis SE, Helidonis E, Jahrsdoerfer RA. Microtia grade as an indicator of middle ear development in aural atresia. Archives of Otolaryngology – Head & Neck Surgery. 1995;**121**(8):885-886

[38] Jahrsdoerfer RA, Kesser BW. Issues on aural atresia for the facial plastic surgeon. Facial Plastic Surgery. 1995;**11**(4):274-277

[39] Eavey RD. Ear malformations. What a pediatrician can do to assist with auricular reconstruction. Pediatric Clinics of North America. 1996;**43**:1233

[40] Brent B. Technical advances in ear reconstruction with autogenous rib cartilage grafts: Personal experience with 1200 cases. Plastic and Reconstructive Surgery. 1999;**104**(2):319

[41] Reiffel AJ, Kafka C, Hernandez KA, Popa S, Perez JL, Zhou S, Pramanik S, Brown BN, Ryu WS, Bonassar LJ, Spector JA. High-fidelity tissue engineering of patient-specific auricles for reconstruction of pediatric microtia and other auricular deformities. PLoS One. 2013;**8**(2):e56506 Epub 2013 Feb 20

[42] Buyse ML. Birth Defect. Encyclopedia Blackwell Scientific Publishing; 1990. p. 590

[43] lubs HA. A marker X chromosome. American Journal of Human Genetics. 1969;**21**:231

[44] Verloes A, Lesenfants S, Philippet B, Iyawa A, Laloux F, Koulischer L. Genetic Counseling. 1996;**7**(4):277-282

[45] Rapini RP, Bolognia JL, Jorizzo JL. Dermatology: 2-Volume Set. St. Louis: Mosby; 2007. ISBN: 1-4160-2999-0

[46] James W, Berger T, Elston D. Andrews' Diseases of the Skin: Clinical Dermatology. 10th ed. Saunders; 2005

[47] Chinnadurai S, Fonnesbeck C, Snyder KM, Sathe NA, Morad A, Likis FE, McPheeters ML. Pharmacologic interventions for infantile hemangioma: A meta-analysis. Pediatrics. February 2016:137

[48] Congenital Dermal Melanocytosis (Mongolian Spots): http://emedicine.medscape.com/article/1068732oveview

[49] Monteagudo B, Labandeira J, León-Muiños E, Carballeira I, Corrales A, Cabanillas M. Prevalence of birthmarks and transient skin lesions in 1000 Spanish newborns. Actas Dermo-Sifiliográficas. 2011 May;**102**(4):264-269

[50] Kanada KN, Merin MR, Munden A, Friedlander SF. A prospective study of cutaneous findings in newborns in the United States: Correlation with race, ethnicity, and gestational status using updated classification and nomenclature. The Journal of Pediatrics. 2012 Aug.;**161**(2):240-245

[51] Ashrafi MR, Shabanian R, Mohammadi M, Kavusi S. Extensive Mongolian spots: A clinical sign merits special attention. Pediatric Neurology. 2006 Feb;**34**(2):143-145

[52] Amitai DB, Fichman S, Merlob P, et al. Cutis marmorata telangiectatica congenita: Clinical findings in 85 patients. Pediatric Dermatology. 2000 Mar-Apr;**17**(2):100-104

[53] Torrelo A, Zambrano A, Happle R. Cutis marmorata telangiectatica congenita and extensive mongolian spots: Type 5 phacomatosis pigmentovascularis. The British Journal of Dermatology. 2003 Feb;**148**(2):342-345

[54] Petrozzi JW, Rahn EK, Mofenson H, et al. Cutis marmorata telangiectatica congenita. Archives of Dermatology. 1970 Jan;**101**(1):74-77

[55] Bormann G, Wohlrab J, Fischer M, et al. Cutis marmorata telangiectatica congenita: Laser doppler fluxmetry evidence for a functional nervous defect. Pediatric Dermatology. 2001Mar-Apr;**18**(2):110-113

[56] Melani L, Antiga E, Torchia D, et al. Cutis marmorata telangiectatica congenita and chronic autoimmune urticaria in a young man. The Journal of Dermatology. 2007 Mar;**34** (3):210-213

[57] Ancillary Techniques in Diagnosing Melanocytic Lesions. Melanocytic Lesions - Springer. DOI: 10.1007/978-1-4939-0891-2

[58] Dysplastic(Atypical)Nevi.MelanocyticLesions-Springer.DOI:10.1007/978-1-4939-0891-2

[59] Benign Neoplasias and Hyperplasias of Melanocytes. Fitzpatrick's Dermatology in General Medicine. Chapter 122. The McGraw-Hill Companies, Inc; 2012. ISBN: 978-0-07-166904-7

[60] Neonatal, Pediatric, and Adolescent Dermatology. Fitzpatrick's Dermatology in General Medicine. Chapter 107. The McGraw-Hill Companies, Inc; 2012. ISBN: 978-0-07-166904-7

[61] Rigel Darrell S, Julie R, Robert F. The evolution of melanoma diagnosis: 25 years beyond the ABCDs. CA: a Cancer Journal for Clinicians. 2016;**60**(5):301-316. ISSN: 1542-4863. PMID: 20671054. DOI: 10.3322/caac.20074

[62] Scope A, Marchetti MA, Marghoob AA, Dusza SW, Geller AC, Satagopan JM, Weinstock MA, Berwick M, Halpern AC. The study of nevi in children: Principles learned and implications for melanoma diagnosis. Journal of the American Academy of Dermatology. 2016;**75**(4):813-823. PMC: 5030195. PMID: 27320410. DOI: 10.1016/j.jaad.2016.03.027

[63] Rypens F, Dubois J, Garel L, et al. Obstetric US: Watch the fetal hands. Radiographics;**26**(3): 811-829. DOI: 10.1148/rg.263055113

[64] Schmitt R, Lanz U, Buchberger W. Diagnostic Imaging of the Hand. Thieme Medical Pub; 2008 ISBN:1588904539

[65] Gupta P, Sharma JB, Sharma R, et al. Antenatal ultrasound and MRI findings of Pena-Shokeir syndrome. Archives of Gynecology and Obstetrics. 2010. DOI: 10.1007/s00404-010-1703-y

[66] Bahabri SA, Suwairi WM, Laxer RM, et al. The camptodactyly-arthropathy-coxa vara-pericarditis syndrome: Clinical features and genetic mapping to human chromosome 1. Arthritis and Rheumatism. 1998;**41**(4):730-735. DOI: 10.1002/1529-0131(199804)41:4<730::AID-ART22>3.0.CO;2-Y

[67] Leung AK, Kao CP. Familial clinodactyly of the fifth finger. Journal of the National Medical Association. 2003;**95**(12):1198-1200

[68] Eggermann T, Begemann M, Spengler S, et al. Genetic and epigenetic findings in silver-Russell syndrome. Pediatric Endocrinology Reviews. 2010;**8**(2):86-93

[69] Flatt AE. The troubles with pinkies. Proceedings (Baylor University Medical Center). 2005;**18**(4):341-344

[70] Castilla EE, Lugarinho da Fonseca R, da Graca Dutra M, et al. Epidemiological analysis of rare polydactylies. American Journal of Medical Genetics. Nov 1996;**65**(4):295-303

[71] Sadler TW. Langman's Embriologie Medicala editia a X a

[72] Kumar P, Burton BK. Congenital malformations, Evidence based Evaluation and Management

[73] Zhou GX, Dai L, Zhu J, et al. Epidemiological analysis of polydactylies in Chinese perinatals. Sichuan Da Xue Xue Bao. Yi Xue Ban. Sep 2004;**35**(5):708-710

[74] Castilla EE, Lugarinho R, da Graca Dutra M, et al. Associated anomalies in individuals with polydactyly. American Journal of Medical Genetics. Dec 1998;**80**(5):459-465

[75] Malik S. Syndactyly: Phenotypes, genetics and current classification. European Journal of Human Genetics. 2012 Aug;**20**(8):817-824. DOI: 10.1038/ejhg.2012.14

[76] Vogels A, Fryns JP. Pfeiffer syndrome. Orphanet Journal of Rare Diseases. 2006;**1**:19. DOI: 10.1186/1750-1172-1-19

[77] Muenke M, Schell U, Hehr A, Robin NH, Losken HW, Schinzel A, et al. A common mutation in the fibroblast growth factor receptor 1 gene in Pfeiffer syndrome. Nature Genetics. 1994;**8**(3):269-274. DOI: 10.1038/ng1194-269

[78] Rutland P, Pulleyn LJ, Reardon W, Baraitser M, Hayward R, Jones B, et al. Identical mutations in the FGFR2 gene cause both Pfeiffer and Crouzon syndrome phenotypes. Nature Genetics. 1995;**9**(2):173. DOI: 10.1038/ng0295-173

[79] Schell U, Hehr A, Feldman GJ, Robin NH, Zackai EH, de Die-Smulders C, et al. Mutations in FGFR1 and FGFR2 cause familial and sporadic Pfeiffer syndrome. Human Molecular Genetics. 1995;**4**(3):323-328. DOI: 10.1093/hmg/4.3.323

[80] Perlyn C, Marsh J. Craniofacial dysmorphology of carpenter syndrome: Lessons from three affected siblings. Plastic and Reconstructive Surgery. March 2008;**121**(3):971-981. PMID: 18317146. DOI: 10.1097/01.prs.0000299284.92862.6c

[81] Nowaczyk MJM, Waye JS. The Smith-Lemli-Opitz syndrome: A novel metabolic way of understanding developmental biology, embryogenesis, and dysmorphology. Clinical Genetics. 2001;**59**(6):375-386. PMID: 11453964. DOI: 10.1034/j.1399-0004.2001.590601.x

[82] D'Souza SW, Robertson IG, Donnai D, Mawer G. Fetal phenytoin exposure, hypoplastic nails, and jitteriness. Archives of Disease in Childhood. 1991 Mar;**66**(3):320-324

[83] DeBaun MR, Ess J, Saunders S. Simpson Golabi Behmel syndrome: Progress toward understanding the molecular basis for overgrowth, malformation, and cancer predisposition. Molecular Genetics and Metabolism. 2001;**72**(4):279-286. PMID: 11286501. DOI: 10.1006/mgme.2001.3150

[84] Committee to Study Fetal Alcohol Syndrome, Division of Biobehavioral Sciences and Mental Disorders, Institute of Medicine. Fetal Alcohol Syndrome: Diagnosis, Epidemiology, Prevention, and Treatment. Washington, D.C.: National Academy Press; 1995. ISBN: 0-309-05292-0

[85] Mankin HJ, Jupiter J, Trahan CA. Hand and foot abnormalities associated with genetic diseases. Hand (New York, N.Y.). 2011 Mar;**6**(1):18-26. Published online 2010 Oct 26. DOI: 10.1007/s11552-010-9302-8

5

Abnormalities of the Umbilical Cord

Sidonia Catalina Vrabie, Liliana Novac,
Maria Magdalena Manolea,
Lorena Anda Dijmarescu, Marius Novac and
Mirela Anisoara Siminel

Abstract

Abnormalities of the umbilical cord, related to morphology, placental insertion, number of vessels and primary tumors, can influence the perinatal outcome and may be associated with other fetal anomalies and aneuploidies. The chapter investigates the most important congenital anomalies of this structure. Single umbilical artery appears to be associated with ventricular septal defects and conotruncal anomalies, hydronephrosis, dysplastic kidneys, esophageal atresia, spina bifida, holoprosencephaly, diaphragmatic hernia, and cystic hygromas. Velamentous insertion of the cord can be associated with trisomy 21, spina bifida, ventricular septal defects, and esophageal atresia. A hypoplastic umbilical artery has an artery-to-artery diameter difference of more than 50%; described anomalies include trisomy 21, polyhydramnios, congenital heart disease, and fetal growth restriction. Pseudocysts are more common than true cysts, and they are strongly associated with chromosomal defects and other congenital anomalies, especially omphalocele, hydrops, and trisomy 18. Other benign masses are teratomas, angiomyxomas, and patent urachus. Alterations in morphology and ultrastructure of the umbilical cord should extend the investigation, since there are associations with chromosomal anomalies.

Keywords: umbilical cord, prenatal ultrasound, congenital anomalies, fetal malformations, outcome

1. Introduction

Umbilical cord makes stable interconnection between fetal well-being and placenta at the fetomaternal interface level. The prenatal ultrasonographic assessment of the umbilical cord offers the possibility to investigate the morphologic characteristics during fetal life, from early to late gestation.

The umbilical cord structure can be demonstrated by conventional real-time ultrasound and the umbilical blood flow patterns can be analyzed by color (power) and pulsed Doppler ultrasound, which relate to its functionality [1]. Second trimester scan is able to assess four characteristics of the umbilical cord: measurement of umbilical cord area, evaluation of the number of vessels, assessment of placental umbilical cord insertion site, and determination of the coiling pattern [2].

Abnormalities of the umbilical cord related to morphology, placental insertion, number of vessels, and primary tumors can influence the perinatal outcome and may be associated with other fetal anomalies and aneuploidies. Many of these conditions are being diagnosed in utero as prenatal ultrasound becomes more sophisticated nowadays.

Using ultrasound, we can depict various congenital abnormalities of the umbilical cord, including cysts, pseudocysts, umbilical vein varix, persistent right umbilical vein, angiomyxomas, aneurysm, single umbilical artery (SUA), velamentous insertion, and teratomas.

2. Abnormal number of vessels

Sometimes, during pregnancy, changes in the number of umbilical vessels may occur. Abnormal number of umbilical cord vessels includes: two-vessel cord (single umbilical artery), four-vessel cord (two veins and two arteries, one vein and three arteries), five and more vessels cord (numerous variations in conjoined twins), umbilical cord that does not keep the same number of vessels at the fetal and placental extremity [3].

2.1. Single umbilical artery

It seems that the first descriptions of the single umbilical artery were made in 1543 by Vesalius in De Humani Corporis [4]. It may be diagnosed with the finding of two vessels on a cross-section of the cord or a vessel seen on only one side of the fetal bladder. These anomalies appear to be more common when the left umbilical artery is absent and may be associated with aneuploid fetuses and renal anomalies in euploid fetuses. Atresia, aplasia, or agenesis of one artery can lead to single umbilical artery syndrome [5].

Single umbilical artery (SUA) is the most common abnormality of the umbilical cord.

There are three theories about the absence of umbilical artery pathogenesis: (1) primary agenesis of an umbilical artery; (2) atrophy or secondary atresia of the previously normally developed umbilical artery; and (3) persistence of the original allantoic artery of the body stalk [6]. It is suggested that from the embryological point of view, the second theory would be a reasonable explanation [7].

In single umbilical artery pregnancies, chromosomal abnormalities were found in 8–11% of fetuses, more commonly trisomy 13 and 18 and less frequently trisomy 21 [8], intrauterine growth restriction (IUGR), preterm birth, placental anomalies, and perinatal mortality [9, 10].

In rare cases, both umbilical arteries are missing and the one arterial vessel is, in fact, a persistent vitelline artery, which branches off the abdominal aorta. [11]. This persistent vitelline artery appears to be associated with serious developmental defects and was classified as type II single umbilical artery (type II SUA) by Blackburn and Cooley. This anomaly accounts for 1.5% cases of single umbilical artery [12]. According to the same authors, the most common form of single umbilical artery (98%) is type I that has one artery and one vein (left), whereas type II SUA has a frequency of 1.5%. Very rare forms are type III with one artery and two veins (left and persistent right umbilical vein) and type IV with one artery and one vein (right).

There is an increased incidence of severe malformations associated with type II SUA with the implication of the caudal body wall (sirenomelia, omphalocele-exstrophy-imperforate anus-spinal defects) and urorectal like exstrophy of the bladder, anal atresia, or urogenital agenesis [13].

Among pregnancies with single umbilical artery associated with various malformations, two-thirds of deaths occur before birth. Regarding the other third of postnatal deaths, an increased incidence of fetal growth restriction and small placental size was found [14].

If no additional chromosomal or structural abnormalities occur, single umbilical artery is defined as an isolated SUA (iSUA) [10], and more than 90% of cases with SUA exhibit an isolated anomaly but without increasing the risk of chromosomal abnormalities [15]. Regarding adverse pregnancy outcomes and perinatal complications, studies show discordant results. A meta-analysis suggests that there is no significant association between iSUA and pregnancy outcomes [16, 17], while another meta-analysis suggests that iSUA is associated with a significant increase in adverse perinatal outcomes [18].

Single umbilical artery can be diagnosed in the first trimester using color Doppler and high-definition ultrasound with a low pulse repetition frequency (PRF) and a high color gain. Visualization of the umbilical arteries is preferable at the level of the fetal urinary bladder (**Figure 1**) by demonstrating the cord's perivesical course [19].

In conclusion, the easiest way to assess the number of arteries by ultrasound is by identifying the intra-abdominal portion of the umbilical artery alongside the bladder with color Doppler and/or by visualizing the cross-section of a free-floating loop of umbilical cord (**Figure 2**) [20]. In a 1991 study, Nyberg's group concluded that prenatal sonography alone was reliable in detecting any associated anomalies. They also recommended no management modification in cases with no concurrent anomalies [7]. The visualization of that anomaly should prompt a detailed sonographic assessment of the cardiovascular and genitourinary systems [3].

Fetal anomalies most commonly associated with single umbilical artery include several anomalies like ventricular septal defects, hydronephrosis, cleft lip, ventral wall defects, esophageal atresia, spina bifida, hydrocephaly, holoprosencephaly, diaphragmatic hernia, cystic hygromas, and polydactyly or syndactyly. In these cases, fetal echocardiography and karyotype analysis should be considered. Usually, there are no specific fetal abnormalities to be associated with the single umbilical artery. In fact, the single umbilical artery is often found in cases with healthy neonates, with a normal size and development at term. Although, to be sure that the infant has no hidden anomalies, the pediatrician should be notified of its existence to

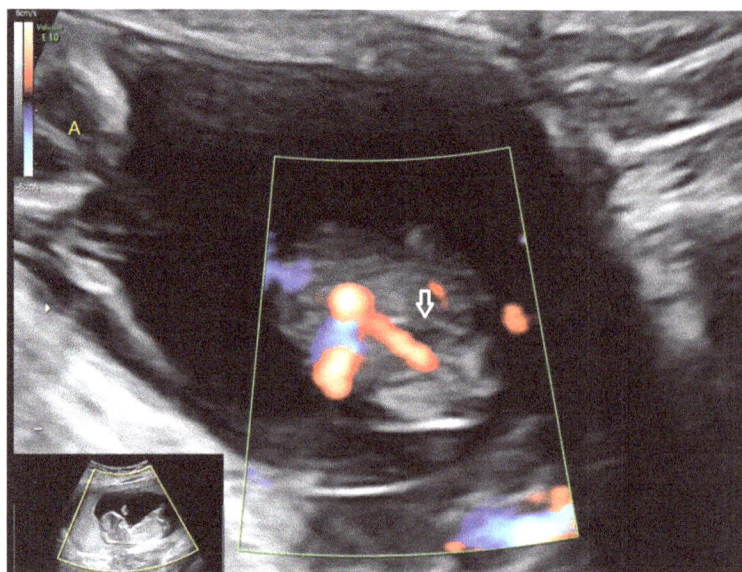

Figure 1. Visualization of the umbilical arteries at the level of the fetal urinary bladder.

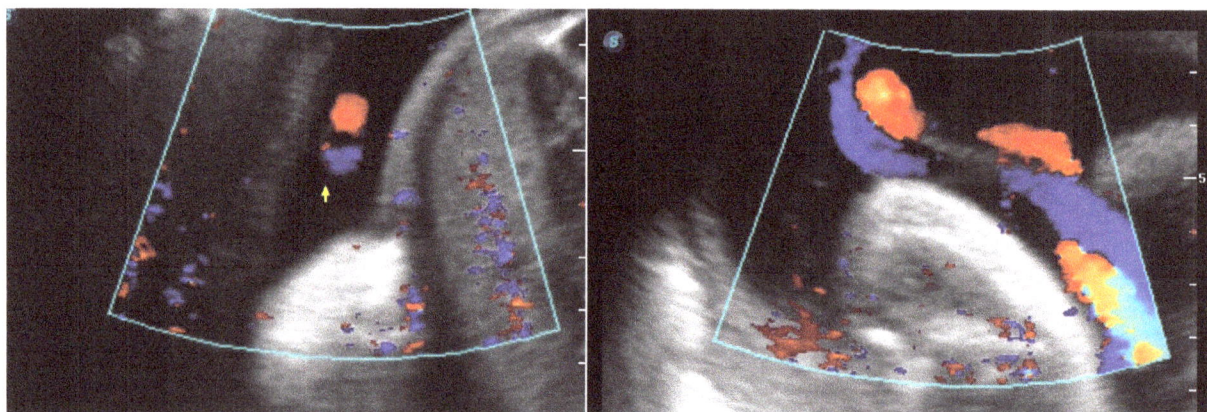

Figure 2. Color Doppler visualization of a free-floating loop of umbilical cord.

have a more detailed physical examination [11, 21]. Ultrasound views of the heart described in FMF's recommendations (minimum four-chamber view, outflow tract, and three-vessel view) can detect 66% of the heart malformations associated with single umbilical artery. The undiagnosed ones are minor and have a favorable outcome [22].

Nonisolated SUA requests invasive testing with chromosomal microarray because the risk of syndromes and chromosomal anomalies are substantially increased (**Figure 3**). Isolated SUA with a normal insertion of the cord does not require special precautions during labor. In these cases, the long-term outcome for children is the same as for children born with three vessels in the umbilical cord [23].

2.2. Persistent right umbilical vein

Unusual persistence of the right umbilical vein with left vein umbilical regression will lead to alteration in the development of embryonic vasculature, knowing that in the normal

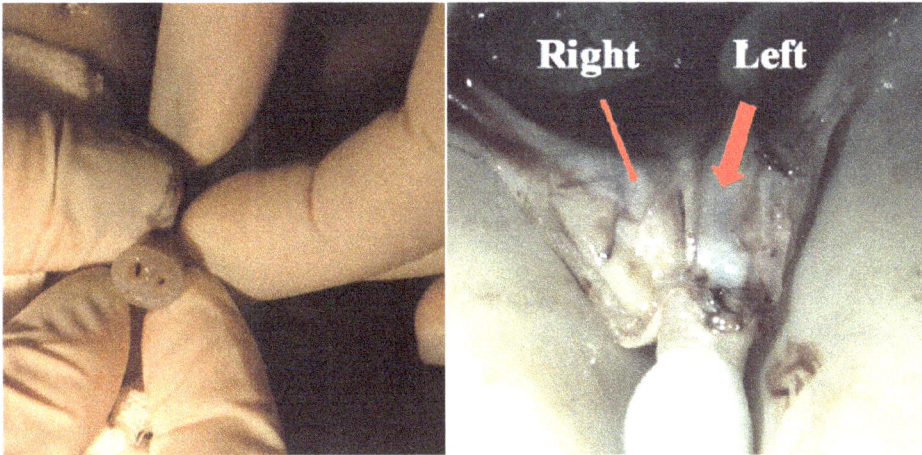

Figure 3. SUA at necropsy.

fetus, the right umbilical vein disappears by the seventh week of gestation. This condition does not alter the formation of ductus venosus, the distribution of blood to the fetus remaining normal [24]. First-trimester folic acid deficiency, teratogens such as retinoic acid or early obstruction of the left umbilical vein from external pressure or occlusion are considered etiologic factors [25].

The ultrasound diagnosis is made in the transverse section of the fetal abdomen. Umbilical vein is abnormally connected to the right portal vein instead to the left portal vein, and fetal gallbladder is located between the umbilical vein and the stomach [26] (**Figures 4** and **5**).

It is associated with congenital anomalies: cardiac anomalies, trisomy 18, abdominal visceral situs inversus, total anomalous pulmonary venous connection, urinary tract malformation like unilateral renal agenesis, umbilical vein varix, skeletal malformations, and others [27].

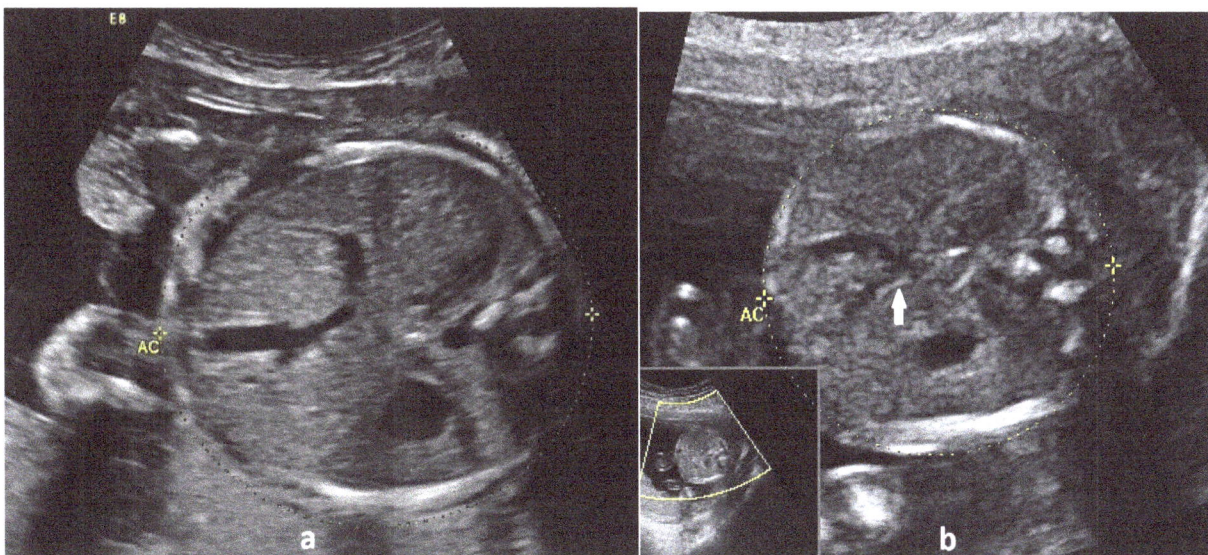

Figure 4. Persistent right umbilical vein: (**a**) Normal section of abdominal circumference and (**b**) section of abdominal circumference with persistent right umbilical vein view.

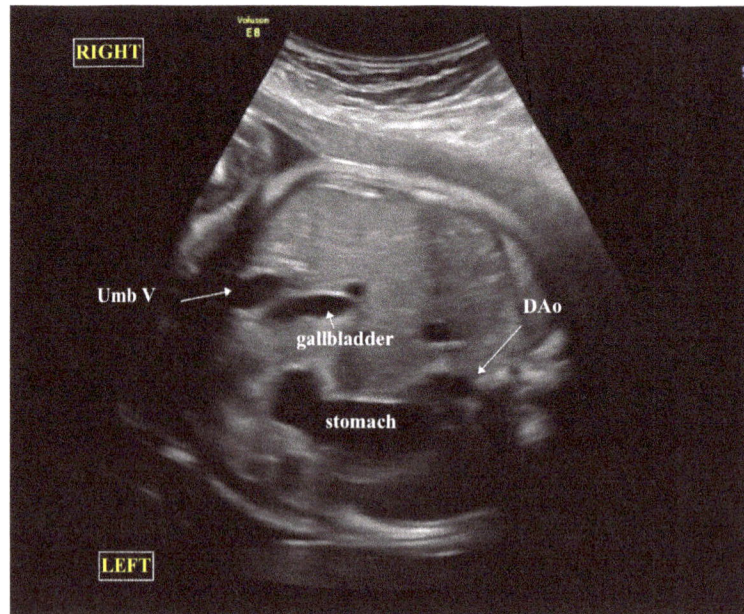

Figure 5. Persistent right umbilical vein (*Dao,* descending aorta).

2.3. Four-vessel umbilical cord

Five percent of umbilical cords exhibit a four-vessel structure due to the persistence of small vitelline arteries, which follow the normal twisting of the main umbilical arteries. [28].

Four umbilical vessels view is an abnormal situation that has been reported to be associated with major congenital anomalies [29]. The presence of three umbilical arteries is the most common situation of four-vessel cord, although in the specialty literature have been reported a few cases of cord with two umbilical veins and two umbilical arteries [30].

3. Abnormal course or connection of vessels

The insertion of umbilical cord can be located following the chorionic plate vessels using color Doppler technique. The placental insertion of the UC is better observed by ultrasound in the first trimester. Later when gestational age increases, visualization becomes difficult, especially when the placenta is posterior. The evaluation of fetal circulation is done by examining the umbilical arteries. The umbilical vascular evaluation provides information on the circulation at the fetomaternal interface level, giving the possibility of early detection of risk to the fetus [19].

3.1. Velamentous insertion of the cord

The umbilical cord insertion is located on the placental mass in about 99% of cases, into the central portion of the placenta. The velamentous insertion is the condition in which the umbilical vessels are configured between amnion and chorion before reaching the placenta on the chorioamniotic membranes [31]. That abnormal insertion occurs when the cord implants in the trophoblast anterior to the decidua capsularis or when placental tissue grows laterally, leaving an area which becomes atrophic. The umbilical cord inserts into the chorion leave at a point away from the placental mass and appears as membranous umbilical vessels at the placental insertion site (velamentous vessels are not protected by Wharton's jelly), the rest of the cord is usually normal. This type of pathological insertion of the cord occurs in 1–2% of singleton pregnancies. In multiple pregnancies, the incidence of velamentous cord insertion is 10-fold higher than in singleton pregnancies [32] (**Figure 6**).

Heinonen et al. [33] in this aberrant attachment, such as at the margins or to the membranes, found an association with higher maternal serum human chorionic gonadotropin (hCG) and lower maternal serum alpha-fetoprotein (AFP). However, until further data is available, no specific recommendations can be made.

Prenatal identification of these pregnancies is an important issue. There is a higher risk for an adverse perinatal outcome like intrauterine growth retardation, preterm birth, placental abruption, vasa previa, low Apgar scores at 1 and 5 min, neonatal death, congenital anomalies, and fetal bleeding [34]. Associated anomalies include trisomy 21, spina bifida, ventricular septal defects, esophageal atresia, obstructive uropathies, congenital hip dislocation, and asymmetrical head shape. It has been noted that a higher rate of deformations occur instead of malformations or disruptions [34]. Velamentous insertion associated with vasa previa appears to have an increased rate of congenital malformations. Also, 13% cases of single umbilical artery are associated with velamentous insertion [14].

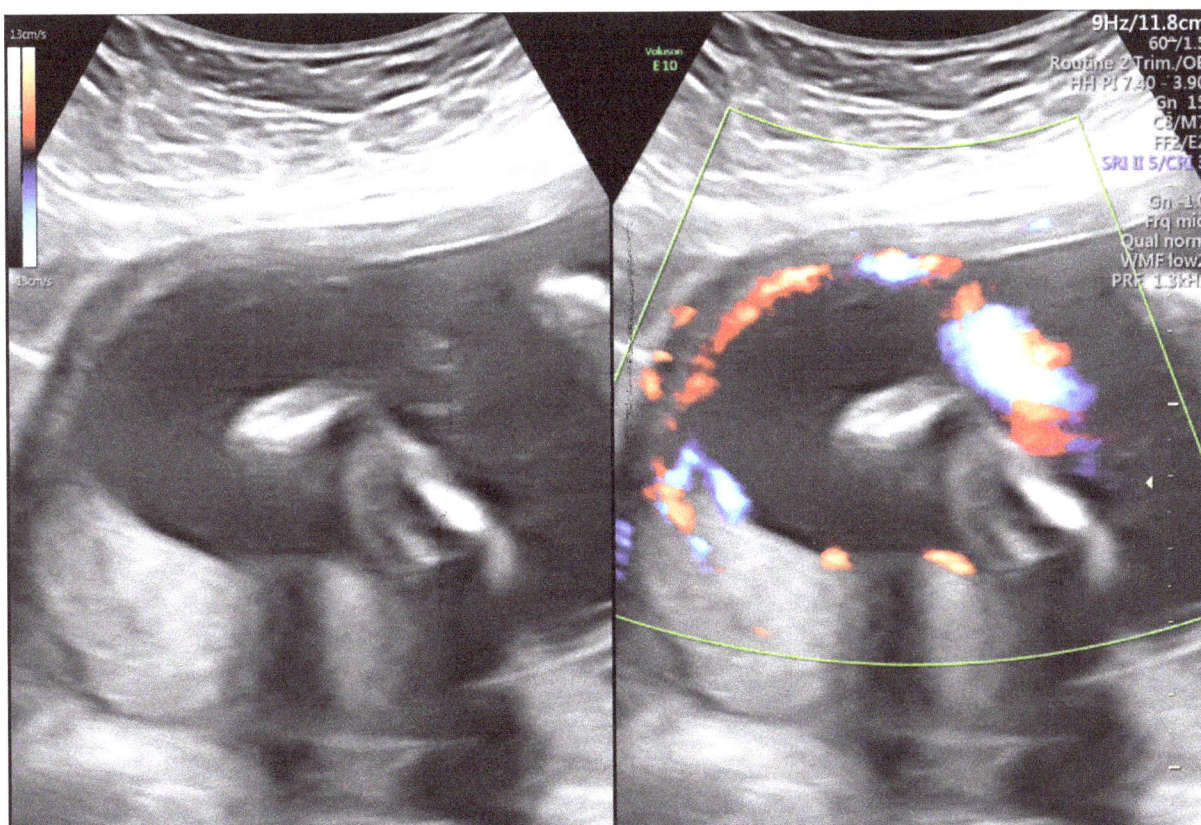

Figure 6. Velamentous cord insertion.

Vasa previa

It is important to be aware that velamentous cord insertion is associated with an increased rate of vasa previa. Vasa previa is a form of velamentous cord insertion in which velamentous vessels pass through the fetal membranes of the lower uterine segment and incidence is estimated to be 0.04% [35]. These fetal vessels may break when membrane rupture occurs and the result is fetal exsanguination. Intrapartum diagnosis is very difficult in this case [36].

4. Abnormal structure or configuration of vessels

4.1. Hypoplastic umbilical artery

A hypoplastic umbilical artery has a smaller diameter than the contralateral artery, showing by ultrasonography an artery-to-artery diameter difference of more than 50% [37] (**Figure 7**).

It seems that the hypoplastic umbilical artery represents a mild form of the single umbilical artery. Described anomalies include trisomy 21, polyhydramnios, congenital heart disease, stillbirth, trisomies, and fetal growth restriction. The presence of discordant umbilical arteries is a sign of different umbilical artery blood flow indices and of placental disease [38]. This condition increases the risk of IUGR, placental infarction, umbilical cord hematoma, and abnormal umbilical cord insertion. It is also known that the fetal prognosis is better for hypoplastic umbilical arteries compared with SUA syndrome [37].

Karyotyping is not indicated in isolated hypoplastic umbilical artery because there is no evidence of increased risk of chromosomal defects.

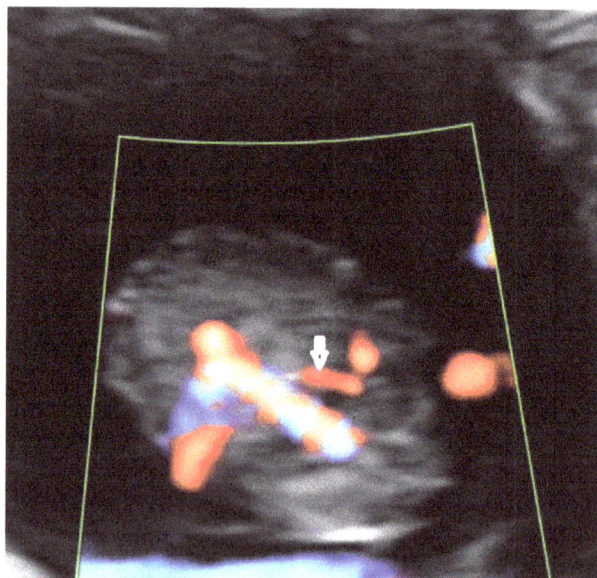

Figure 7. Hypoplastic umbilical artery.

4.2. Umbilical vein varix

Umbilical vein varix is a rare condition which occurs in the intrahepatic portion of the umbilical vein presents an incidence of 2.8:1000 [39]. Ultrasound scan usually discovers a circular vessel dilation ≥ 9 mm, 59 or more than 50% over the diameter of the intrahepatic UV [40]. The condition is associated with chromosomal anomalies in up to 12% of cases, especially trisomy 21and poor fetal outcome with emergent cesarean delivery [41].

Complete follow-up includes karyotyping, regular fetal testing, and third trimester interval growth studies [42]. Because the incidence is very low, the clinical significance remains controversial.

4.3. Umbilical artery aneurysm

Umbilical artery aneurysm is an extremely rare vascular anomaly usually associated with high risk of fetal aneuploidy, IUGR, and fetal demise. Fetal demise is a result of compression of the dilated artery on the umbilical vein, thrombus formation, or due to associated fetal anomaly like trisomy 18 [43]. This condition is a vascular anomaly which appears as an anechoic cyst close to cord insertion with a hyperechogenic rim in which color flow and spectral Doppler examinations show nonpulsatile and turbulent blood flow within the artery [44].

It is important to consider karyotype analysis given the high incidence of aneuploidy associated with umbilical artery aneurysm.

Tumors of the Umbilical Cord

4.4. Cord cysts

Cord cysts have no clinical relevance and develop from the remnants of the allantois or the omphalomesenteric duct. The finding of an isolated umbilical cord cystic mass should lead to further detailed sonographic evaluation and karyotype testing should be done when IUGR or other anomalies are found [45]. The majority of first-trimester cysts are transient ultrasound findings that have no influence on pregnancy outcome [46]. The prognosis of persistent cysts appears to be similar to that of second-trimester cysts [47].

Several studies concluded that morphologic features of cord cyst (single, multiple) correlate with fetal abnormalities like abdominal wall defects and patent urachus [48].

Umbilical cord cysts are classified as true cysts or pseudocysts. True cysts have an incidence of 3.4% in first trimester of pregnancy and have no clinical significance, and are sometimes associated with fetal structural anomalies and aneuploidy [45]. True cysts are derived from the embryological remnants of either the allantois or the omphalomesenteric duct, are located typically toward the fetal insertion of the cord and range from 4 to 60 mm in size [49].

The exact cause of umbilical cyst is not known, but it is thought to be due to raised hydrostatic pressure in the umbilical vessels (**Figure 8**).

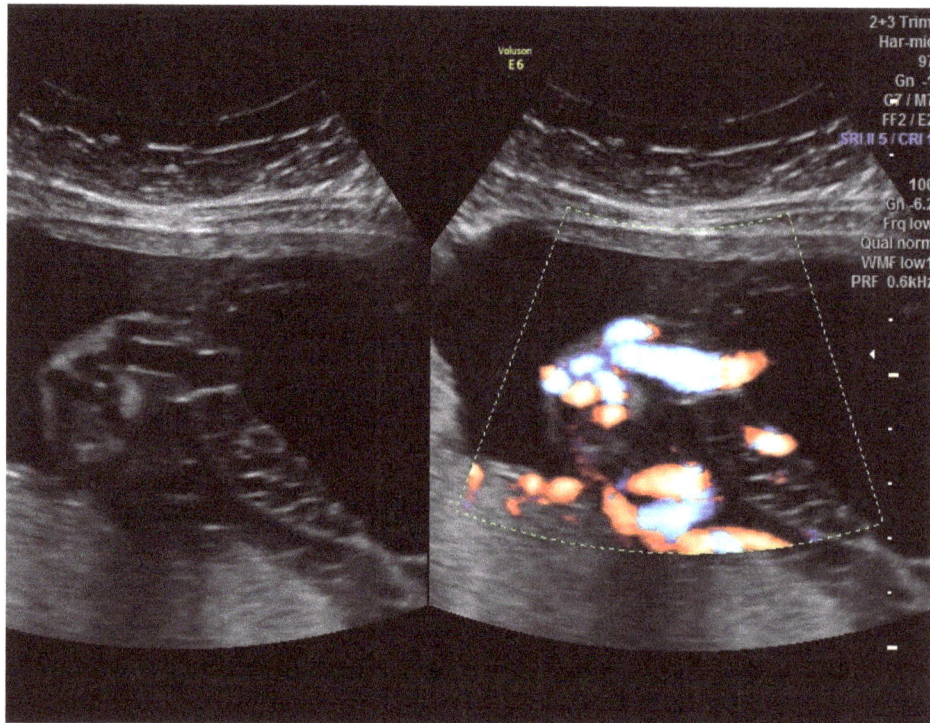

Figure 8. Large umbilical cyst in the second trimester.

Pseudocysts are more common than true cysts and can be located anywhere along the cord; they have no epithelial lining and represent localized edema and liquefaction of Wharton's jelly (known as Wharton jelly cysts). It is rarely possible to differentiate between true cysts and pseudocysts on ultrasound imaging [50]. But differentiation between the two entities is not very important because both are associated with anomalies. Pseudocysts are more common than true cysts and they are strongly associated with chromosomal defects and other congenital anomalies, especially omphalocele, hydrops, and trisomy 18 [51]. Usually, ultrasonography monitoring is sufficient, invasive tests not being typically needed. A higher risk of fetal anomalies is associated with the following: detection of cysts in the second or third trimester, persistence after the first trimester, large size, and location near fetal or placental end. Also, trisomy 18, 13, and 21 are known to be associated, in such cases, chromosomal analysis may be warranted [52].

They might be associated with omphalocele, Meckel's diverticulum, patent urachus, and hydronephrosis. False cysts are most commonly found at the fetal end of the cord, do not have an epithelial lining and might be associated with omphalocele, patent urachus, and chromosomal anomalies [53]. Twenty percent of cord cysts, no matter what type they are, are associated with structural or chromosomal anomalies [54].

When the umbilical cyst is detected antenatally, especially in second or third trimesters, it is recommended a detailed ultrasonographic examination of the fetus, and it should be carefully looked for any associated defects. In case of any suspicion should be done the karyotyping analysis.

4.5. Umbilical cord teratomas

They are rare benign lesions, only 12 cases reported in the literature, which may lead to adverse fetal outcomes. These tumors are the only true neoplasms of the umbilical cord which have a very polymorphic presentation and should be evaluated when the lesion contains calcifications [55].

It can also be associated with severe fetal anomalies such as anencephaly, intestinal anomalies, and abdominal wall defects. The outcome in extragonadal teratomas can be affected by the presence of associated anomalies and surgical complications after correction of the congenital malformations [56].

Angiomyxomas are benign solid masses which may be associated with fetal demise. Associated complications are premature delivery, cardiovascular anomalies, nonimmune hydrops fetalis, hydatidiform mole, polyhydramnios, and stillbirth [57]. The management of pregnancy with angiomyxoma in the third trimester is not well defined.

5. Patent urachus

Urachus represents a vestigial structure formed by the bladder dome and the obliterated umbilical arteries. Patent urachus represents 10–15% of all urachal anomalies in the literature [58] and may lead to urination through umbilicus and infections. It is a rare condition because urachal lumen typically closes at week 17 post-conception [59]. Alterations in the morphology of the umbilical cord should extend the investigation, since there are associations with chromosomal anomalies. It has been associated with bladder exstrophy and anterior abdominal wall defects.

6. Congenital hernia of the umbilical cord

Congenital hernia of the umbilical cord (CHUC) is a rare congenital entity recognized as a distinct entity since the 1920s but is often misdiagnosed as a small omphalocele. During the first 5th–6th week of gestation, the bowel herniates into the developing umbilical cord and withdraws into the abdominal cavity until the 10th–12th week of gestation [60]. Return of

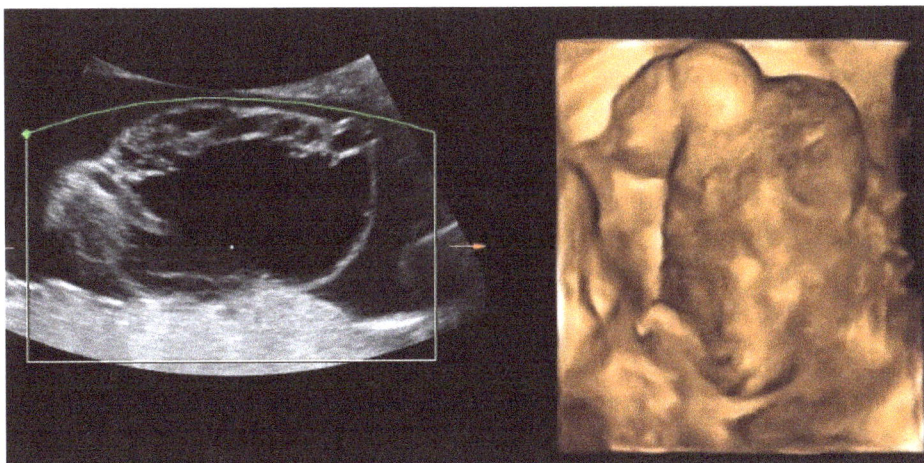

Figure 9. Large umbilical cyst 3D view.

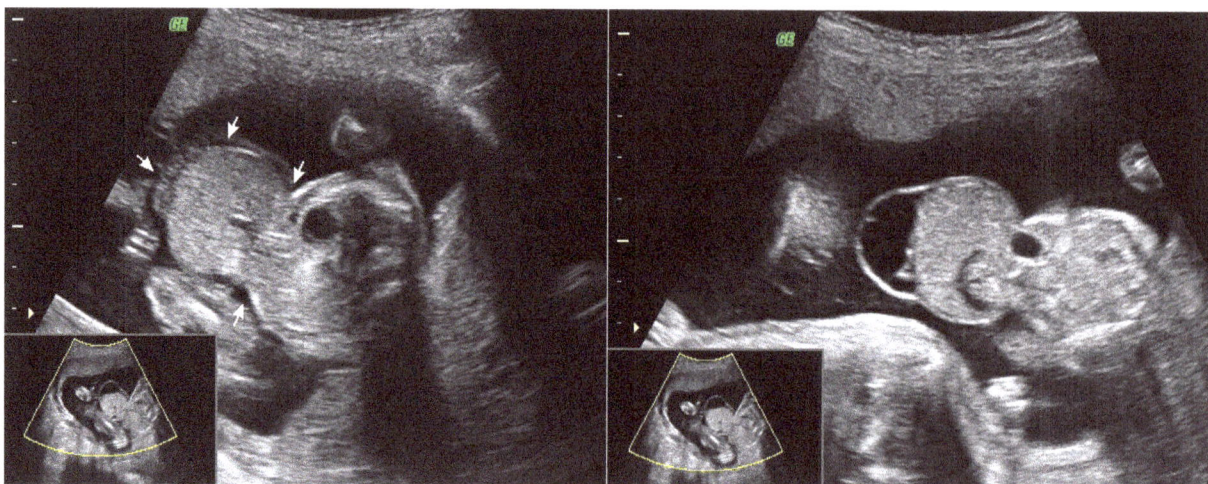

Figure 10. Congenital hernia of the umbilical cord.

physiologically herniated bowel or failed closure of umbilical ring (**Figures 8** and **9**). A review of the literature described associated malformations like pulmonary stenosis, cleft lip and palate, ear tag, small and large bowel atresia and stenosis, short bowel syndrome, tetralogy of Fallot, Meckel's diverticulum, persistent cloaca, and congenital glaucoma [61] (**Figure 10**).

7. Congenital umbilical arteriovenous malformation

The literature reported extremely rare cases of congenital umbilical arteriovenous malformation, less than 10 cases communicated in literature because congenital arteriovenous malformations are found most commonly in the brain, liver, and extremities. Congenital umbilical arteriovenous malformation is congenital lesions presented as a multitude of arteries and veins connected by a fistula. This condition can be asymptomatic but can also lead to congestive heart failure and massive hemorrhagic shock [62].

8. Conclusion

Invasive (diagnostic and therapeutic) procedures implying the puncture of the umbilical circulation are widely guided by ultrasound. Therefore, perinatal management may be enhanced by a prenatal ultrasonographic depiction of the morphology of the umbilical cord. In early pregnancy should be undertaken targeted examination because many details of cord development become difficult to identify on ultrasound with increasing gestational age. It is known also the association with structural (especially cardiovascular) and chromosomal anomalies, and for that further extended investigation should be needed in case of detection of abnormalities in the number, structure, or course of cord vessels. Most cases with isolated congenital anomalies of UC have a favorable outcome. Particular attention should be paid to umbilical cord insertions, both fetal and placental one. In apparently isolated single umbilical artery, further ultrasound scans during the late pregnancy and continuous fetal-heart-rate monitoring during labor should be offered. The single umbilical artery assumes an additional risk and the parents should be advised of the need for extra surveillance; they have to be also aware regarding the possibility of detection of some possible associated abnormality only after delivery.

Author details

Sidonia Catalina Vrabie[1]*, Liliana Novac[1], Maria Magdalena Manolea[1], Lorena Anda Dijmarescu[1], Marius Novac[2] and Mirela Anisoara Siminel[3]

*Address all correspondence to: sidocatalina@yahoo.com

1 Department of Obstetrics and Gynecology, University of Medicine and Pharmacy, Craiova, Romania

2 Department of Anesthesiology and Intensive Care, University of Medicine and Pharmacy, Craiova, Romania

3 Department of Neonatology, University of Medicine and Pharmacy, Craiova, Romania

References

[1] Predanic M, Kolli S, Yousefzadeh P, Pennisi J. Disparate blood flow patterns in parallel umbilical arteries. Obstetics and Gynecology. 1998;**9**:757-760

[2] Sepulveda W, Amy E, Wong E, Gomez L, Alcalde J. Improving sonographic evaluation of the umbilical cord at the second – Trimester anatomy scan. Journal of Ultrasound in Medicine. 2009;**28**:831-835

[3] Moshiri M, Zaidi SF, Robinson TJ, Bhargava P, Siebert JR, Dubinsky TJ, Katz DS. Comprehensive imaging review of abnormalities of the umbilical cord. Radiographics. 2014;**34**:179-196. DOI: https://doi.org/10.1148/rg.341125127

[4] Jauniaux E. The single artery umbilical cord: It is worth screening for antenatally? Ultrasound in Obstetrics & Gynecology. 1995;**5**:75-76

[5] Predanic M. Sonographic assessment of the umbilical cord. Donald School Journal of Ultrasound in Obstetrics and Gynecology. 2009;**3**(2):48-57

[6] Geipel A, Germer U, Welp T, Schwinger E, Gembruch U. Prenatal diagnosis of single umbilical artery: Determination of the absent side, associated anomalies, Doppler findings and perinatal outcome. Ultrasound in Obstetrics & Gynecology. 2000;**15**:114-117

[7] Nyberg DA, Mahony BS, Luthy D, Kapur R. Single umbilical artery: Prenatal detection of concurrent anomalies. Journal of Ultrasound in Medicine. 1991;**10**:247-253

[8] Saller DN, Keene CL, Sun CJ, Schwartz S. The association of single umbilical artery with cytogenetically abnormal pregnancies. American Journal of Obstetrics and Gynecology. 1990;**163**:922-925

[9] Ashwal E, Melamed N, Hiersch L, Edel S, Bardin R, Wiznitzer A, Yogev Y. The impact of isolated single umbilical artery on labor and delivery outcome. Prenatal Diagnosis. 2014;**34**:581-585. DOI: 10.1002/pd.4352

[10] Tulek F, Kahraman A, Taskın S, Ozkavukcu E, Soylemez F. Determination of risk factors and perinatal outcomes of singleton pregnancies complicated by isolated single umbilical artery in Turkish population. Jounal of the Turkish German Gynecological Association. 2015;**16**:21-24. DOI: 10.5152/jtgga.2015.15115. eCollection 2015.

[11] Bryan EM, Kohler HG. The missing umbilical artery. I. Prospective study based on a maternity unit. Archives of Disease in Childhood. 1974;**49**:844-852

[12] Blackburn W, Cooley W. Umbilical cord. In: Stevenson RE, Hall JG, Goodman R, editors. Human Malformations and Related Anomalies. Vol. II. New York: Oxford University Press; 1993. pp. 1275-1350

[13] Nalluri HB, Sirikonda P, Leela V. Origin, course and associated congenital anomalies of type 2 single umbilical artery: A fetal anatomic study. International Journal of Anatomy Research. 2016;**4**(1):2041-2046. DOI: 10.16965/ijar.2016.143

[14] Heifetz SA. Single umbilical artery. A statistical analysis of 237 autopsy cases and review of the literature. Perspectives in Pediatric Pathology. Winter 1984;**8**(4):345-378

[15] Hildebrand E, Selbing A, Blomberg M. Comparison of first and second trimester ultrasound screening for fetal anomalies in the southeast region of Sweden. Acta Obstetricia Gynecologica Scandinavica. 2010;**89**(11):1412-1419

[16] Xu Y, Ren L, Zhai S, Luo X, Hong T, Liu R, Ran L, Zhang Y. Association between isolated single umbilical artery and perinatal outcomes: A meta-analysis. Medical Science Monitor. Apr 30, 2016;**22**:1451-1459

[17] Tudorache S, Iliescu DG, Comanescu A. OP21.04: First trimester diagnosis of SUA – Feasibility of the marker, importance in screening for aneuploidies. Ultrasound in Obstetrics & Gynecology. 2011;**38**:117. DOI: 10.1002/uog.9456

[18] Kim HJ, Kim J-H, Chay DB, Park JH, Kim M-A. Association of isolated single umbilical artery with perinatal outcomes: Systemic review and meta-analysis. Obstetrics & Gynecology Science. May 2017;**60**(3):266-273. DOI: 10.5468/ogs.2017.60.3.266

[19] Bosselmann S, Mielke G. Sonographic assessment of the umbilical cord. Geburtshilfe und Frauenheilkunde. Aug 2015;**75**(8):808-818. DOI: 10.1055/s-0035-1557819

[20] Timofeev J, Holland M, Ganheart CC, Landy HJ, Tefera E, Driggers RW. Assessment of the number of umbilical cord vessels at the time of nuchal translucency screening. International Jounal of Obstetrics and Gynecology. 2014;**1**(2):00009. DOI: 10.15406/ogij.2014.01.00009

[21] Byrne J, Blanc WA. Malformations and chromosome anomalies in spontaneously aborted fetuses with single umbilical artery. American Journal Obstetrics Gynecology. 1985;**151**:340

[22] DeFigueiredo D, Dagklis T, Zidere V, Allan L, Nicolaides KH. Isolated single umbilical artery: Need for specialist fetal echocardiography? Ultrasound in Obstetrics & Gynecology. Nov 2010;**36**(5):553-555. DOI: 10.1002/uog.7711

[23] Chetty-John S, Zhang J, Chen Z, Albert P, Sun L, Klebanoff M, Grewal U. Long-term physical and neurologic development in newborn infants with isolated single umbilical artery. American Journal of Obstetrics and Gynecology. Oct 2010;**203**(4):368.e1-7. DOI: 10.1016/j.ajog.2010.06.031

[24] Weichert J, Hartge D, Germer U, Axt-Fliedner R, Gembruch U. Persistent right umbilical vein: A prenatal condition worth mentioning? Ultrasound in Obstetrics & Gynecology. 2011;**37**:543-548. DOI: 10.1002/uog.7764

[25] Barnett CP. Congenital abnormalities: Prenatal diagnosis and screening. In: Khong T, Malcomson R, editors. Keeling's Fetal and Neonatal Pathology. Cham: Springer; 2015. pp. 183-217. DOI: https://doi.org/10.1007/978-3-319-19207-9_8

[26] Yagel S, Kivilevitch Z, Cohen SM, Valsky DV, Messing B, Shen O, Achiron R. The fetal venous system, Part II: Ultrasound evaluation of the fetus with congenital venous system malformation or developing circulatory compromise. Ultrasound in Obstetrics & Gynecology. 2010;**36**:93-111. DOI: 10.1002/uog.7622

[27] Puvabanditsin S, Garrow E, Bhatt M, Kathiravan S, Gowda S, Wong R, Nagar M. Four-vessel umbilical cord associated with multiple congenital anomalies: A case report and literature review. Fetal and Pediatric Pathology. 2011;**30**(2):98-105. DOI: 10.3109/15513815.2010.524687

[28] Schimmel MS, Eidelman AI. Supernumerary umbilical vein resulting in a four-vessel umbilical cord. American Journal of Perinatology. May 1998;**15**(5):299-301. DOI: 10.1055/s-2007-993947

[29] Du X, Yuan Q, Li Z, Li Y. Three umbilical arteries resulting in a four-vessel umbilical cord in a stillbirth. International Journal of Clinical and Experimental Medicine. 2015;**8**(3):4682-4685

[30] Abuhamad AZ, Shaffer W, Mari G, Copel JA, Hobbins JC, Evans AT. Single umbilical artery: Does it matter which artery is missing? American Journal of Obstetrics Gynecology. 1995;**173**:728-732

[31] Heinonen S, Ryynanen M, Kirkinen P, Saarikoski S. Perinatal diagnostic evaluation of velamentous umbilical cord insertion: Clinical, Doppler, and ultrasonic findings. Obstetrics and Gynecology. 1996;**87**:112-117

[32] Hasegawa J, Matsuoka R, Ichizuka K, Sekizawa A, Okai T. Velamentous cord insertion: Significance of prenatal detection to predict perinatal complications. Taiwanese Journal of Obstetrics and Gynecology. 2006;**45**(1):21-25. DOI: 10.1016/S1028-4559(09)60185-6

[33] Heinonen S, Ryynanen M, Kirkinen P, Saarikoski S. Elevated midtrimester maternal serum hCG in chromosomally normal pregnancies is associated with preeclamp-
sia and velamentous umbilical cord insertion. American Journal of Perinatology. Oct
1996;13(7):437-441. DOI: 10.1055/s-2007-994384

[34] Eddleman KA, Lockwood CJ, Berkowitz GS, Lapinski RH, Berkowitz RL. Clinical significance and sonographic diagnosis of velamentous umbilical cord insertion. American
Journal of Perinatology. 1992;9(2):123-126. DOI: 10.1055/s-2007-994684

[35] Oyelese Y, Catanzarite V, Prefumo F, Lashley S, Schachter M, Tovbin Y, Goldstein V,
Smulian JC. Vasa previa: The impact of prenatal diagnosis on outcomes. Obstetrics and
Gynecology. 2004;103:937-942. DOI: 10.1097/01.AOG.0000123245.48645.98

[36] Catanzarite V, Maida C, Thomas W, Mendoza A, Stanco L, Piacquadio KM. Prenatal
sonographic diagnosis of vasa Previa: Ultrasound findings and obstetric outcome in
ten cases. Ultrasound in Obstetrics & Gynecology. 2001;18:109-115. DOI: 10.1046/j.1469
-0705.2001.00448.x

[37] Petrikovsky B, Schneider E. Prenatal diagnosis and clinical significance of hypoplastic
umbilical artery. Prenatal Diagnosis. 1996;16(10):938-940. DOI: 10.1002/(SICI)1097-0223
(199610)16:10<938::AIDPD964>3.0.CO;2-S

[38] Raio L, Ghezzi F, Di Naro E, Gomez R, Saile G, Bruhwiler H. The clinical significance
of antenatal detection of discordant umbilical arteries. Obstetrics and Gynecology. Jan
1998;91(1):86-91

[39] Lee SW, Kim MY, Kim JE, Chung JH, Lee HJ, Yoon JY. Clinical characteristics and outcomes of antenatal fetal intra-abdominal umbilical vein varix detection. Obstetrics and
Gynecology Science. 2014;57:181-186. DOI: 10.5468/ogs.2014.57.3.181

[40] Nyberg D. Varix of the umbilical vein. In: Nyberg DA, McGahan JP, Pretorius DH, Pilu G,
editors. Diagnostic Imaging of Fetal Anomalies. Philadelphia, PA: Lippincott Williams
& Wilkins; 2003. pp. 114-115

[41] Sepulveda W, Mackenna A, Sanchez J, Corral E, Carstens E. Fetal prognosis in varix of
the intrafetal umbilical vein. Journal of Ultrasound in Medicine. Mar 1998;17(3):171-175

[42] Weissmann-Brenner A, Simchen MJ, Moran O, Kassif E, Achiron R, Zalel Y. Isolated
fetal umbilical vein varix – Prenatal sonographic diagnosis and suggested management.
Prenatal Diagnosis. Mar 2009;29(3):229-233. DOI: 10.1002/pd.2219

[43] Shen O, Reinus C, Baranov A, Rabinowitz R. Prenatal diagnosis of umbilical artery aneurysm: A potential lethal anomaly. Journal of Ultrasound in Medicine. 2007;26:251-253

[44] Berg C, Geipel A, Germer U, Gloeckner-Hofmann K, Gembruch U. Prenatal diagnosis of umbilical cord aneurysm in a fetus with trisomy 18. Ultrasound in Obstetrics &
Gynecology. Jan 2001;17(1):79-81

[45] Zangen R, Boldes R, Yaffe H, Schwed P, Weiner Z. Umbilical cord cysts in the second and third trimesters: Significance and prenatal approach. Ultrasound in Obstetrics & Gynecology. 2010;**36**:296-301. DOI: 10.1002/uog.7576

[46] Sepulveda W, Leible S, Ulloa A, Ivankovic M, Schnapp C. Clinical significance of first trimester umbilical cord cysts. Journal of Ultrasound in Medicine. 1999;**18**:95-99

[47] Ross JA, Jurkovic D, Zosmer N, Jauniaux E, Hacket E, Nicolaides KH. Umbilical cord cysts in early pregnancy. Obstetrics and Gynecology. 1997;**89**:442-445

[48] Smith GN, Walker M, Johnston S, Ash K. The sonographic finding of persistent umbilical cord cystic masses is associated with lethal aneuploidy and/or congenital anomalies. Prenatal Diagnosis. 1996;**16**:1141-1147

[49] Marino T. Ultrasound abnormalities of the amniotic fluid, membranes, umbilical cord, and placenta. Obstetrics and Gynecology Clinics of North America. 2004;**31**(1):177-200

[50] Kiran H, Kiran G, Kanber Y. Pseudocyst of the umbilical cord with mucoid degeneration of Wharton's jelly. European Journal of Obstetrics Gynecology and Reproductive Biology. 2003;**111**(1):91-93

[51] Kinare A. Fetal environment. The Indian Journal of Radiology and Imaging. Nov 2008; **18**(4):326-344. DOI: 10.4103/0971-3026.43848

[52] Szpejankowski K, Guzik P, Chechlinski P, Jach R, Ostrowski B. Pseudocyst of the umbilical cord-case report. Przeglad Lekarski. 2015;**72**(7):394-396

[53] Ratan SK, Rattan KN, Kalra R, Maheshwari J, Parihar D, Ratan J. Omphalomesenteric duct cyst as a content of omphalocele. Indian Journal of Pediatrics. May 2007;**74**(5):500-502

[54] Kilicdag EB, Kilicdag H, Bagis T, Tarim E, Yanik F. Large pseudocyst of the umbilical cord associated with patent urachus. The Journal of Obstetrics and Gynaecology Research. Dec 2004;**30**(6):444-447

[55] Khong TY, Dilly SA. Calcification of umbilical artery: Two distinct lesions. Journal of Clinical Pathology. Sep 1989;**42**(9):931-934

[56] Kreczy A, Alge A, Menardi G, Gassner I, Gschwendtner A, Mikuz G. Teratoma of the umbilical cord. Case report with review of the literature. Archives of Pathology & Laboratory Medicine. Sep 1994;**118**(9):934-937

[57] Cheng HP, Hsu CY, Chen CP, Su TH. Angiomyxoma of the umbilical cord. Taiwanese Journal of Obstetrics & Gynecology. Dec 2006;**45**(4):360-362. DOI: 10.1016/S1028-4559(09)60262-X

[58] Cuda SP, Vanasupa BP, Sutherland RS. Nonoperative management of a patent urachus. Urology. Dec 2005;**66**(6):1320. DOI: 10.1016/j.urology.2005.06.121

[59] Bunch PT, Kline-Fath BM, Imhoff SC, Calvo-Garcia MA, Crombleholme TM, Donnelly LF. Allantoic cyst: A prenatal clue to patent urachus. Pediatric Radiology. Oct 2006;**36**(10): 1090-1095

[60] Pal K. Congenital hernia of the umbilical cord associated with extracelomic colonic atresia and perforation of gut in a newborn. African Journal of Paediatric Surgery. 2014; **11**:74-76

[61] Mirza B, Ali W. Distinct presentations of hernia of umbilical cord. Journal of Neonatal Surgery. 2016;**5**(4):53. DOI: 10.21699/jns.v5i4.400

[62] Shibata M, Kanehiro H, Shinkawa T, et al. A neonate with umbilical arteriovenous malformation showing hemorrhagic shock from massive umbilical hemorrhage. American Journal of Perinatology. 2009;**26**(8):583-586. DOI: 10.1055/s-0029-1220778

6

Congenital Abnormalities of the Fetal Face

Maria Șorop-Florea, Roxana-Cristina Dragușin,
Ciprian Laurențiu Pătru, Lucian George Zorilă,
Cristian Marinaș, Virgiliu-Bogdan Șorop,
Cristian Neamțu, Alina Veduța,
Dominic Gabriel Iliescu and Nicolae Cernea

Abstract

Even at the early stages of gestation, the fetal face can be examined. There have been observations of the normal anatomy, such as orbits and the forehead, starting with the 12th week of gestation. However, nowadays, ultrasound equipment still cannot distinguish the soft tissues of the face, which are too thin. Yet, after the age of 14 weeks, we can easily examine the forehead, orbits, nose, lips, and ears. Recently, three-dimensional ultrasound (3D) images of the fetus can also be obtained. However, two-dimensional (2D) ultrasonographic (US) images are more easily, rapidly, efficiently, and accurately obtained. At the first stage of embryogenesis, the main part in the development of the fetal face is taken by the genetic factors. Later, the influence of the environment becomes more important. It is known that the outcome of chromosomal aberrations and of teratogenic factors is the facial malformation. Therefore, examining the facial dimorphism may get us useful hints in revealing chromosomal or genetic abnormalities. This chapter focuses on the fetal face anomalies more frequently found while performing the prenatal diagnosis. It is divided into anomalies of the orbits, nose, lip, palate, and mandible.

Keywords: fetal face, facial malformation, ultrasound, prenatal diagnosis, congenital abnormalities

1. Introduction

The study of the fetal face may be performed during the early stages of gestation. Depending on the gestational age, we can identify various elements of anatomy, such as the orbits or the forehead, from the 12th week. Yet, after that time, we can easily identify and study the forehead, the nose, the lips, the ears, and the orbits of the fetus [1]. Prenatal recognition of facial abnormalities during pregnancy has many benefits. It can lead to the diagnosis of multiple genotypic syndromes and chromosomal anomalies. Also, it allows more adequate counseling and preparation of the parents. Considering that the sonographic assessment of the fetal face is a major part of the anatomic survey of the fetus, sagittal, axial, and coronal planes are used when examining the fetus.

The facial anomalies are divided into nose, orbit, lip, mandible, and palate anomalies. The US method may reveal also benign and less frequent anomalies, for example, lacrimal duct cysts, hemangiomas, and so on.

1.1. Sagittal planes

In order to assess the normality of the fetus profile, sagittal planes of the face are used (**Figure 1**).

One of the US parameters used to obtain an exact measurement of the position of the anterior end of the maxilla to the forehead is the angle between the surface of the palate and the frontal bone examined in a mid-sagittal view of the fetal face, called the frontomaxillary facial angle [2]. This angle is increased in fetuses with trisomy 21, and it is believed that the reason for this is the hypoplasia or posterior displacement of the palate [2, 3].

Ears are well visualized in parasagittal scans tangential to the calvarium. In late gestation, significant details of the anatomy of the external ear can be seen.

1.2. Axial planes

Orbits may be visualized simultaneously, by means of an axial plane, slightly caudal to the one used to measure the biparietal diameter (**Figures 2–4**) [4].

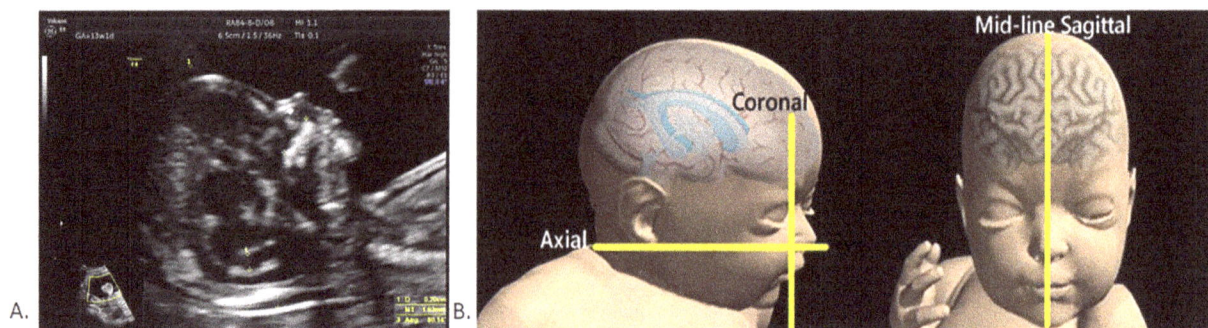

Figure 1. (A). Normal fetal profile at 12–13 weeks. (B). Schematic representation of the scanning planes to be used for obtaining axial and coronal views of the fetal face.

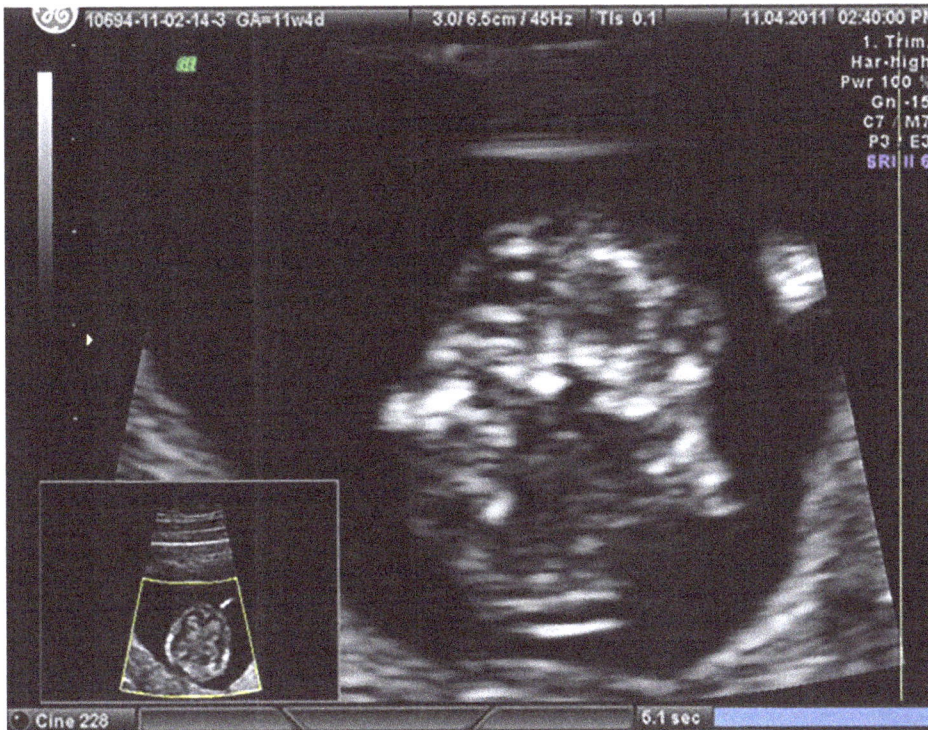

Figure 2. Axial scan passing through the orbits of a normal second trimester fetus.

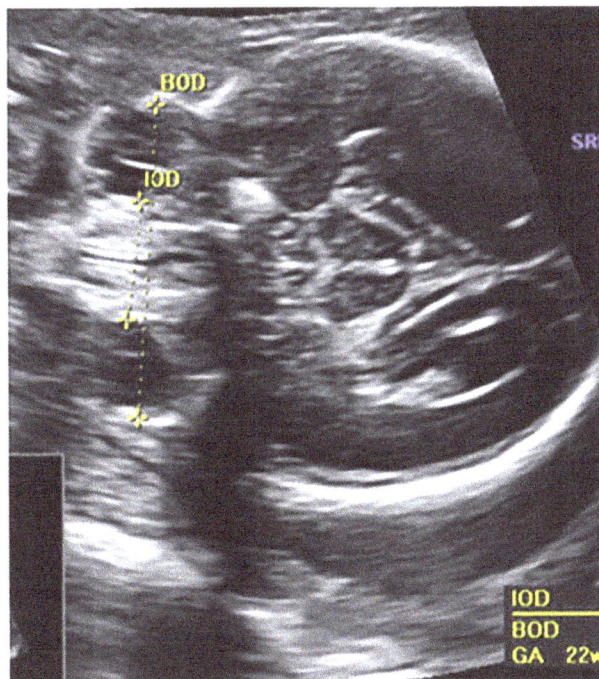

Figure 3. The interocular distance (IOD) and binocular distance (BOD) are demonstrated in this scan. The lens is visible inside the orbit.

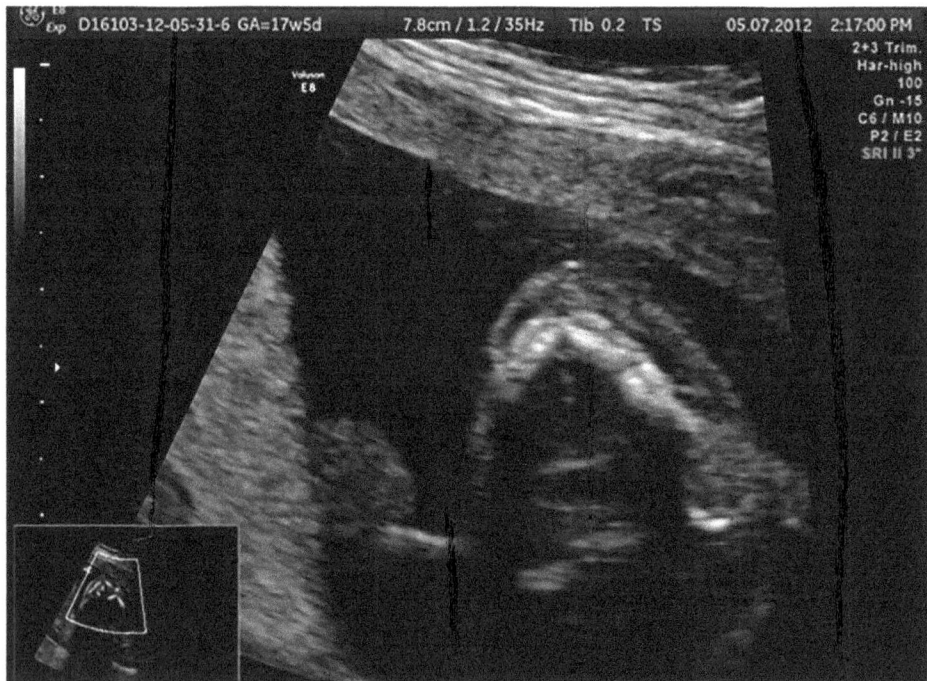

Figure 4. Axial scan of the lower fetal face demonstrating the upper lip and the anterior palate.

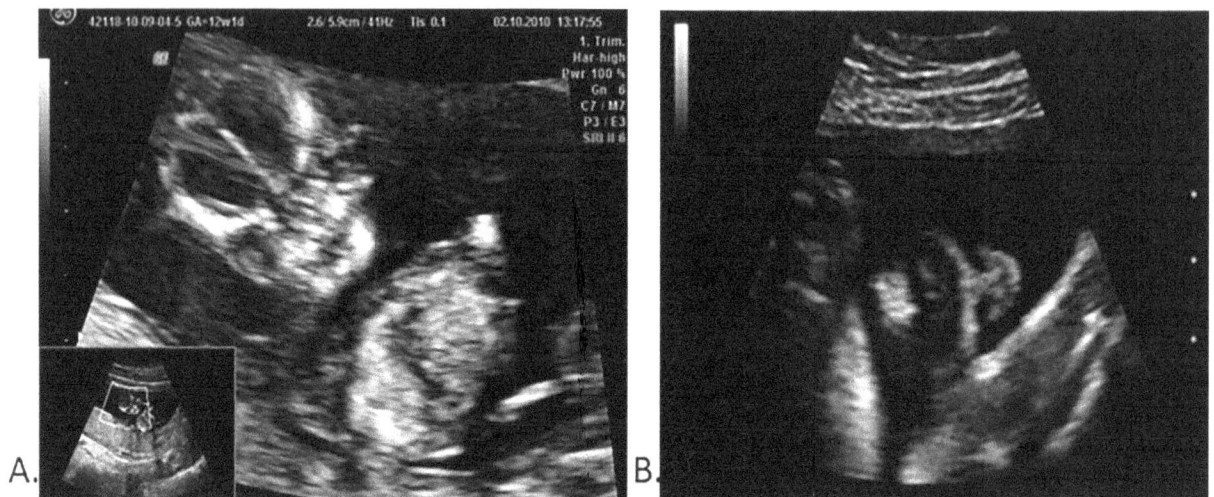

Figure 5. A. Coronal anterior plane in a late first trimester (FT) fetus: The lens inside the corpus vitreum B. The tip of the nose, the alae nasi, and the columna are seen above the upper lip. The nostril typically appears as two little anechoic areas.

1.3. Coronal planes

Evaluation of the integrity of the facial anatomy is assessed by visualizing the eyelids, orbits, lips, forehead, and nose, whose nostrils usually appear as two little anechoic areas. For these features, coronal planes are more important than the previous one (**Figure 5**).

1.4. Fetal face profile

One of the most common "soft sonographic sings" providing essential clues of congenital syndromes [1] is the deviations from the proportions normally found during a sagittal fetal

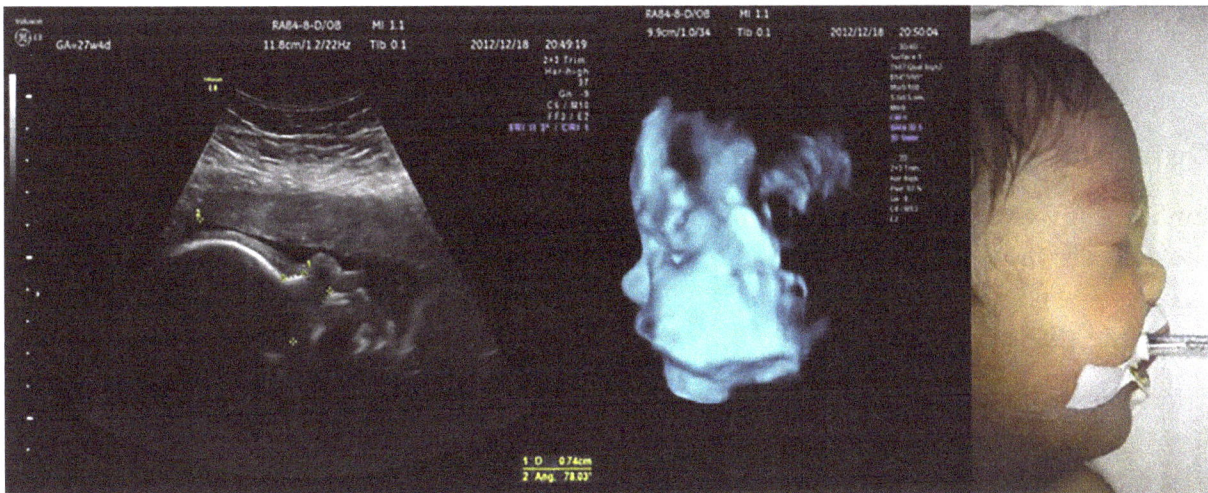

Figure 6. Sonographic pictures of fetal bossing forehead at 24 weeks of gestation. The postnatal aspect of the neonates with bossing forehead.

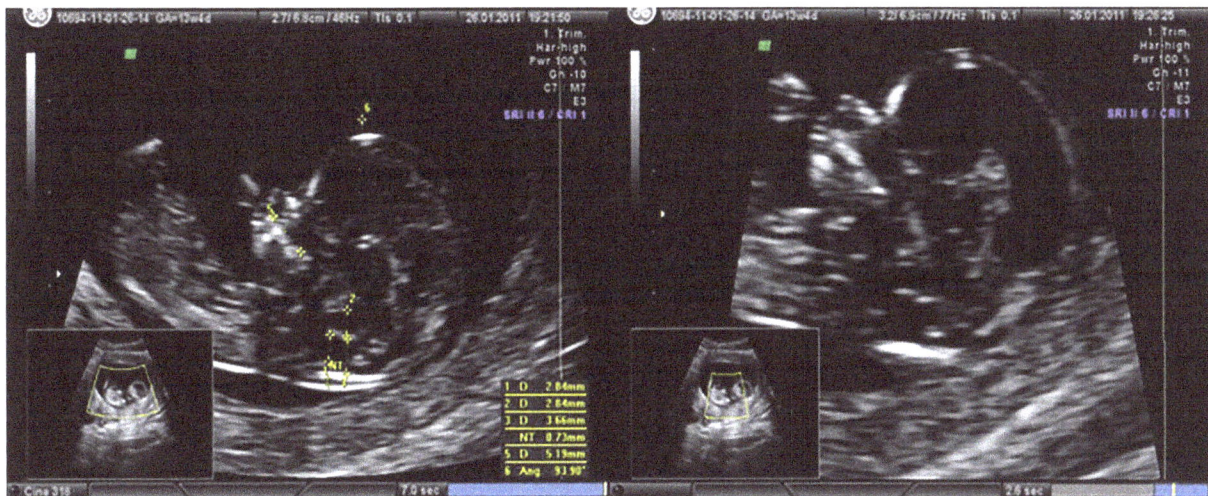

Figure 7. Sagittal scan of a fetus at 13–14 weeks of gestation shows FT bossing forehead.

face examination (**Figures 6**, **7**). Apert or Carpenter syndromes are ruled out by examining the bridge of the nose. [5] The cleft lip is excluded when the normal prominent lips are visible. [1]. As for micrognathia or prognathia, these can be noticed in the subjective abnormal appearance of the jaw [6].

2. The fetal eyes

From the late FT or in the early second trimester onward, we should consider the visualization of the fetal orbit and lens. The orbits will appear as echolucent circles on the upper fetal face, whereas the lens will be visualized inside these structures, as circular hyperechogenic rings. These images can be obtained during almost all scans, beginning with the late first trimester. Any deviation from the relative size might suggest congenital malformations of the orbits and lens. To assess them, coronal and especially axial planes of the fetal head are the best approach.

2.1. Anomalies of the orbits

2.1.1. Hypertelorism

Definition: Hypertelorism is an increased interocular distance.

Embryology and pathogenesis: At the first stage of the development of the human embryo, the eyes are to be found laterally, like in animals with panoramic vision. As the pregnancy evolves, the fetal eyes migrate toward the midline, thus generating the conditions for the stereoscopic vision to develop (**Figure 8**).

There are at least two theories as to why hypertelorism may appear. The first theory states that there are several mechanisms causing it: the forward migration of the first half of the eyes, a midline tumor, meningoencephalocele for instance, causing the second half, or skull bones with abnormal growth vectors. The second theory links a splanchnocranium, which presents an abnormal growth, to the undeveloped bones which derive from the first branchial arches [8].

Pathology: Three parameters are used to measure the fetuses' ocular spacing: interpupillary distance, canthal distance, and interorbital distance. Hypertelorism is bilateral most of the times, with little incidents of unilateral cases associated with plagiocephaly and proboscis lateralis. Also, this condition is either isolated or accompanied by other malformations or clinical syndromes such as the median cleft syndrome and craniosynostoses. In craniosynostoses, hypertelorism syndromes such as Apert, Crouzon, and Carpenter are usually present [9].

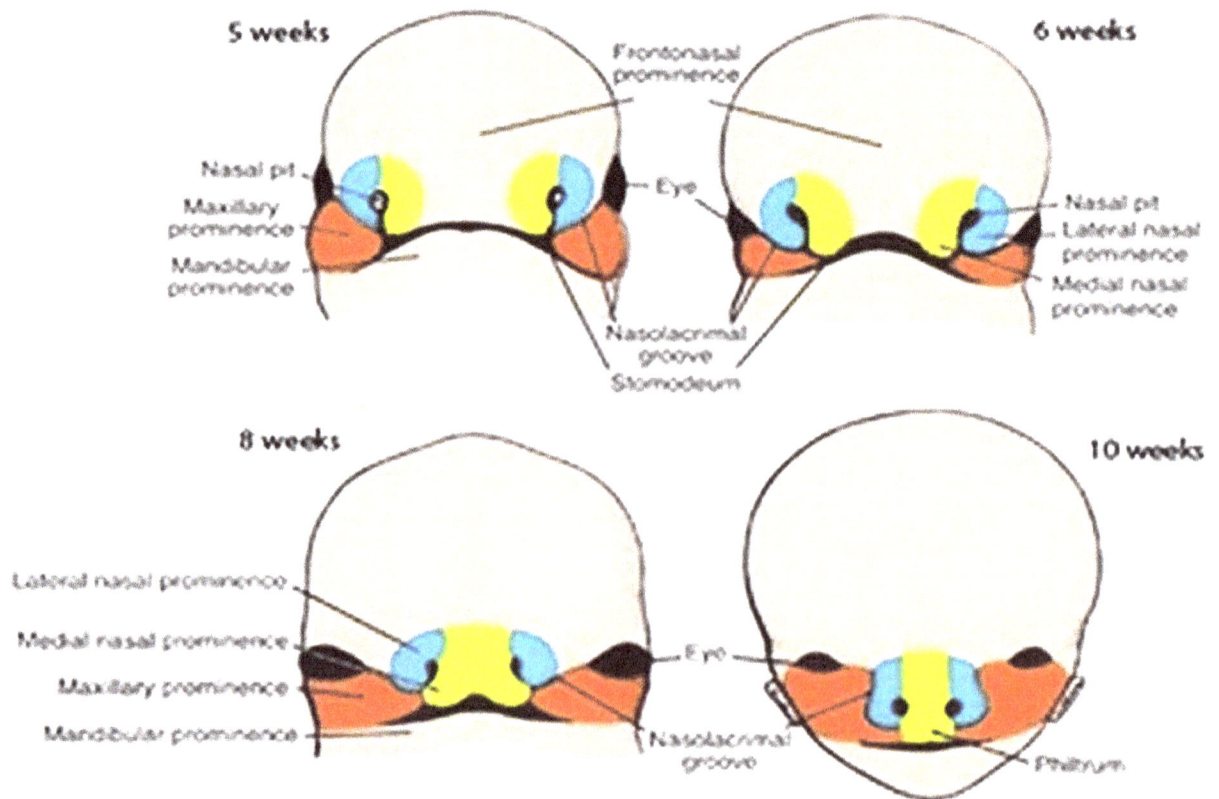

Figure 8. The facial structures development, represented schematically between the 5th and the 10th week of gestation. During the early stages, we can notice the primitive eyes on both sides of the cephalic pole. However, they move toward the median line as gestation goes on [7].

Ultrasound diagnosis: Interorbital diameter is larger than 95th. The accuracy of ultrasound exam in the hypertelorism diagnosis has not been established.

Investigations: Detailed ultrasound examination for associated defects. Invasive testing for karyotyping and array.

Follow up: Standard follow-up in isolated cases. Any underlying syndrome antenatal care should be adjusted, considering the additional risk of the condition.

Delivery: Standard obstetric care and delivery.

Isolated: It is good, even if there might be esthetic implications in severe cases as well as impaired stereoscopic binocular vision. For these cases, there are several operative procedures such as canthoplasty, orbitoplasty, surgical positioning of the eyebrows, and rhinoplasty.

Syndromic: The prognosis of hypertelorism is usually poor, and it does have a risk of mental retardation. However, normal life span and normal intellect are to be expected in the case of medial facial cleft syndrome [8]. The esthetic aspect should not be underestimated.

Recurrence: Isolated: no increased risk of recurrence.

2.1.2. Hypotelorism

Definition: Hypotelorism is a decreased interorbital distance.

Prevalence: 1 in 20,000 births.

Etiology: Hypertelorism is almost always associated with other severe abnormalities, especially with the sequence of holoprosencephalic abnormality.

Embryology and Pathogenesis: Out of the mesenchymal mass there comes the craniofacial skeleton. This mass has two points of origin: the mesoderm and the neutral crest, the latter migrating to the region. The development of the median facial structures (forehead, nose, interorbital structures and upper lip) is closely linked to the forebrain differentiating process. It is possible that these two development steps are induced by the tissue, which lies between the prosencephalon and the stomodeum (the root of the primitive mouth), namely the prechordal mesenchyma. Thus, defects of the facial midline, for example, hypotelorism, are often linked to cerebral abnormalities, most often with holoprosencephaly. Hypotelorism can be found in association with trigonocephaly, microcephaly, Meckel syndrome and chromosome aberrations [10, 11].

Ultrasound diagnosis: It is based on the documentation of a reduced interocular distance. The interorbital diameter is lower than <5th and, together with the almost always present holoprosencephaly (**Figure 9**), is to be found among the midline migration defects; in this case, the hypotelorism can be extreme, as in cyclopia [10].

Associated abnormalities: In half of the cases, we encounter chromosomal defects, especially trisomy 13, as well as genetic syndromes [9].

Investigations: A thorough ultrasound examination should be conducted, including neurosonography, in order to find associated defects as well as invasive testing for karyotyping and array.

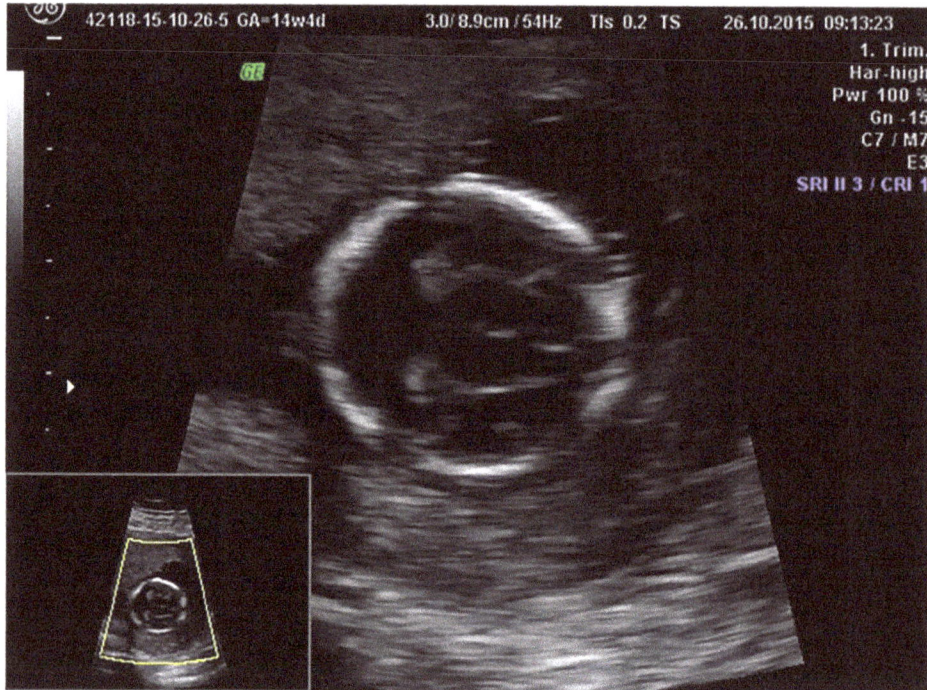

Figure 9. Axial scan a fetus at 14–15 weeks with alobar holoprosencephaly.

Prognosis: The prognosis and the management are decided on the accompanying malformations. Usually, the prognosis is poor, with high levels of mortality. In cases with normal karyotype, there is a high risk of mental retardation, depending on the degree of holoprosencephaly.

Recurrence: Isolated: no increased risk. One percentage risk of trisomy and 13.25% risk of being part of an autosomal recessive condition [11].

2.1.3. Microphthalmia/Anophthalmia

Definition: Microphthalmia refers to the decreased size of the eyeball, whereas anophthalmia refers to absence of the eye. However, the pathologist should demonstrate not only the absence of the eye but also of the optic nerves, chiasma, and tracts.

Prevalence: While it is difficult to define, it accounts for 1 in 20,000 births, and for 4% of the cases of congenital inheritable blindness.

Etiology/Pathology: Microphthalmia is usually associated with other anomalies. Microphthalmia is either as a sporadic disorder or as a condition inherited with an autosomal dominant, recessive, or X-linked pattern. We use the term "cryptophthalmia" to define fused eyelids, a condition often associated [9, 10].

Ultrasound diagnosis: Microphthalmia and anophthalmia can be unilateral or bilateral. Diagnosis can be suspected by demonstrating an orbital diameter below the fifth percentile for gestational age (**Figure 10**). If the diagnosis is suspected, a thorough search for associated anomalies (microtia, micrognathia, syndactyly, camptodactyly, median cleft, feet abnormalities, such as rocker bottom and talipes, hemivertebrae, and congenital heart defects) should be performed.

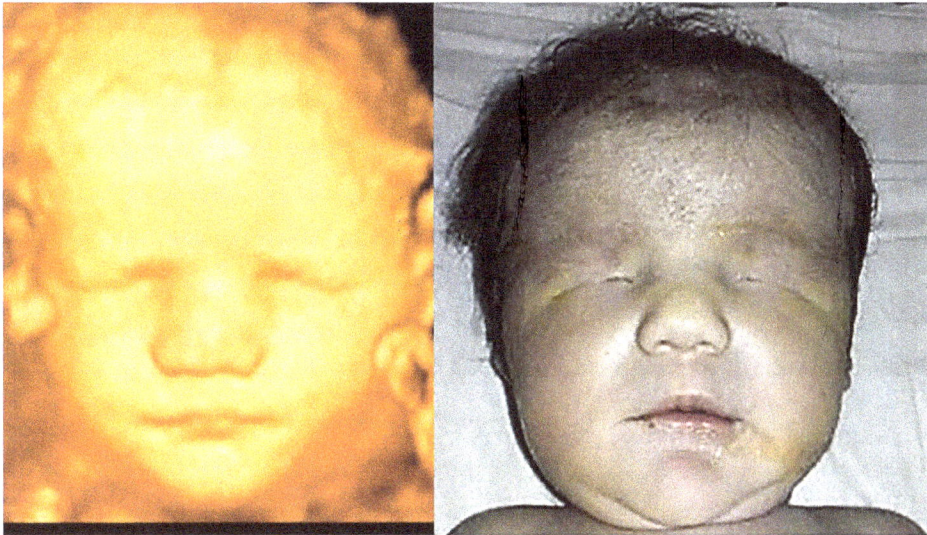

Figure 10. This picture shows a case of anophthalmia, prenatal and postnatal aspects.

Associated abnormalities: Chromosomal defects, especially trisomy 13, are found in more than 50% of the cases. The most common include: Goldenhar syndrome (1:3000 births), Fraser syndrome, Fryns syndrome and Meckel-Gruber [9].

Investigations: Besides detailed ultrasound, karyotyping and array should be offered. Also, a fetal brain MRI may be useful to diagnose abnormalities (e.g., the absence of the optic nerve).

Prognosis and obstetrical management: Isolated: good, with an altered life quality because of the esthetic aspect of the lesion: plastic surgery might be considered. Syndromic: prognosis is very poor. Management depends on the specific syndrome [11].

Recurrence: Isolated: no increased risk. Part of an autosomal recessive condition: 25%.

2.1.4. Dacryocystocele

Definition: Dacryocystocele is a congenital obstruction of the nasolacrimal duct, resulting in cystic dilatation of the proximal part of the duct. (**Figure 11**).

Prevalence: 1 in 4000.

Ultrasound diagnosis: Cyst (75% unilateral and 25% bilateral) between the lower part of the orbit and the nose. About 90% of the cases are due to delayed canalization of the lacrimal duct beyond 32 weeks gestation.

The differential diagnosis: includes an anterior cephalocele, hemangiomas, and dermoid cyst. Usually, hemangiomas have a solid appearance or multiple septae, and they are shown as exophytic lesions with an echogenicity, similar to the placenta. Among the complications of hemangiomas, we should include ulceration, bleeding, infection, and scar formation. The dermoid cysts have often a superolateral location. It is difficult to differentiate anterior cephaloceles from these lesions. If hydrocephaly is present, we should suspect a cephalocele [12, 13].

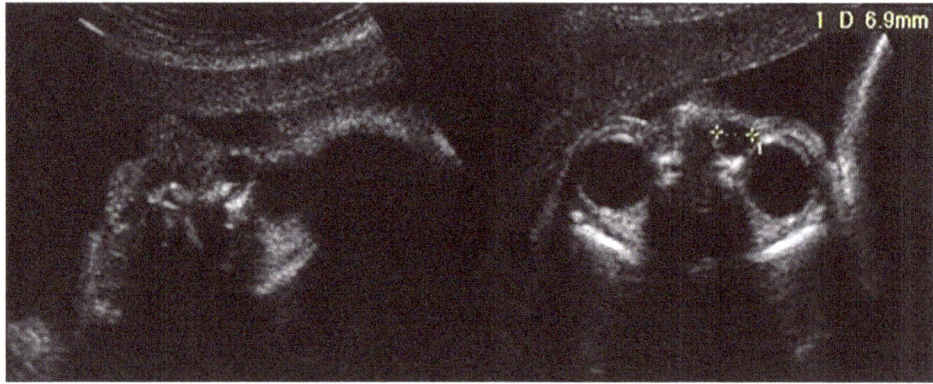

Figure 11. Ultrasonographic aspect of the congenital dacryocystocele.

Associated abnormalities: Not associated with chromosomal or other abnormalities.

They resolve spontaneously in 78% of the cases by 3 months, 91% by 6 months, or during the third semester.

2.1.5. Cyclopia

Definition: Cyclopia is another type of anomaly, in which the fetus has only one single orbital fossa, with bulbs, eyelids and lacrimal apparatus fused to a variable degree. In many cases, there is one single eye or one partially divided eye, in a single orbit and arhinia with proboscis (**Figure 12**), [14, 15].

Incidence: Cyclopia results from the incomplete cleavage of the prosencephalon into right and left hemispheres, a process which should be occurring between the 18th and the 28th day of pregnancy, and it is a lethal human malformation, relatively complex, but also quite rare. Moreover, holoprosencephaly occurs in 1/16,000 live births [16].

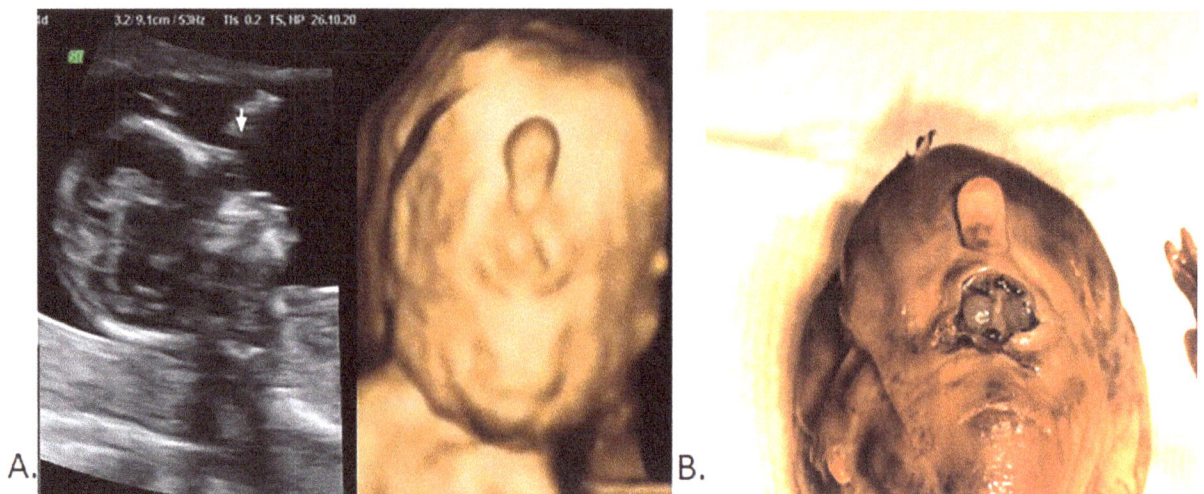

Figure 12. A. Axial and sagittal scans of a fetus at 15 weeks of gestation show cyclopia and proboscis. B. Ethmocephaly — Postmortem demonstrating hypotelorism and proboscis.

The etiology of this rare syndrome incompatible with life is still not known in detail, because most cases are sporadic, even if the implication of heterogeneous risk factors has been proven. Among risk factors, we include maternal diabetes (the only formally recognized environmental factor, with a 1% risk and a 200-fold increase in fetal holoprosencephaly), infections during pregnancy (TORCHs), active drugs during pregnancy physical agents (ultraviolet light), and chromosomal (mostly trisomy 13) and genetic causes (familial occurrences in twins and in consanguineous marriages [17].

In order to get **the differential diagnosis** of these cases, we must distinguish between ethmocephaly and cebocephaly. In other words, we must be able to trace extreme hypotelorism, arhinia and blinded proboscis located between the eyes as opposed to hypotelorism and a single nostril nose without midline cleft. In case the image shows united palatine and lacrimal bones, as well as no sign of nasal bones, maxilla and nasal septum, then the diagnosis is ethmocephaly [15].

2.1.6. Cataracts

Definition: any opacity of the eye lens.

The incidence of cataract is as follows: 1–6 newborn infants every 10,000 births [18] for congenital cataracts in newborn babies, whereas 8.3–25% is considered to be inherited.

Etiology: There are several ways in which a fetus might inherit congenital cataracts: autosomal dominant, autosomal recessive, or X-linked fashion. However, the most frequent and the strongest penetration is the autosomal dominant. A series of other complications are associated with cataracts: genetic syndromes, congenital infections, metabolic disorders, and chromosomal abnormalities. The genetic cause is present in 30% of the unilateral cataracts and in 50% of the bilateral ones [19].

During the examination of the fetal cataracts solid, either some echogenic discs or echogenicity areas within an echolucent orbit will be noticed (**Figure 13**), having either unilateral or bilateral

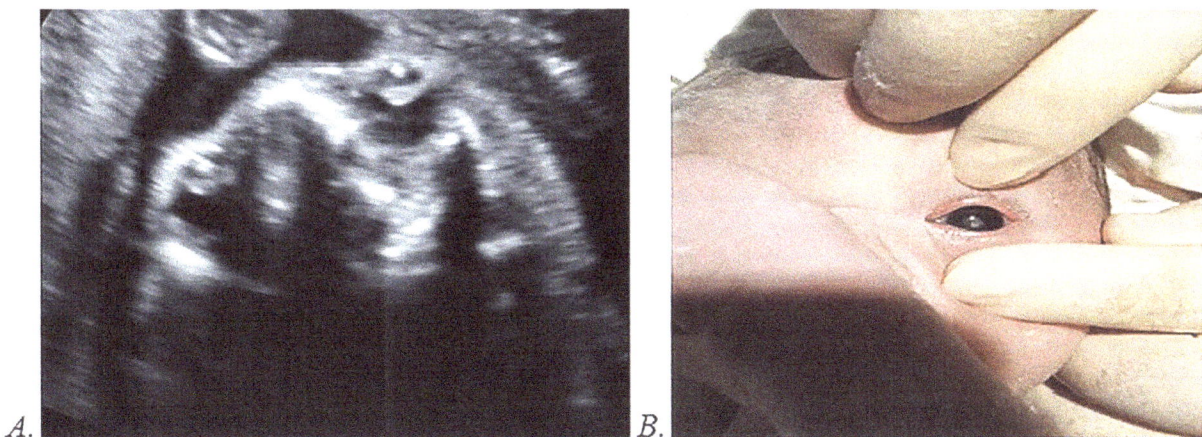

A.

B.

Figure 13. A. Sonographic pictures of fetal cataracts at 24 weeks of gestation. Coronal views of echogenic lens. B. The postnatal aspect of the lens.

opacity of the lens. Usually, the bilateral lesions are generally syndromic, with a poor prognosis; as for unilateral lesions, they are generally linked to a fetal infection. The genetic aspect of cataracts can be linked to microphthalmia.

Associated abnormalities: there is not any high risk of chromosomal abnormalities. It is in only 10% of the cases that genetic syndromes are found, and these include the chromosomal defects. In about 10% of the cases, genetic syndromes are found, and the most common include: Walker-Warburg syndrome and chondrodysplasia punctata. Only a fifth of the congenital cataracts cases are linked to infections such as rubella, toxoplasmosis, or CMV [20].

Investigations: ultrasound, karyotyping, array and TORCH.

Prognosis: Usually good for isolated cases. Postpartum ophthalmologic surgeries have good results, which do not affect the quality of life. Prognosis is quite poor for syndromic cataract, though.

3. The ear

The most frequent clinical characteristic in diagnosing the Down syndrome has been the short ear length. Sonographic studies implied that measurements of the short ear length could be a useful predictor of fetal anomalies. In late gestation, important details of the anatomy of the external ear became accessible. In good conditions for scanning, and using high-resolution systems, the helix, scaphoid fossa, triangular fossa, concha, antihelix, tragus, antitragus, intertragic incisure, and lobule are sometimes visualized [21].

4. The nasal bone and nostrils

A small nose is very commonly seen during postnatal examination of fetuses or neonates who also present trisomy 21 as well as for more than 40 other genetic problems. The nasal bone can be measured using a mid-sagittal profile for normal singleton fetuses between the 14th and 34th week of gestation. Thus, the length of the nasal bones increase from 4 mm at 14 weeks to 12 mm at 35 weeks gestation. A possible improvement in screening for trisomy 21 by examining the fetal nasal bone with ultrasound at 11–14 weeks of gestation has been considered [22].

4.1. Anomalies of the nose

4.1.1. Arhinia

Definition: Absence of the nose.

Etiology: Unknown. It can either be an isolated malformation or be part of a malformation complex, such as holoprosencephaly or mandibulofacial dysostosis (Treacher Collins syndrome) [23].

Embryology: Around the 6th week of gestation, the primitive nasal and oral cavities communicate freely using an opening, which will close progressively when the palate starts developing.

When the lateral palatine processes fuse with the nasal septum in the middle, the oral and the two nasal cavities are formed and separated; this takes place around the 12th week of gestation. The external nose starts at the lower portion of the frontonasal prominence, merging on both sides with the maxillary processes (**Figure 9**). If the frontonasal prominence does not fully develop, the result is partial or complete nasal aplasia. This anomaly is part of a more complex spectrum of midfacial defects, which, in the holoprosencephalic sequence, are considered to appear from a primitive defect of the prechordal mesenchyma, the tissue responsible for the induction of both facial and cerebral structures [24, 25].

Prognosis depends on the associated anomalies; however, isolated arhinia is not life incompatible.

4.1.2. Proboscis

Definition: A proboscis is a trunk-like appendage, with one or two internal openings, and it is usually associated with the absence of the nose.

Incidence: Cyclopia and cebocephaly, two of the main conditions for a proboscis to be present, occur in 1:40,000 and 1:16,000 births, respectively [26].

Embryology: The presence of a proboscis is frequently associated with holoprosencephaly. Apparently, a primary disorder in the prechordal mesenchyma develops into an abnormal induction of the midfacial structures. If the nasal prominences develop abnormally, this may lead to a fusion of the olfactory placodes and to the formation of a proboscis [27].

Pathology and associated anomalies: Usually there is a single central opening in the proboscis, and it does not have any connection to the choanae. The ethmoid, the nasal conchae, and the nasal and lacrimal bones are absent. Usually, in cyclopia, ethmocephaly, and cebocephaly, the cleft of the lip and the palate are absent. The presence of a proboscis is seldom found in the absence of holoprosencephaly. In rare cases, a bilateral proboscis can be noticed [28].

Diagnosis: The diagnosis relies on the demonstration of a trunk-like structure, usually with a single central opening either occupying the normal position of the nose or hanging above the orbits [29] (**Figure 8**).

5. The tongue

Fetal macroglossia and microglossia are associated with several chromosomal defects.

5.1. Macroglossia

Prevalence: Depends on the underlying disorder (present in 97.5% of Beckwith-Wiedemann syndrome cases: incidence 0.73:10,000 live births, congenital hypothyroidism: incidence 2.5:10,000 live births) [30].

Etiology: If it is isolated, it is usually sporadic and it relates to the underlying disorder; there have been only two families with autosomal dominant transmission.

Pathogenesis: In cases of Beckwith-Wiedemann syndrome, it is part of the generalized viscero-megaly probably secondary to fetal hyperinsulinism. The most common cause of Beckwith-Wiedemann syndrome is the uniparental paternal disomy, a result which was found using 11p15.5 markers. It is the same region in which the code for insulin-like hormones is found [30].

Diagnosis: Considering the imaginary line between the mandible and the maxilla on the sagittal scanning plane, the diagnosis is confirmed by the protruding tip of the tongue past that line; if we consider the axial scan, the diagnosis is confirmed by the protruding tip of the tongue past the lower lip.

Associated anomalies: It is diagnosed by prenatal ultrasound in cases of Beckwith-Wiedemann syndrome, in association with hydramnios (due to impaired fetal swallowing and possibly to increased urine production), omphalocele, nephromegaly, gigantism (sometimes hemihypertrophy), hepatomegaly, genital anomalies, cystic adrenal glands, and heart defects. In the absence of an omphalocele, a careful search for markers of trisomy 21 is indicated [31].

6. Anomalies of the lip and palate

Facial cleft

Synonyms: The Cleft lip and the cleft palate.

Definition: This term refers to a wide spectrum of lateral clefting defects, usually involving the upper lip (**Figure 14**), the palate (**Figure 15**) or both.

Incidence: Facial clefting is the second most common congenital malformation, around 13% of all anomalies. It is usually encountered in 1 in 1000 live births; however, it can be higher for fetuses, many of them having other malformations as well. The occurrence of the cleft palate is 1 of 2500 white births, cleft lip being more common to boys, and cleft palate being more

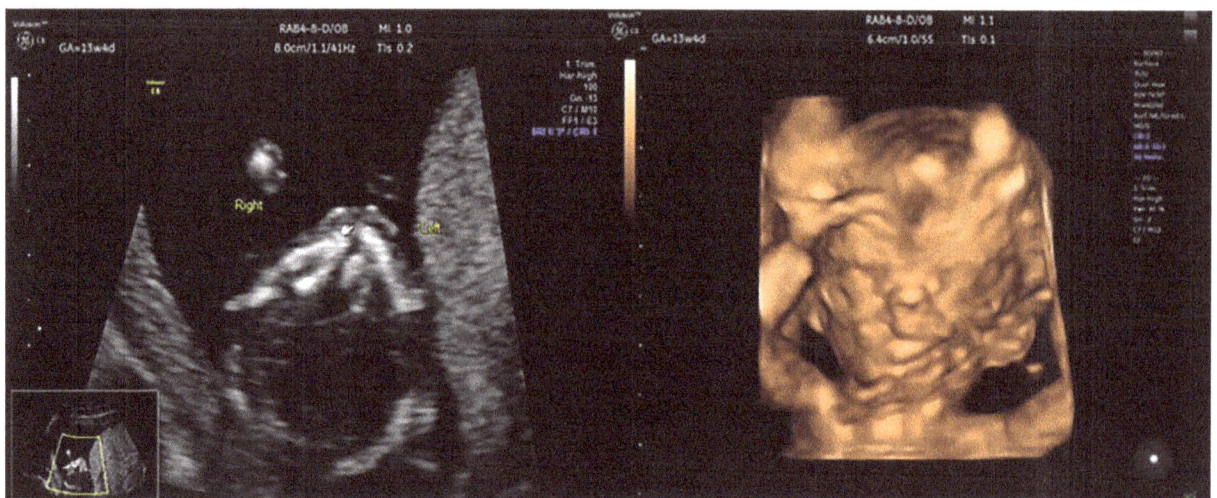

Figure 14. 2D and 3D ultrasonographic pictures of cleft lip.

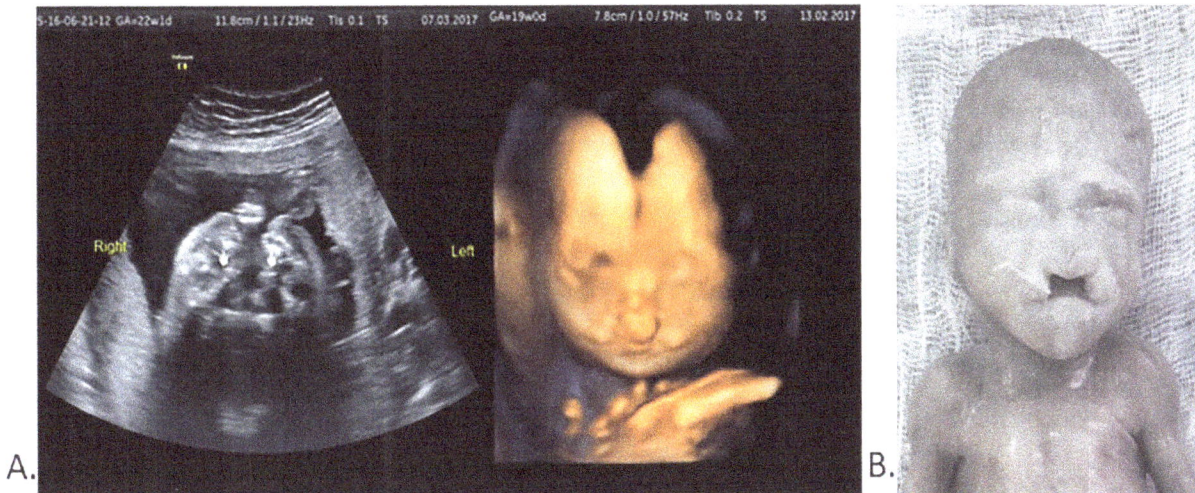

Figure 15. A. Sonographic pictures of the bilateral cleft palate (22 weeks of gestation). B. The postnatal aspect of the cleft palate.

common to girls. In 50% of cases, both the lip and palate are affected, in 25% only the lip and in 25% only the palate. The condition is unilateral in 75% of cases (more common on the left side) and bilateral in 25% [1, 32].

Etiology: The cleft lip is one or more splits (clefts) in the upper lip, ranging from a small indentation in the lip to a split in the lip, which may extend up into one or both nostrils. In the clear majority of patients, the cleft lip (CL) and the cleft palate (CP) have a multifactorial etiology, including genetic and environmental factors. CL (with or without CP) and isolated CP are two different anomalies. CL-CP and isolated CP can be noticed as a component of a well-defined syndrome in 3% of the cases (syndromic) and in 97% of cases (nonsyndromic). CL-CP can develop either as a result of a multifactorial defect or the combination of an autosomal dominant with incomplete expressivity and penetrance (25%) or a sporadic disorder (75%). If the affected parent is the mother, the recurrence risk is decreased, and if it is the father, the recurrence risk is increased. The opposite is true for CL-CP. Chromosomal abnormalities are present in less than 1% of clefting abnormalities [33].

Embryology: The cleft lip results from the persistence of the grooves between the frontonasal, maxillary, and mandibular prominences and develops in about the 6th to 8th week of gestation, when the structures of the upper jaw do not fuse properly and the upper lip does not completely merge. The formation of the cleft is due to the collapse of the mesenchymal tissue under the groove [12]. At times, usually between the 7th and the 12th week of gestation, the cleft palate bones and tissues do not join totally during fetal growth. This leads to the nasal cavity, palate and upper teeth to be affected by the roof of the mouth that remains opened. The cleft palate varies in severity and type according to the place on the palate where the cleft occurs and whether the layers of the palate are affected completely. Sometimes, if some tissues cover the cleft, a milder form of cleft palate will not be visible. A more severe form of the cleft palate, the complete one, involves tissues from all layers of the soft palate, encompasses the hard palate as well, and it might continue to the lip and nose. From time to time, the cleft palate problems also include deformities of the nasal cavities [33].

Pathology: Facial clefts encompass a large spectrum of severity, from minimal defects, such as a bifid uvula, linear indentation of the lip, or submucous cleft of the soft palate, to large, deep, defects of the facial bones and soft tissues (**Figure 16**).

Diagnosis: To set a diagnosis, both transverse and coronal planes can be used. The accuracy of ultrasound in detecting small lesions has not been established; however, color Doppler might be useful to demonstrate the flow across the palate in the case of the cleft palate. Diagnosis of isolated cleft palate is difficult. Diagnosis of the cleft lip and palate at 11–13 weeks gestation can be obtained using axial planes at the level of the bony palate. In rare cases, the retronasal triangle in a coronal view and the maxillary gap in the standard mid-sagittal view of the face may be helpful [35].

Associated anomalies: There have been found associated anomalies in 50% of the patients with isolated CP and 13% of those with CL-CP In cases of isolated CL or CP, the most frequent anomaly is clubfoot, whereas in cases of CL-CP, it is polydactyly. It is particularly important to notice the association with congenital heart disease [36].

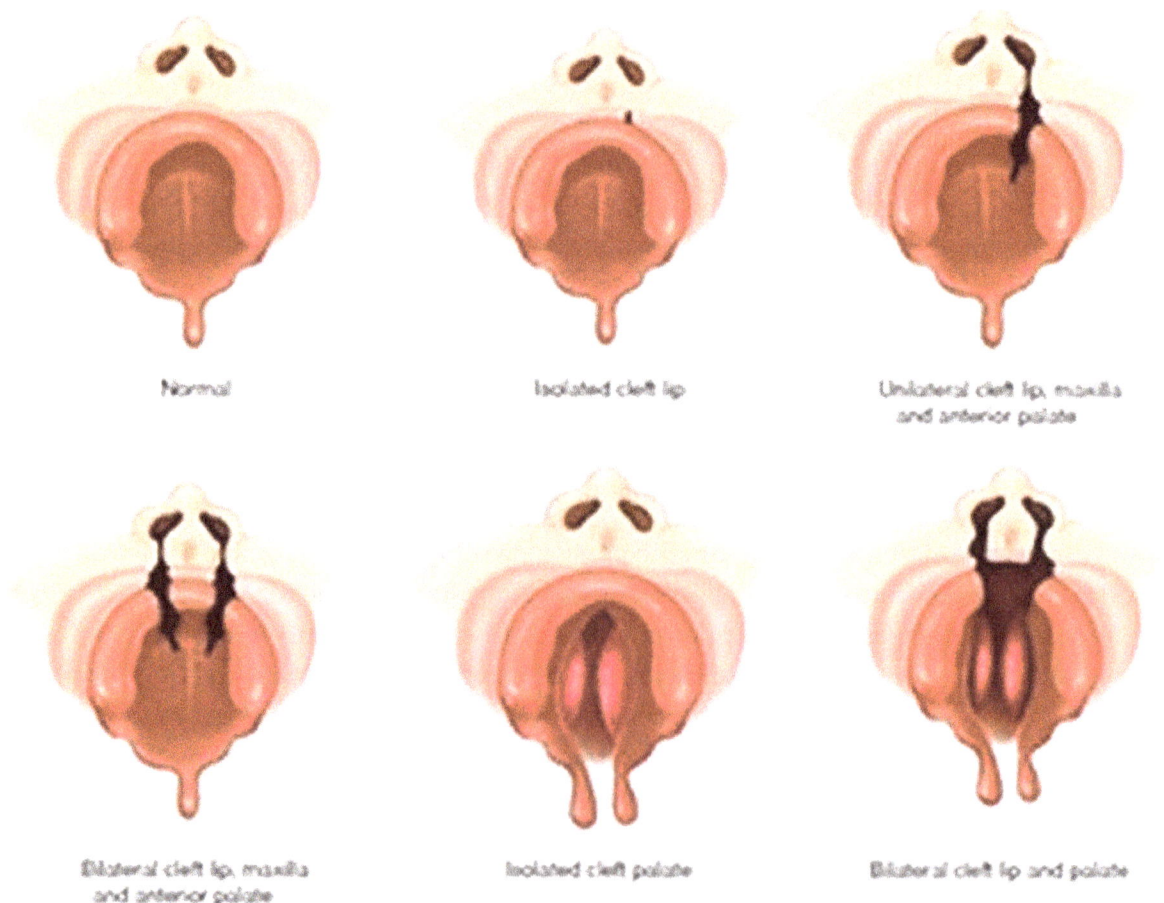

Figure 16. Schematic representation of various types of the cleft lip and the cleft palate. (A) Normal, (B) Isolated cleft lip, (C) Unilateral cleft lip, maxilla and anterior palate, (D) Bilateral cleft lip, maxilla and anterior palate, (E) Isolated cleft palate, and (F) Bilateral cleft lip and palate [34].

Prognosis: If the defects are minimal, as is the case with the lineal indentations of the lips or submucosal cleft of the soft palate, surgical correction may not be required. If the defects are larger and cause esthetic, swallowing, and respiratory problems, then surgical correction is a must, and recent advances in surgical techniques have had good results. Anyhow, the prognosis depends primarily on the presence and type of associated anomalies [37].

The advisability of karyotype is controversial due to the low incidence of chromosomal anomalies in clefting defect. Fetuses should be delivered in a tertiary center because of the possibility of respiratory and feeding problems.

6.1. Median cleft lip

Synonyms: Complete median cleft lip, pseudomedian cleft lip, and premaxillary agenesis.

Definition: A quadrangular or triangular median defect of the upper lip, which could extend to the posterior of the nose (**Figure 17**) [38].

Incidence: Median cleft lip (MCL) is noticed in 0.2–0.7% of all cases of the cleft lip [39].

Embryology: The maxillary prominences are joined by the frontonasal prominence, from where the maxilla and the median region of the upper lip start (**Figure 9**). It is the exact area which is left underdeveloped or absent in the median cleft lip cases. There is a strong link between the development of the midline facial structures and the process by which the forebrain is differentiated. The prechordal mesenchyma, the tissue interposed between the prosencephalon, and the roof of the primitiva mouth (stomodeum) are likely to induce both events [40]. Cerebral anomalies, such as holoprosencephaly, are often linked with the midline abnormalities of the face.

Etiology and pathology: MCL is described only as part of two distinct syndromes: MCL with orbital hypotelorism, in itself a synonym for holoprosencephaly, and MCL with orbital hypertelorism. In the former case, the premaxillary bone, nasal septum, nasal bones, and crista galli

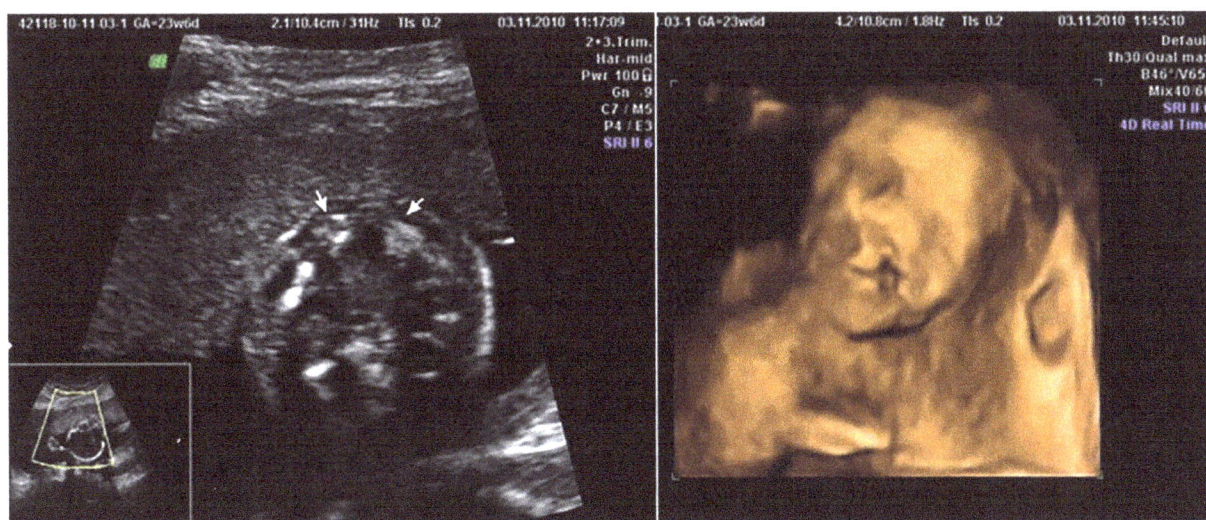

Figure 17. Axial scan of the median cleft lip.

are absent. The ethmoid bone (that set the interorbital distance) is hypoplastic. The secondary palate may or may not be involved. MCL with hypertelorism (also known as "median cleft face syndrome" or "frontonasal dysplasia") is characterized by the presence of a bifid nose and cranium bifidum occultum, as well as of the premaxilla, while the brain is normal in most cases.

Diagnosis: The defect, involving both the upper lip and the palate, is better seen in axial scans of the palate (**Figure 17**). A useful hint in this process is the visualization of the tongue in a position within the oral cavity, which is higher than normal. The sonographer should be alerted to a possible pitfall in the diagnosis of MCL because sometimes the defect may be masked by the tongue, giving a false impression of an intact palate [41].

Prognosis and obstetrical management: Prognosis depends entirely on the association with other anomalies. MCL syndrome is associated in 80% of cases with normal intelligence. Radical cosmetic surgery is required. If alobar holoprosencephaly present, it is uniformly lethal [42].

6.2. Epignathus

Definition: A teratoma that arises from the oral cavity or pharynx.

Incidence: 2% of all pediatric teratomas occur in the nasopharyngeal area (including oral, tonsillar, and basicranial areas). The majority of cases occur in newborn [43, 44].

Pathology: Tumors arise mainly from the sphenoid bone; they rarely arise from other areas (the hard and soft palate, the pharynx, the tongue, and jaw). These tumors grow into the oral or nasal cavity or intracranially. Obstruction of the mouth is responsible for polyhydramnios. Most tumors are benign, consisting histologically of tissues derived from any of the three germinal layers. They can fill the mouth and airways and lead to acute asphyxia immediately after birth [44].

Ultrasound diagnosis: Solid tumor arising from the sphenoid bone, hard and soft palate, the pharynx, the tongue, and the jaw. The tumor may grow into the oral or nasal cavity or intracranially. Calcifications and cystic components may also be noticed. The differential diagnosis will include neck teratomas, encephaloceles, conjoined twins, and other tumors of the facial structures. Polyhydramnios (due to pharyngeal compression) is usually present.

Associated abnormalities: This is a sporadic condition, with no increased incidence of chromosomal defects or genetic syndromes; only 6% of these tumors have associated anomalies, and the facial ones being attributed to the mechanical effects of the tumor on developing structures [45].

Investigations: Scans every 4 weeks to monitor the growth of the tumor and assess the amniotic fluid. If polyhydramnios develops, amniodrainage may be balanced. Fetal MRI is recommended at 32 weeks to assess the spatial relation of the tumor to adjacent structures.

Prognosis: It depends on the size of the lesion and the involvement of vital structures. The lesions are usually very large, and the polyhydramnios associates a poor prognosis. The major cause of neonatal death is asphyxia due to airway obstruction. Surgical resection is possible at times. There are no reported cases of malignancies [46–49].

Fetuses with large tumors are best delivered by cesarean section, and an expert pediatric team must be available to intubate of the infant.

7. Abnormalities of the mandible

7.1. Robin anomalad

Synonyms: Cleft palate, micrognathia and glossoptosis, and Pierre Robin syndrome.

Definition: This anomaly is associated with micrognathia and glossoptosis, with a posterior cleft palate or a high arched palate.

Incidence: The frequency is 1:30,000 [50].

Etiology: In 40% of the cases, the anomaly is isolated and mostly sporadic, although sometimes familiar cases suggest both autosomal recessives and autosomal dominant patterns of transmission. It is most frequently seen in association with other anomalies or with recognized genetic and nongenetic syndromes [51].

Embryology: The mandible starts at the point in which the two mandibular prominences join to delimit the inferior part of the stomodeum. The fusion of the three palatine processes forms the palate. Finally, the frontonasal prominence creates the median, and the maxillary processes create the two lateral ones. It is apparent that the three components of this defect are related to one another. Possibly, an early hypoplasia of the mandible creates this defect, as it leads to the tongue being displaced toward the posterior region, which prevents the posterior palatine processes to close as they should in a normal situation [52].

Associated anomalies: The Robin anomaly is found as an isolated lesion in 39% of all patients. In 36%, one or more associated anomalies are present. In 25% of patients, a known syndrome is found.

Robin anomaly is to be suspected when polyhydramnios is associated with micrognathia (**Figure 18**). Congenital heart disease occurs in 10% of affected neonates, so fetal echocardiography is recommended [53].

Prognosis: The Robin anomaly is a neonatal emergency in many cases. Glossoptosis may lead to the obstruction of the airways and suffocation.

It is mandatory that a pediatrician be present in the delivery room and be prepared to intubate the infant. Karyotype should be considered [54].

7.2. Otocephaly

Definition: Otocephaly is a grotesque anomaly, characterized by the absence or hypoplasia of the mandible, proximity of the temporal bones, and abnormal horizontal position of the ears. This malformation is considered to be the result of an improper development of the mandible, probably caused by a defect in the migration of the neural crest cells. The ears position

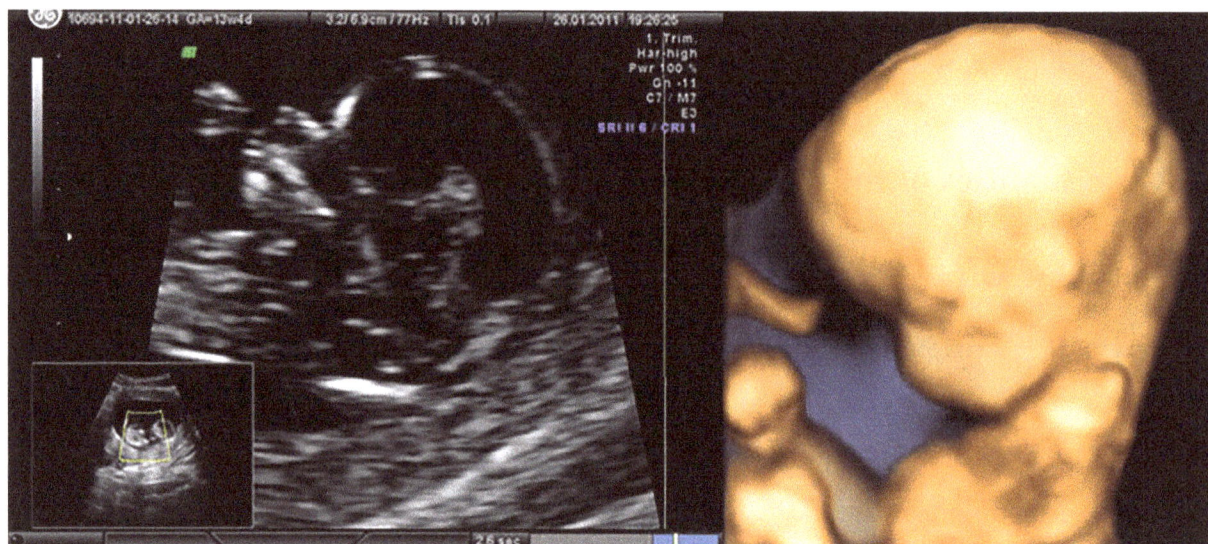

Figure 18. Sagittal scan a fetus at 13 weeks of gestation shows prominent forehead and retrognathia (polyploidy).

themselves horizontally, with the lobules closer to the midline, most certainly because of either absence or extreme hypoplasia of the mandible (**Figure 8**).

The anatomic lesions range from ears closely opposed to the midline (synotia), agnathia, absence of the mouth to varying degrees of micrognathia and low set ears (melotia).

Otocephaly may be part of very severe malformation complexes, such as conjoined twins and holoprosencephaly [55].

Associated anomalies: Holoprosencephaly, neural tube defects, cephaloceles, midline proboscis, hypoplastic tongue, tracheoesophageal fistula, cardiac anomalies, and adrenal hypoplasia [56].

Diagnosis: This anomaly is to be suspected when the jaw cannot be visualized and the ears are noticed in a very low position. Fetuses with extremely severe anomalies, such as anencephaly, holoprosencephaly, and cephaloceles, also present this defect. In cases of milder anomalies, it is difficult to distinguish the otocephaly from other conditions characterized by very low set ears, for instance Treacher Collins syndrome, during a prenatal ultrasound examination [57, 58].

Prognosis and obstetrical management: This condition is incompatible with life. Pregnancy termination could be offered any time in a pregnancy when a confident diagnosis is made [57].

8. The chin: Micrognathia-retrognathia or prognathia

Abnormal size of the chin, micrognathia and macrognathia, and abnormal length of the philtrum (short or long) are morphological features in numerous syndromes.

8.1. Micrognathia-retrognathia

Prevalence: 1: 1500 births.

Ultrasound diagnosis: Subjective finding of prominent upper lip and receding chin in the mid-sagittal view of the face (**Figure 18**). These findings might be due to micrognathia (short mandible) or retrognathia (backward displacement of the mandible). Severe micrognathia is associated with polyhydramnios (>25 weeks gestation), due to glossoptosis (normal tongue obstructing small oral cavity).

Associated abnormalities: Chromosomal abnormalities, mainly trisomy 18 and triploidy, are found in about 30% of cases. Any one of >50 genetic syndromes are found in most fetuses. Micrognathia is usually associated with >50 genetic syndromes, including Pierre-Robin anomaly, Treacher Collins syndrome, otocephaly [59].

Investigations: ultrasound including echocardiography, karyotyping and array.

Follow up: Ultrasound scans every 4 weeks to monitor growth and amniotic fluid.

Delivery: In hospital with facilities for neonatal intensive care, while a pediatrician is present in the delivery room and be prepared to intubate the neonate.

Prognosis: Neonatal mortality >80% due to associated abnormalities. In Pierre–Robin anomaly, the survival rate is good.

Recurrence: Genetic syndromes: 25–50%. Trisomies: 1%. Isolated: no increased risk of recurrence.

Author details

Maria Șorop-Florea[1], Roxana-Cristina Dragușin[1], Ciprian Laurențiu Pătru[1], Lucian George Zorilă[1], Cristian Marinaș[2], Virgiliu-Bogdan Șorop[3], Cristian Neamțu[4], Alina Veduța[5], Dominic Gabriel Iliescu[1]* and Nicolae Cernea[1]

*Address all correspondence to: dominic.iliescu@yahoo.com

1 Department of Obstetrics and Gynecology, Prenatal Diagnostic Unit, University Emergency County Hospital, University of Medicine and Pharmacy Craiova, Romania

2 Department of Anatomy, University of Medicine and Pharmacy Craiova, Romania

3 Department of Obstetrics and Gynecology, University of Medicine and Pharmacy "Victor Babeș" Timișoara, Romania

4 Department of Pathophysiology, University of Medicine and Pharmacy Craiova, Romania

5 Department of Obstetrics and Gynecology, University of Medicine and Pharmacy "Carol Davila" Bucharest, Romania

References

[1]   Benacerraf BR. Ultrasound of Fetal Syndromes. New York, London, Philadelphia, San Francisco: Churchill Livingstone.1998; pp. 83-223

[2]   Sonek J, Borenstein M, Dagklis T, Persico N, Nicolaides KH. Frontomaxillary facial angle in fetuses with trisomy 21 at 11-13(6) weeks. American Journal of Obstetrics Gynecology. 2007;**196**:271.e1-271.e4

[3]   Borenstein M, Persico N, Kagan KO, Gazzoni A, Nicolaides KH. Frontomaxillary facial angle in screening for trisomy 21 at 11+0 to 13+6 weeks. Ultrasound in Obstetrics & Gynecology. 2008;**32**:5-11

[4]   Jeanty P, Dramaix-Wilmet M, Van Gansbeke D, et al. Fetal ocular biometry by ultrasound. Radiology. 1982;**143**:513

[5]   Smith D, Jones KL. Smith's Recognizable Patterns of Human Malformation. 4th ed. Philadelphia: WB Saunders Company; 1988

[6]   Sivan E, Chan L, Mallozzi-Eberle A, Reece EA. Sonographic imaging of the fetal face and the establishment of normative dimensions for chin length and upper lip width. American Journal of Perinatology. 1997 April;**14**:191-194

[7]   Langman's Medical Embryology: 12th ed - Ch. 17 (Head & Neck). pp. 276-277

[8]   Goldstein I, Tamir A, Weiner Z, Jakobi P. Dimensions of the fetal facial profile in normal pregnancy. Ultrasound in Obstetrics & Gynecology. (February), 2010;**35**(2):191-194

[9]   Bergsma, D. Birth Defects Compendium. 2nd ed. Macmillan; 1979

[10] Jeanty P, Cantraine F, Consaert E, Romero R, Hobbins JC. The binocular distance: A new way to estimate fetal age. Journal of Ultrasound in Medicine. 1984 June;**3**(6):241-243

[11] Mayden KL, Totora M, Berkowitz RL, Bracken M, Hobbins JC. Orbital diameters: A new parameter for prenatal diagnosis and dating. American Journal of Obstetrics & Gynecology. 1982;**1**;144(.3) October:pp. 289-297

[12] Schlenck B, Unsinn K, Geley T, Schon A, Gassner I. Sonographic diagnosis of congenital dacryocystocele. Ultraschall in der Medizin. 2002;**23**:181-184

[13] Shashy RG, Durairaj V, Holmes JM, Hohberger GG, Thompson DM, Kasperbauer JL. Congenital dacryocystocele associated with intranasal cysts: Diagnosis and management. Laryngoscope. 2003;**113**:37-40

[14] Tonni G, Ventura A, Centini G, De Felice C. First trimester three-dimensional transvaginal imaging of alobar holoprosencephaly associated with proboscis and hypotelorism (ethmocephaly) in a 46, XX fetus. Cong Animal. 2008;**48**:51-55

[15] Goldstein I, Weissman A, Brill-Zamir R, Laevsky I, Drugan A. Ethmocephaly caused by de novo translocation 18; 21 – Prenatal diagnosis. Prenatal Diagnosis. 2003 October; **23**(10):788-790

[16]   Christele D, Claude B, Laurent P, et al. Holoprosencephaly. Orphanet J Rare Dis. 2007;2:8. Published online 2007 February; doi: 10.1186/1750-1172-2-8

[17]   Johnson CY, Rasmussen SA. Non-genetic risk factors for holoprosencephaly. American Journal of Medical Genetics. 2010;**154C**(1):73-85

[18]   Francis PJ, Berry V, Bhattacharya SS, et al. The genetics of childhood cataract. Journal of Medical Genetics. 2000;**37**:481-488

[19]   Hejtmancik J. Congenital cataracts and their molecular genetics. Seminars in Cell & Developmental Biology. 2008;**19**:134-149

[20]   Lee JO, Jung JL, Kim MJ, et al. Prenatal ultrasonographic diagnosis of congenital cataract: A case report. Korean Journal of Ultrasound Obstetrics Gynecology. 2012;**55**:839-842

[21]   Chitkara U, Lee L, Oehlert JW, Bloch DA, Holbrook RH, El-Sayed YY, Druzin ML. Fetal ear length measurement: A useful predictor of aneuploidy? Ultrasound in Obstetrics & Gynecology. 2002 February;**19**(2):131-135

[22]   Cicero S, Curcio P, Papageorghiou A, Sonek J, Nicolaides K. Absence of nasal bone in fetuses with trisomy 21 at 11-14 weeks of gestation: An observational study. Lancet. 2001 November 17;**358**(9294):1665-1667

[23]   Olsen E, Gjelland K, Reigstad H, Rosendahl K. Congenital absence of the nose: A case report and literature review. Pediatric Radiology. 2001;**31**:225-232

[24]   McGlone L. Congenital arhinia. Journal of Pediatrcis Child Health. 2003;**39**:474-476

[25]   Cusick W, Sullivan CA, Rojas B, Poole AE, Poole DA. Prenatal diagnosis of total arhinia. Ultrasound Obstetrics Gynaecology. 2000;**15**:259-261

[26]   Lim AS, Lim TH, Kee SK, et al. Holoprosencephaly: An antenatally-diagnosed case series and subject review. Annals of the Academy of Medicine, Singapore. 2008;**37**:594-597

[27]   Chen CP, Shih JC, Hsu CY, Chen CY, Huang JK, Wang W. Prenatal three-dimensional/four-dimensional sonographic demonstration of facial dysmorphisms associated with holoprosencephaly. Journal of Clinical Ultrasound. 2005;**33**:312-318

[28]   Chen CP, Chern SR, Lin CJ, Lee CC, Wang WA. Comparison of maternal age, sex ratio and associated anomalies among numerically aneuploid, structurally aneuploid and euploid holoprosencephaly. Genetic Counseling. 2005;**16**:49-57

[29]   Papageorghiou AT, Avgidou K, Spencer K, Nix B, Nicolaides KH. Sonographic screening for trisomy 13 at 11 to 13 + 6 weeks of gestation. American Journal of Obstetrics and Gynecology. 2006;**194**:397-401

[30]   Eckmann-Scholz C, Jonat W. 3-D ultrasound imaging of a prenatally diagnosed Beckwith-Wiedemann syndrome. Archives of Gynecology and Obstetrics. 2011;**284**:1051-1052

[31]   O'Connor C, Levine D. Case 49: Beckwith-Wiedemann syndrome. Radiology. 2002;**224**:375-378

[32] Walker SJ, Ball RH, Babcook CJ, Feldkamp MM. Prevalence of aneuploidy and additional anatomic abnormalities in fetuses and neonates with cleft lip with or without cleft palate: A population-based study in Utah. Journal of Ultrasound in Medicine. 2001; **20**:1175-1180

[33] Sohan K, Freer M, Mercer N, Soothill P, Kyle P. Prenatal detection of facial clefts. Fetal Diagnosis and Therapy. 2001;**16**:196-199

[34] Bianchi DW, Crombleholme TM, D'Alton ME, Malone FD. Diagnosis and Management of the Fetal Patient, 2nd ed

[35] Campbell S, Lees CC. The three-dimensional reverse face. Obstetrics and Gynecology. 2003;**22**:552-554

[36] Hanikeri M, Savundra J, Gillett D, Walters M, McBain W. Antenatal transabdominal ultrasound detection of cleft lip and palate in Western Australia from 1996 to 2003. The Cleft Palate-Craniofacial Journal. 2006;**43**:61-66

[37] Cohen MM. Etiology and pathogenesis of orofacial clefting. Oral and Maxillofacial Surgery Clinics of North America. 2000;**12**:379-397

[38] Mossey PA, Julian L, Mungar R, Dixon MJ, Shaw WC. Cleft lip and palate. Lancet. 2009;**374**:1773-1785

[39] Saraf S. Median cleft of the lip: A rare facial anomaly. Internet. Journal of Plastic Surgery. 2006;**2**

[40] Ewings EL, Carstens MH. Neuroembryology and functional anatomy of craniofacial clefts. Indian Journal of Plastics Surgery. 2009;**42**(Suppl):S19-S34

[41] Collares MP, Pinto RA. False vs true media cleft lip: Report of two cases and differential management. Brazil Journal of Cranio-Maxillo-Facial Surgery. 2001;**4**(2):25-31

[42] Urata MM, Kawamoto HK Jr. Median clefts of the upper lip: A review and surgical management of a minor manifestation. The Journal of Craniofacial Surgery 2003 Sep;14(5):749-755

[43] Şorop-Florea M, Iliescu DG, Tudorache S, Simionescu C, Cernea N, Novac LV, Tanase F, Cotarcea S, Comanescu a, Dragusin R, Patru C, Carbunaru O, Zorila L, Cernea D. The importance of perinatal autopsy. Review of the literature and series of cases. Romanian Journal of Morphology and Embryology 2017;**58**(2):323-337

[44] Ahmadi M, Dalband M, Shariatpanahi E. Oral teratoma (epignathus) in a newborn: A case report. Journal of Oral and Maxillofacial Surgery, Medicine Pathology. 2012;**24**:59-62

[45] Shah A, Latoo S, Ahmed I, Malik A. Head and neck teratomas. Journa of Maxillofacial and oral Surgery. 2009;**8**(1):60-63

[46] Tsitouridis I, Sidiropoulos D, Michaelides M. Sonographic evaluation of [12] epignathus. The Hip. 2009;**13**(1):55-57

[47] Iliescu D, Tudorache S, Comanescu A, Antsaklis P, Cotarcea S, Novac L, Cernea N, Antsaklis A. Improved detection rate of structural abnormalities in the first trimester using an extended examination protocol. Ultrasound in Obstetrics & Gynecology. 2013 Sep;**42**(3):300-309. DOI: 10.1002/uog.12489

[48] Tudorache Ș, Gabriel D Iliescu Parental attitude to participate in follow-up research studies of their children's development after diagnosis of fetal abnormalities in a tertiary center in Romania Obstetrica și Ginecologia, nr.4, 2016

[49] Hu R, Jiang RS. The recurrence of a soft palate teratoma in a neonate: A case report. Head & Neck Oncology. 2013;**5**(2):16

[50] Printzlau A, Andersen M. Pierre Robin sequence in Denmark: A retrospective population-based epidemiological study. The Cleft Palate-Craniofacial Journal. 2004;**41**(1):47-52

[51] Selvi R, Mukunda Priyanka AR. Role of SOX9 in the etiology of Pierre-Robin syndrome. Iranian Journal of Basic Medical Sciences. 2013;**16**(5):700-704

[52] Jakobsen LP, Knudsen MA, Lespinasse J, et al. The genetic basis of the Pierre Robin sequence. The Cleft Palate-Craniofacial Journal. 2006;**43**(2):155-159

[53] Bronshtein M, Blazer S, Zalel Y, Zimmer EZ. Ultrasonographic diagnosis of glossoptosis in fetuses with Pierre Robin sequence in early and mid pregnancy. American Journal of Obstetrics and Gynecology 2005;**193**(4):1561-1564

[54] Smith MC, Senders CW. Prognosis of airway obstruction and feeding difficulty in the Robin sequence. International Journal of Pediatric Otorhinolaryngology. 2006; **70**(2):319-324

[55] Gekas J, Li B, Kamnasaran D. Current perspectives on the etiology of agnathia-otocephaly. European Journal of Medicine Genetics. 2010;**53**:358-366

[56] Iliescu D, Cara M, Tudorache S, Antsaklis P, Ceausu I, Paulescu D, Novac L, Cernea N, Antsaklis A. Challenges in sonographic detection of fetal major structural abnormalities at the first trimester anomaly scan. Donald School Journal of Obstetrics Gynecology. 2015;**9**(3):239-259. DOI: 10.5005/jp-journals-10009-1411

[57] Dragusin R, Florea M, Iliescu D, Cotarcea S, Tudorache S, Novac L, Cernea N. The contribution and the importance of modern ultrasound techniques in the diagnosis of major structural abnormalities in the first trimester. Current Health Sciences Journal. 2012;**38**:1

[58] Wagner JH, Hérbene JFM, Edward AJ, Jurandir PP. Agnathia-otocephaly: Prenatal diagnosis by two- and three-dimensional ultrasound and magnetic resonance imaging. Case report. Medical Ultrasonography. 2014;**16**(4):377-379

[59] Gull I, Wolman I, Merlob P, Jaffa AJ, Lessing JB, Yaron Y. Nomograms for the sonographic measurement of the fetal philtrum and chin. Fetal Diagnosis and Therapy. 2005 March–April;**20**(2):127-131

7

Prenatal Biochemical and Ultrasound Markers in Chromosomal Anomalies

Eusebiu Vlad Gorduza,
Demetra Gabriela Socolov and
Răzvan Vladimir Socolov

Abstract

The unbalanced chromosomal anomalies generate an abnormal pattern of development and usually determine miscarriage. The most frequent prenatal chromosomal anomalies are X monosomy, trisomies of chromosomes 21, 18, 13, 16, 8, triploidy and tetraploidy. Identification of chromosomal anomalies can be done by prenatal screening and diagnosis. Prenatal screening is biochemical, sonographic or molecular (detection of fetal DNA in maternal blood). Biochemical screening can be done in the first or second trimester. First-trimester screening is based on the detection in maternal serum of beta-hCG (β-hCG) and pregnancy-associated plasma protein-A (PAPP-A). Biochemical screening in the second trimester requires the detection of alpha-fetoprotein (aFP) hGC, unconjugated estriol (μE) and inhibin A. The sonographic examination can be used in the first or second trimesters. In the first trimester, an ultrasound can identify soft markers like nuchal translucency, nasal bone and ductus venous flow. In the second trimester the sonographic examination can identify congenital anomalies or different soft markers. Prenatal chromosomal diagnosis requires an invasive procedure to obtain embryonic or fetal material. Such procedures are represented by chorionic villus sampling amniocentesis or cordocentesis. The fetal cells are used for cell cultures (in cytogenetic methods) or for molecular analyses (FISH, QF-PCR, MLPA, array-CGH).

Keywords: chromosomal anomalies, chromosomal syndromes, prenatal screening, biochemical screening, ultra-sonographic screening

1. Introduction

Chromosomal anomalies represent large genomic modifications that could be identified using light microscope. Apart from these characteristics, many chromosomal anomalies produce severe changes in the phenotypes of carriers that induce a high rate of miscarriage (>50% of spontaneous abortions are produced by a chromosomal anomaly) and chromosomal disorders in neonates and infants (global incidence in newborns is 1%). Early identification of chromosomal anomalies during the prenatal period has become the purpose of prenatal screening and diagnosis. Prenatal screening allows discovery of pregnancies at risk using non-invasive methods that do not harm the pregnant woman and fetus. An abnormal prenatal screening imposes the confirmation by using a prenatal diagnosis method. Prenatal screening methods could be biochemical, ultra-sonographic and genomic. Biochemical methods imply detection of some serum constituents in maternal blood like hCG, β-hCG, aFP, μE3, PAPP-A, and so on. Ultra-sonographic methods imply the use of ultrasound for the assessment of morphologic features of the fetus. Genomic prenatal screening allows the detection of free fetal DNA in maternal blood. Prenatal diagnosis imposes the use of the invasive methods that allow the harvesting of these fetal cells (trophoblastic cells, amniotic cells or blood cells). The major inconvenience of invasive methods is the risk of miscarriage or fetal damage. Fetal cells could be used for cytogenetic or molecular genetics investigations that allow a prenatal diagnosis [1].

2. Chromosomal anomalies

Chromosomal anomalies are produced by genomic or chromosomal mutations. Chromosomal anomalies could be numerical and structural. Numerical chromosomal anomalies produce an important genomic imbalance and the phenotype of carriers is severely affected. Numerical chromosomal anomalies are represented by aneuploidies (trisomies, monosomies, etc.) and polyploidies (triploidy and tetraploidy). These are generated by errors during meiosis, fertilization or first mitosis of embryo. The most common error is chromosomal non-disjunction during the first meiosis that generates an aneuploidy (trisomy or monosomy) and is associated with advanced maternal age. Structural chromosomal anomalies are generated by changes of structure of one or multiple chromosomes and could be divided into unbalanced and balanced anomalies. Unbalanced structural chromosomal anomalies are characterized by absence (partial monosomy) or supplementary (partial trisomy) chromosomal segment(s) and produce a genomic imbalance that induces an abnormal phenotype. Balanced chromosomal anomalies are characterized by changes in the position of some chromosomal segments, but the quantity of genetic material remains unchanged. The phenotype of carriers is usually normal, but they could present a malsegregation of derivative chromosomes during meiosis that generates formation of gametes with genomic imbalances. Fertilizing such gametes results in embryos with unbalanced chromosomal anomalies [1].

Unbalanced chromosomal anomalies produce a severe modification of phenotype and generate chromosomal diseases. The majority of such anomalies do not permit survival of the embryo and the pregnancy ends in miscarriage. Other anomalies—gonosomal trisomies (XXX, XXY, XYY), some autosomal trisomies (21, 18, 13), some cases with X monosomy, some partial monosomies or partial trisomies—are compatible with life, but children have a chromosomal disease [1].

The epidemiological studies showed that the frequency of chromosomal anomalies will be reduced during pregnancy, from 1/4 at conception to 1/100 at birth (**Table 1**). The aneuploidies are the most frequent of these anomalies. The most common chromosomal disorders are Down syndrome (trisomy 21—**Figure 1**, birth prevalence 1/700–1/800) [2, 3], Klinefelter syndrome (trisomy XXY—**Figure 2**, birth prevalence 1/1000), triplo X syndrome (trisomy X—**Figure 3**, birth prevalence 1/1000), Turner syndrome (monosomy X—**Figure 4**, birth prevalence 1/2000 girls), Edwards syndrome (trisomy 18—**Figure 5**, birth prevalence 1/6500) and Patau syndrome (trisomy 13—**Figure 6**, birth prevalence 1/12,500). The risk of a couple having an affected child with a major trisomy (13, 18 and 21) is associated with advancing maternal age. In the last decade, the age of women at first pregnancy increases such that the birth prevalence for trisomy 21 in the USA has increased from 1 in 740 in 1974 to 1 in 504 by 1997 [4, 5].

The majority of chromosomal disorders has a high lethality rate during pregnancy and thus in the first trimester there are a significant number of fetuses affected than at full term. For example, in the case of trisomy 21, there is a 40% fetal loss between 12 weeks and full term and a 30% fetal loss between 16 weeks and full term. For trisomies 13 or 18, the loss is more important with an 80% fetal loss between 12 weeks and full term and a 40% fetal loss between 16 weeks and full term [6].

The incidence of the main chromosomal disorders in neonates is present in **Table 2**.

For trisomy 21, the risk at 12 weeks of gestation is 1/1000 for a woman aged 20 years and 1/250 for a woman aged 35 years. The risk of delivering an affected baby with Down syndrome is 1/1500 for a woman aged 20 years and 1/350 for a woman aged 35 years. For trisomy 18, the risk at 12 weeks of gestation is 1/2500 (for a woman aged 20 years) and 1/600 (for a woman aged 35 years) [7].

Ontogenetic period: disorder	Incidence of chromosomal anomalies
1. gametes	10-25%
2. biochemical miscarriages	unknown, probably 33-6-7%
3. spontaneous miscarriages during first trimester of pregnancy	50-70%
4. intrauterine death	5%-10%
5. newborns	1%
6. severe congenital anomalies	4%
7. plurimalformative syndromes	5,5%

Table 1. Incidence of chromosomal anomalies in prenatal and perinatal period (adapted from Gorduza [1]).

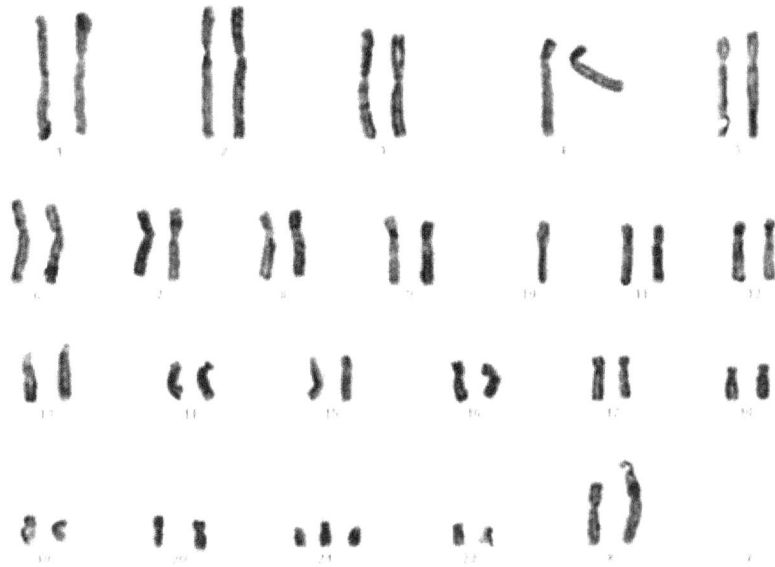

Figure 1. Trisomy 21 (collection of cytogenetic laboratory, "Grigore T. Popa" University of Medicine and Pharmacy Iaşi, Romania).

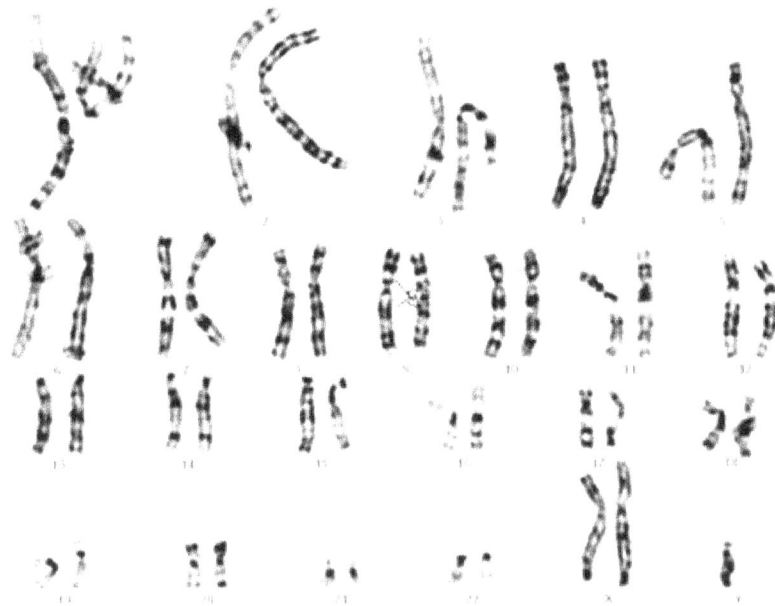

Figure 2. Trisomy XXY (collection of cytogenetic laboratory, "Grigore T. Popa" University of Medicine and Pharmacy Iaşi, Romania).

The risk of delivering an affected baby with Edwards syndrome is 1/18,000 for a woman aged 20 years and 1/4000 for a woman aged 35 years. For trisomy 13, the risk at 12 weeks of gestation is 1/8000 (for a woman aged 20 years) and 1/1800 (for a woman aged 35 years). The risk of delivering an affected baby with Patau syndrome is 1/42,000 for a woman aged 20 years and 1/10,000 for a woman aged 35 years [7].

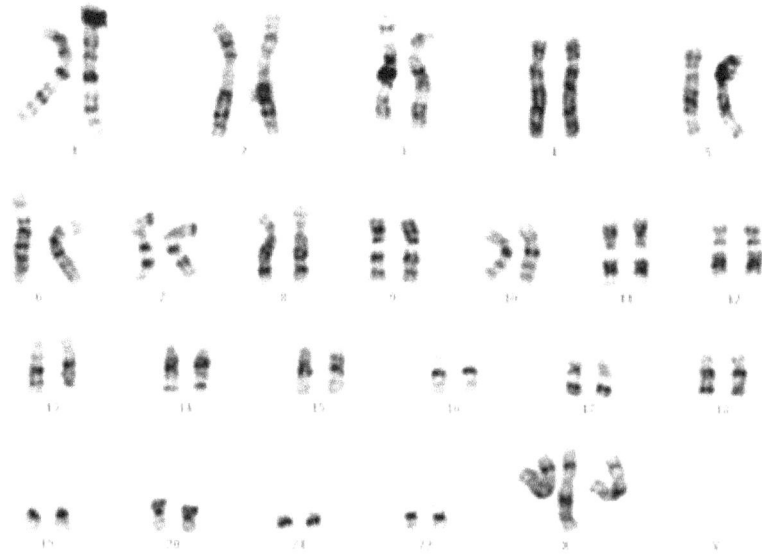

Figure 3. Trisomy X (collection of cytogenetic laboratory, "Grigore T. Popa" University of Medicine and Pharmacy Iași, Romania).

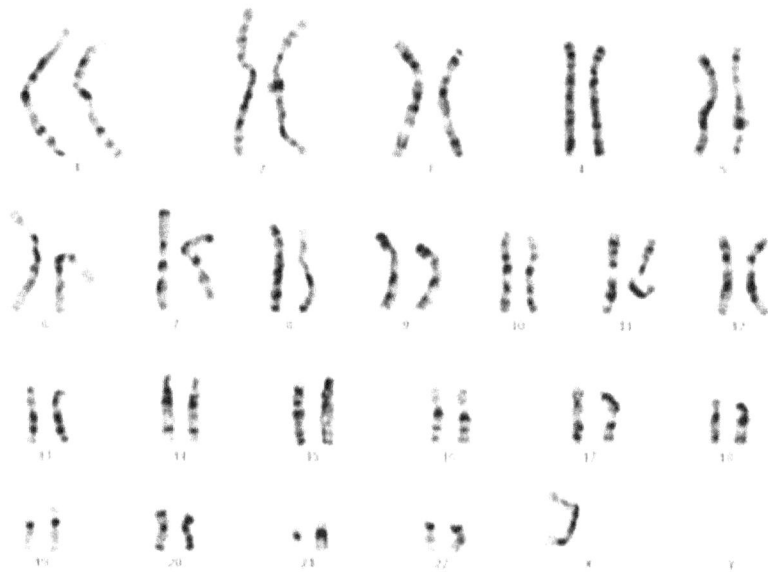

Figure 4. Monosomy X (collection of cytogenetic laboratory, "Grigore T. Popa" University of Medicine and Pharmacy Iași, Romania).

In the case of gonosomal aneuploidies the risks are not correlated with advanced maternal age, and with the exception of monosomy X, the chromosomal anomaly does not modify the viability of the fetus. In monosomy X, the prevalence of anomaly is about 1/1500 at 12 weeks of gestation and 1/4000 at 40 weeks. For the gonosomal trisomies (47,XXX, 47,XXY and 47,XYY), the overall prevalence of 1/500 does not decrease with gestation [7].

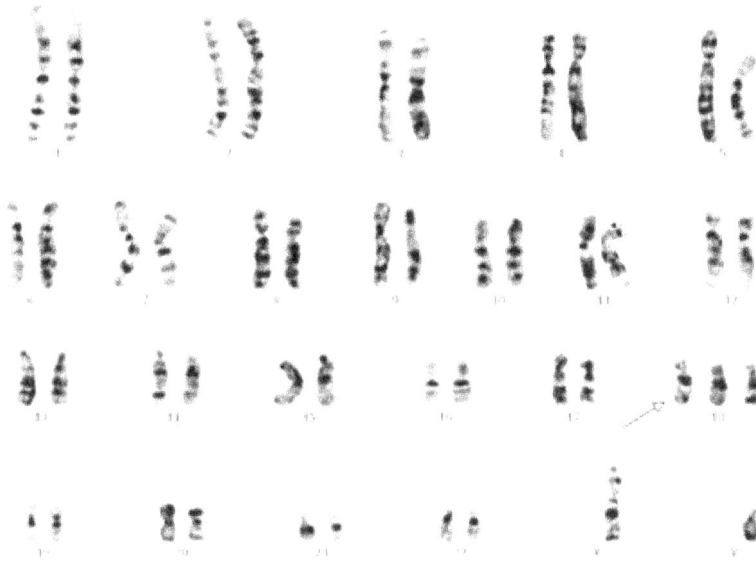

Figure 5. Trisomy 18 (collection of cytogenetic laboratory, "Grigore T. Popa" University of Medicine and Pharmacy Iaşi, Romania).

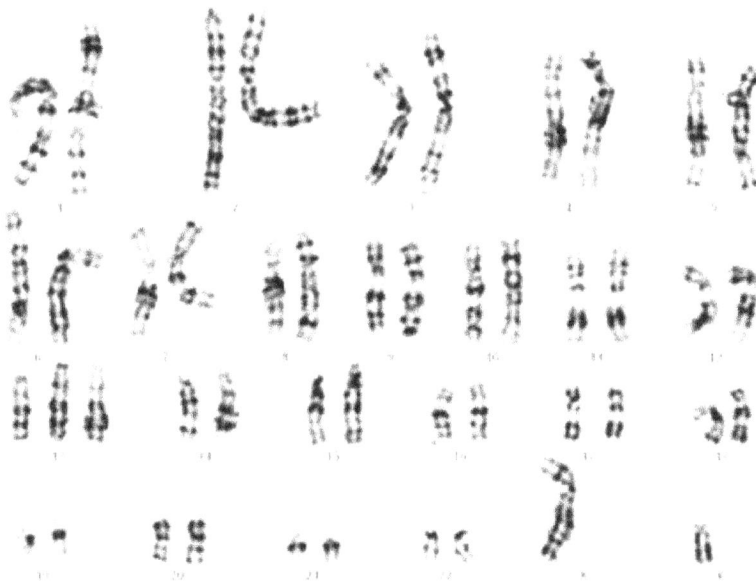

Figure 6. Trisomy 13 (collection of cytogenetic laboratory, "Grigore T. Popa" University of Medicine and Pharmacy Iaşi, Romania).

Triploidy is unrelated to maternal age and the prevalence is about 1/2000 at 12 weeks, but the majority of affected fetuses die by 20 weeks and the born babies are mosaics 46/69 [7].

The birth of a child is an important event in the life of every family and represents the end of a long period of uncertainty generated by fear that the future child will be abnormal. The high incidence of chromosomal anomalies during prenatal life and the severity of phenotype of chromosomal anomalies that allow survival, imposed the development of methods of prenatal

Autosomal trisomies	13 –Patau syndrome	$0.08^{0}/_{00}$	Global 1.4$^{0}/_{00}$
	18 –Edward syndrome	$0.15^{0}/_{00}$	
	21 –Down syndrome	$1.2^{0}/_{00}$	
Triploidies			$0.02^{0}/_{00}$
Gonosomal aneuploidies in boys	47,XXY –Klinefelter syndrome	$1^{0}/_{00}$	Global 2.75$^{0}/_{00}$
	47,XYY –double Y syndrome	$1^{0}/_{00}$	
	other	$0.74^{0}/_{00}$	
Gonosomal aneuploidies in girls	monosomy X –Turner syndrome	$0.3^{0}/_{00}$	Global 1.8$^{0}/_{00}$
	47,XXX –triplo X syndrome	$1.1^{0}/_{00}$	
	other	$0.37^{0}/_{00}$	
Unbalanced structural chromosomal anomalies			$0.7^{0}/_{00}$
Unbalanced chromosomal anomalies (numerical and structural)			$4^{0}/_{00}(1/250)$
Balanced structural chromosomal anomalies	Reciprocal translocations	$2.5^{0}/_{00}$	Global 4.3$^{0}/_{00}$
	Robertsonian translocations	$1^{0}/_{00}$	
	Inversions	$0.8^{0}/_{00}$	

Table 2. Incidence of chromosomal anomalies in neonates (adapted from Gorduza [1]).

screening and diagnosis. Different such methods were developed during the last decades and now it is possible to discover the chromosomal pathology of the embryo in a couple at risk.

3. Methods of prenatal screening and diagnosis

The main procedures of prenatal screening are biochemical screening and ultrasound that allow the identification of pregnancies with increased genetic risk. The prenatal screening methods were introduced in medical practice in the1980s, based on the association between incidence of trisomy 21 (Down syndrome) and advanced maternal age. A decade later both the maternal serum biochemistry and detailed ultra-sonographic examination in the second trimester were developed and allowed the identification of high-risk pregnancies. In the 1990s, the prenatal screening shifted to first trimester by a combination of maternal age, fetal nuchal translucency (NT) thickness and maternal serum-free β-hCG and PAPP-A. In the last 10 years, the prenatal screening methods changed again by the introduction of genomic screening that searches free fetal DNA in maternal blood [8].

The prenatal diagnosis imposes the obtaining of embryonic or fetal cells by using invasive methods like chorionic villus sampling (CVS), amniocentesis or cordocentesis. All these methods present risks for spontaneous miscarriages, obstetrical hemorrhages and fetal damages. The embrionar or fetal cells are used for cytogenetic or molecular diagnosis.

3.1. Biochemical screening

Biochemical screening is based on the determination of maternal serum markers that are associated with an increased risk of chromosomal diseases. Biochemical screening could be applied during the first or the second trimester of pregnancy. The presence of a fetal aneuploidy is associated with changes of maternal serum concentrations of some fetoplacental products: aFP, free ß-hCG, inhibin A, μE3 and PAPP-A. In normal pregnancies, aFP concentration in maternal serum increases from 11.3 ng/ml in the 8th week of gestation to 250 ng/ml in the 32nd week of pregnancy. After that, it then declines slightly until term. In normal pregnancies, hCG in the maternal serum increases in first trimester of pregnancy and reaches a peak in weeks 7–9 (100.000 IU/ml). After that, it reduces continuously until around 20 weeks of pregnancies, when reduction is stopped and plasma levels remain constant until term. In normal pregnancies, inhibin A increases from the 6th week of pregnancy to the 9th week of pregnancy and reaches a peak (~550 pg/ml). After that, the values decline continuously to the 14th week of pregnancy. In normal pregnancies, μE3 is first detectable at 9 weeks of gestation (0.05 ng/ml) and after that it increases continuously to about 30 ng/ml at term. In normal pregnancies, PAPP-A is first detected in maternal serum after 4 weeks of pregnancies. PAPP-A concentration increases exponentially in the first trimester. After that, the rise occurs slowly, but it continues until delivery [9–12].

In biochemical screening, the measured concentration of the markers is converted into a multiple of the median (MoM) of unaffected pregnancies at the same gestation. The Gaussian distributions of log10 (MoM) in trisomy 21 and unaffected pregnancies are then derived, and the ratio of the heights of the distributions at a particular MoM represents the likelihood ratio for a trisomy [7].

3.1.1. First-trimester prenatal screening

During the first trimester of pregnancy, different serological components present variations, but only free β-hCG and PAPP-A were associated with the presence of a trisomy 21. Other serological marker could be ADAM-12.

3.1.1.1. Human chorionic gonadotropin

The first attempts of using the hCG in detection of trisomy 21 in the first trimester of pregnancy gave controversial results. Use of total hCG in the first-trimester screening is inadequate because this marker becomes elevated only after 11 weeks of gestation [13]. In opposition, β-hCG is substantially elevated at 8–14 weeks of gestation in trisomy 21 pregnancies [14]. At a 5% false positive rate, the association between β-hCG and maternal age allows the detection of 42–46% of cases with trisomy 21 [15, 16].

3.1.1.2. Pregnancy-associated plasma protein-a

Pregnancy-associated plasma protein-A (PAPP-A) is produced by placental trophoblasts, but its function still unclear. The level of maternal serum PAPP-A is low during the first trimester in pregnancies with trisomy 21 and thus this marker could be used in prenatal screening of first trimester [17]. By using a protocol that associates PAPP-A in combination with maternal age, at a 5% false positive rate, the detection rate of cases with trisomy 21 ranges from 48 to 52%. After 15 weeks of gestation, the efficacy of this marker is low and its use in second-trimester screening is without benefits [15, 16].

3.1.1.3. Other biochemical markers

The serum marker used in second-trimester screening (aFP, μE3 and inhibin-A [INH-A]) shows minimal differences in trisomy 21 pregnancies and thus could not be used in first-trimester screening [14].

ADAM 12 is a glycoprotein synthesized by the placenta and secreted through pregnancy. ADAM 12 presents proteolytic functions and has a low level in first-trimester cases with trisomy 21 or trisomy 18. This reduction is more pronounced in earlier gestation, with best results at around 8–10 weeks. ADAM 12 in combination with PAPP-A (both measured at 8–9 weeks), nuchal translucency (NT) and free β-hCG measured at 12 weeks allow a detection rate of 97% at a 5% false positive rate and thus could be the best protocol for prenatal screening in the first trimester of pregnancy [18, 19].

3.1.1.4. Screening of other aneuploidies

The screening of other aneuploidies in the first trimester of pregnancy is also possible and has a good rate of detection. Low maternal serum PAPP-A was identified in trisomy 18, trisomy 13, triploidy and monosomy X. Low levels of free β-hCG were discovered in trisomy 18, trisomy 13 and in some cases of triploidy [20–23]. However, all these disorders have a high rate of spontaneous miscarriages (minimum 80%) and any conversion of the observed detection rates to true detection rates is, therefore, associated with a substantial degree of uncertainty [13].

3.1.2. Second-trimester prenatal screening

Second-trimester serum markers are represented by alpha-fetoprotein, human chorionic gonadotropin, unconjugated estriol and inhibin-A.

Screening for aneuploidies was initially focused on the second trimester of pregnancy and demonstrated a substantial improvement in detection rates of trisomy 21, compared with screening using only maternal age. At a false positive rate of 5%, the detection rate improves from 30% in screening by maternal age alone to 60–65% by combining maternal age with serum AFP and free ß-hCG (double test), 65–70% with the addition of μE (triple test) and 70–75% with the addition of inhibin A (quadruple test). In the case of hCG, it is better to search for free ß-hCG than total hCG [24–27].

3.1.2.1. Alpha-fetoprotein

The first report concerning the association between low level of maternal serum alpha-fetoprotein and fetal trisomy 21 was made in 1984, by Merkatz et al. [9]. At a risk cut-off of 1:270 for trisomy 21 (equivalent to the maternal age of 35), using this parameter alone would allow the detection of 55% of cases with trisomy 21 [28, 29].

The aFP is produced by fetal liver, but its biological functions and the reason why the aFP level is lower in Down syndrome pregnancies remain unclear. Placentas of affected pregnancies show a high level of aFP suggesting a defect in the secretion of AFP into the maternal circulation [30].

3.1.2.2. Human chorionic gonadotropin

In 1987, Bogart et al. showed that human chorionic gonadotropin (hCG) levels are generally higher in the maternal serum of women with Down syndrome pregnancies. They noted that hCG appeared to be superior to aFP in detecting fetal chromosome abnormalities, and association of maternal age with hCG as the screening method allows the identification of about 60% of pregnancies with trisomy 21 [31].

hCG is a glycoprotein produced by the placenta, composed of two subunits: α and β. Maternal serum contains intact hCG but also free α, free β and degradation products. At 8–10 weeks of gestation, intact hCG and free β-hCG show peak concentrations. Similar high levels of these compounds are found during the second trimester of pregnancy [32].

The anomalies of the placenta, characterized by disturbance in fluid homeostasis, like fetal hydrops and/or a cystic placenta, are associated with high levels of hCG in maternal serum. Such anomalies are present in hydropic Down syndrome, triploidy, Turner syndrome or other causes of hydrops fetalis. Even in the absence of hydrops, in cases with trisomy 21, there is a fluid accumulation that causes enlarged nuchal translucency and thickening and this could be related to the increase of hCG [33–35].

3.1.2.3. Unconjugated estriol

The presence of a low level of estriol in maternal urine in the case of a pregnancy with trisomy 21 was first reported by Jørgansen and Trolle [36]. Other studies confirmed this particularity and μE3 could be used as a marker in the prenatal screening of Down syndrome [37, 38].

The placenta uses 16 alpha-hydroxydehydroepiandrosterone sulfate (DHEAS) as the precursor of μE3. In Down syndrome pregnancies, both μE3 and DHEAS present lower levels in different tissues, including placenta [39]. During the second trimester the concentration of μE3 rises quickly and this marker can identify pregnancies with a small or underdeveloped fetus at the time of screening [27].

3.1.2.4. Inhibin-A

The possible application of inhibin in Down syndrome prenatal screening was suggested by Van Lith et al. [10]. Inhibin is a glycoprotein synthesized by gonads and placenta. The functional protein is dimeric with two subunits, α and β. The subunit α could be coupled with two different β subunits (βA or βB) and forms inhibin-A or inhibin-B. Inhibin-A (INH-A) is increased in pregnancies with trisomy 21 and presents an interdependent secretion with hCG. INH-A allows a good distinction between affected and unaffected pregnancies, alone or in combination with hCG [40–42]. INH-A has not got variations in relation with gestational age and thus the accuracy of testing is better by comparison with other serological markers [43].

3.1.2.5. Multiple marker screening in the second trimester of pregnancy

Second-trimester serum screening could be applied between 14 and 22 weeks of gestation, but usually it is carried out at 15–18 weeks of pregnancy. The serum markers could be combined in different ways but the most commonly used tests are double test (association between aFP and hCG), triple test (association between aFP, µE3 and hCG), and quadruple test (association between aFP, µE3, hCG and INH-A) [42, 44, 45]. The values obtained by these tests are combined based on a multivariate Gaussian model and finally a risk algorithm is obtained [46].

A very important parameter is the age of gestation and this must be established using an ultrasound determination of gestational age (best results with crown-rump measurement between 8 and 11 weeks) [47]. The risk algorithm must include other variables like maternal weight, ethnicity, maternal diseases (diabetes, systemic lupus erythematosus), multiple gestation, smoking, in vitro fertilization, sex of the fetus or maternal rhesus blood type [48–56]. In unaffected twins' pregnancy, the concentrations of maternal serum markers are twofold higher than that seen in unaffected singleton pregnancies and thus the algorithm needs an adjustment by using a "pseudo-risk" [51].

3.1.2.6. Screening of other aneuploidies

In case of a pregnancy with trisomy 18, all serum markers (aFP, µE3, hCG and INH-A) for the second trimester are characterized by low concentrations [57]. The risks are calculated using a multivariate normal model and the detection rates for this aneuploidy are similar to those of trisomy 21 screening [58]. For other autosomal trisomies (13, 16, 20) and for triploidy different protocols for the second-trimester biochemical screening were tried but without specific features [27].

Among the sex chromosome aneuploidies, only one presents a bad prognosis: monosomy X with fetal hydrops. In this case, the biochemical prenatal screening shows an association between low aFP and µE3 and elevated hCG and INH-A. In pregnancies with monosomy X without hydrops, all serological markers are lower than normal concentrations [59].

3.2. Ultrasound screening

Ultrasound examination represents a good tool for the detection of morphological abnormalities in fetuses with chromosomal aberrations. In aneuploidies we could identify structural defects and non-structural findings (sonographic markers). Sonographic markers of fetal aneuploidy (SMFAs) are insignificant by themselves because they are nonspecific and often transient [60]. The sensitivity of sonography for detecting these abnormalities varies with a number of factors: type of chromosomal abnormality, gestational age, quality of the sonography and the experience of the sonographer. During the first trimester only the SMFA could be identified in pregnancies with aneuploid fetuses. During the second trimester, major/structural abnormalities could be observed in 20% of fetuses with trisomy 21 and in the majority of fetuses with trisomies 18 and 13. By combining SMFA and structural defects, the sonography allows the identification of 50% of fetuses with trisomy 21, 80% of fetuses with trisomy 18 and 90% of fetuses with trisomy 13 [61, 62].

3.2.1. First-trimester screening

During the first trimester of pregnancy many sonographic markers of fetal aneuploidy were described, but the most used are nuchal translucency and nasal bone (NB). Also, some major congenital anomalies could be identified but usually such changes are diagnosed during the second trimester of pregnancy.

3.2.1.1. Nuchal translucency

Nuchal translucency (NT) was introduced in medical practice in the 1990s and it is the sonographic appearance of a subcutaneous collection of fluid in the region of fetal neck [63]. Using a fixed cut-off for the NT measurement of 3 mm, it was possible to identify 64% of chromosomally abnormal cases, while only 4.1% of normal fetuses showed similar NT values [64]. It was proved that cut-off value was variable depending on gestational age, and it developed a Gaussian model for the NT variable that allowed this test to be readily combined with other markers [65].

The measurement of fetal NT thickness is done at the 11–14th week of gestation. This sonographic scan has been combined with maternal age to provide an effective method of screening for trisomy 21—at 5% false positive rate, about 75% of trisomic pregnancies can be identified by this method [63].

The explanations of NT are multiple but the most plausible are cardiovascular defects which cause over-perfusion of the head and neck and abnormal or delayed development of the lymphatic system. Thus, NT marker could be associated also with other chromosomal anomalies that produce fluid accumulation in the neck region. Also, NT can be a transient phenomenon that appears in a normal fetus and it spontaneously resolves in the second trimester [66].

3.2.1.2. Nasal bone

Cicero et al. were the first who evaluated the absence of the nasal bone (NB) in pregnancies and showed that it was present in 73% of trisomy 21 fetuses versus 0.5% of unaffected fetuses. They concluded that in trisomy 21, the absence of the nasal bone is not related to the nuchal translucency thickness, and thus both sonographic markers could be combined to provide an effective method of early screening for trisomy 21 [67]. This combined screening allows an increase of sensitivity from about 57 to 86% at a fixed false positive rate of about 1%. If the biochemical screening in the first trimester is added, a sensitivity of more than 90% could probably be achieved at a false positive rate of 1% [5, 67]. The analysis of nasal bone in aneuploidy versus euploidy, made by Kagan et al., showed that the nasal bone was absent in 2.6% of the euploid fetuses, in 59.8% with trisomy 21, 52.8% with trisomy 18, 45.0% with trisomy 13 and in none of the fetuses with Turner syndrome [68]. In contrast, Cicero et al. indicated that trisomy 21 was associated with the absence of nasal bone in 68.8% of cases, trisomy 18 in 54.8% of cases, trisomy 13 in 34.2% of cases, monosomy X in 10.9% of cases, gonosomal aneuploidies (XXX, XXY, XYY) in 5% of cases and other types of autosomal aneuploidies in 16.7% of cases, but none of the 19 cases with triploidy presented the absence of nasal bone [69].

3.2.1.3. Other sonographic markers in the first trimester

Another potential marker for trisomy 21 in the first trimester of pregnancy is tricuspid regurgitation (TR) observed by pulsed wave Doppler ultra-sonography. Falcon et al. indicated a tricuspid regurgitation in 67.5% of fetuses with trisomy 21, 33.3% of fetuses with trisomy 18 and only 4.4% of euploid fetuses [70]. Kagan et al. reported this anomaly in 55.5% of fetuses with trisomy 21, 33.3% of fetuses with trisomy 18, 30% of fetuses with trisomy 13, 37.5% of fetuses with monosomy X and only 0.9% of euploid fetuses. The free β-hCG and PAPP-A present an independent variation in relation with tricuspid regurgitation and by combining all these parameters it would be expected to achieve a detection rate of 95% at a 5% false positive rate or 90% at a 2% false positive rate [71].

Borrell et al. measured the pulsatility index for veins and found an abnormal blood flow through the ductus venosus (DV) in the Down fetus. ***They indicated that with a 4–5% false positive rate, the detection rate for trisomy 21 is 65–75%. The use of this marker in association with NT increased the detection rate to 75–80%. Combining these two markers with serum biochemical markers measured at 10 weeks provided a detection rate of 92% at a 5% false positive rate [72].

Abele et al. analyzed retrospectively the NB, TR and DV. For normal children NB was identified in 2.0% of cases, TR was identified in 1.7% of cases and DV was identified in 3.5% of cases. In opposition, in cases with trisomy 21, NB was identified in 61.3% of cases, TR was identified in 61.3% of cases and DV was identified in 60.2% of cases. The normal children presented at least one of the markers in 5.9% of cases while more than 95% of the fetuses with trisomy 21 presented minimum 1 of these markers. The use of such combined prenatal screening (maternal age + NT + NB + TR + DV) during the first trimester could offer a detection rate of 95% with 1.5% false positive rate at a risk cut-off of 1:50 [73].

The assessment of each of these ultrasound markers can be incorporated into first-trimester combined screening by maternal age, fetal NT and serum-free ß-hCG and PAPP-A, resulting in the improvement of the performance of screening with an increase in detection rate from 93 to 96% and a decrease in false positive rate to 2.5% [68, 71, 74].

3.2.2. Second-trimester screening

During the second trimester of pregnancy different sonographic markers could be identified, as well as major congenital anomalies. The most common markers in the second trimester are nuchal thickening, hyperechoic bowel, shortened extremities, renal pyelectasis, echogenic intracardiac foci (EIF) and choroid plexus cysts. The discovery of such a marker is important especially in cases with trisomy 21 because many cases with Down syndrome do not present major congenital anomalies. In other aneuploidies and also in triploidy, usually the visceral anomalies are common, and identification of a congenital defect imposes an invasive procedure, followed by a chromosomal diagnosis [62].

3.2.2.1. Trisomy 13

Trisomy 13 is a severe disorder, characterized by the presence of different malformations in the brain (holoprosencephaly, agenesis of the corpus callosum, Dandy-Walker malformation, vermian agenesis and neural tube defects), face (cyclopia, hypotelorism, cleft lip and palate), kidneys (renal cystic dysplasia and hydronephrosis) and heart (aterial septal defect, ventricular septal defect and patent ductus arteriosus). Also, cystic hygroma, polydactyly and club or rocker-bottom feet could be identified. All these anomalies can be observed easily by ultrasound examination in the second trimester of pregnancy. Also in the cases of trisomy 13 some sonographic markers can be discovered, but they are nonspecific. Such markers are intrauterine growth restriction (IUGR), mild dilatation of the lateral cerebral ventricles, hyperechoic bowel and echogenic intracardiac foci. The most commonly identified marker is echogenic intracardiac foci. A specific association that can be considered is the one between echogenic intracardiac foci and the hypoplastic left side of the heart [62].

3.2.2.2. Trisomy 18

Trisomy 18 is a severe disorder characterized by a lot of congenital anomalies that could be identified by ultrasound examination during the second trimester of pregnancy. These anomalies involve the central nervous system (hydrocephalus, spina bifida, vermian agenesis), lymphatic system (cystic hygroma, nonimmune hydrops), cardiovascular malformations (ventricular and atrial septal defects, patent ductus arteriosus and polyvalvular disease), thorax and abdomen (diaphragmatic hernia, tracheoesophageal fistula, omphalocele), genitourinary system and skeletal system (clenched hands, club feet, radial aplasia, limb shortening). Also, the ultrasound examination shows an intrauterine growth restriction associated with polyhydramnios [75, 76].

Some subtle anomalies discovered by ultrasound examination were considered markers for trisomy 18. Such anomalies are choroid plexus cysts, brachycephaly, "strawberry-shaped" head and single umbilical artery [62]. Choroid plexus cysts are a relatively common variant during the second trimester. It is transient, and if the karyotype is normal it does not have an adverse outcome. The median prevalence of choroid plexus cysts in the general population has been reported as 1–2%. The importance of this marker is limited. Snijders et al. discovered only two cases of chromosomal anomalies in a cohort of 107 fetuses with isolated choroid plexus cysts who had karyotyping. On the other hand, the same authors found no chromosomal anomaly among the 174 children with choroid plexus cysts who did not have amniocentesis [77]. However, Nyberg et al. noted that choroid plexus cysts are observed in 30–40% of fetuses with trisomy 18 before 20 weeks, but usually this marker was associated with other major anomalies specific to trisomy 18 [62]. The presence of isolated choroid plexus cysts is associated with higher likelihood ratios for trisomy 18. Thus, Ghidini et al. [78] found a likelihood ratio of 7.1 and Yoder et al. [79] found a likelihood ratio of 13.8 for trisomy 18 in the presence of isolated choroid plexus cysts. Nyberg et al. concluded that fetal karyotyping should be offered only in cases when all the following conditions are met: maternal age at delivery is over 36 years, the biochemical risk for trisomy 18 is more than 1/3000 and choroid plexus cysts are large. However, the detection of isolated choroid plexus cysts imposes an ultrasound follow-up that can show other abnormalities that were previously missed [62].

3.2.2.3. Trisomy 21

During the second trimester of pregnancy, congenital anomalies in trisomy 21 fetuses are not frequently discovered. Before 20 weeks, the detection of such anomalies in trisomy 21 is around 16% and this value reflects the low sensitivity of sonography for detection of cardiac defects. The most frequent anomalies are cardiac defects, hydrops, cystic hygroma and duodenal atresia associated with esophageal atresia [62]. However, a sonographic scan at

24 weeks of gestation performed by a competent specialist could discover around 50% of congenital anomalies (including subtle ventricular septal defects) in trisomy 21 fetuses [80].

The markers for trisomy 21 in the second trimester of gestation are nuchal thickening, hyperechoic bowel, shortened limbs, pyelectasis, echogenic intracardiac foci, widened pelvic angle, shortened frontal lobes, clinodactyly, pericardial effusion, right–left disproportion of the heart and small ears [81, 82].

Each marker taken alone has a low sensitivity, but the presence of more than one marker is detected in minimum half of the pregnancies with trisomy 21. The presence of only one marker is discovered in around 22.6% of fetuses with trisomy 21 but also in 11% of normal fetuses. In opposition, identification of more than two markers is present in one-third of pregnancies with trisomy 21, while only 2% of normal pregnancies show such a characteristic. The risk for trisomy 21 is twofold higher if one marker is detected, but the risk becomes 10-fold higher when two markers are present and gets more than 100-fold when three markers are identified. The search of these markers is widely referred to as a "genetic sonogram". The results of a genetic sonogram depend on gestational age, quality of the apparatus and competence of the sonographer and the type of marker, but the minimum sensitivity of this method is around 60% [62]. The big inconvenience of this screening is the high false positive rate associated with the use of multiple sonographic markers that generates anxiety among low-risk patients and imposes an invasive procedure to deny the presence of trisomy 21 [83].

To improve the use of sonographic markers in detection of trisomy 21, Bromley et al. proposed a scoring index, and amniocentesis is offered only to those with a score of 2 or higher. A major congenital anomaly, nuchal thickening and an age bigger than 40 years are noted with 2 points each. Hyperechoic bowel, shortened femur, shortened humerus, pyelectasis, echogenic intracardiac foci and age between 35 and 40 years are noted with 1 point. The authors showed that a score ≥ 2 is associated with 75.5% of 21 trisomic pregnancies, while in normal pregnancies such a score is discovered in only 5.7% of cases [84]. An improvement of sonographic screening is the combination of this with biochemical screening, because the sonographic features are independent of biochemical analytes [85].

3.2.2.4. Nuchal thickening

Redundant skin on the neck is a clinical feature of infants with trisomy 21 and it was first reported by Benacerraf et al. as nuchal thickening during the second trimester [86]. Nuchal thickening is one of the most important markers of trisomy 21 during the second trimester. The sensitivity of this criterion is 20–40%. First, a threshold ≥6 mm after 15 weeks of pregnancy was associated with a high risk of trisomy 21, but now a nuchal thickening of greater than 5 mm up to 20 weeks is considered an adequate value [87]. The normal nuchal thickness varies with gestational age. Thus, the better choice is the use of multiple-of-the-median data, comparing the nuchal measurement with the expected measurement. In these conditions, the calculation of likelihood ratios would permit integration with maternal serum biochemical markers for a combined risk [88].

3.2.2.5. Hyperechoic bowel

Hyperechoic bowel is detected with increased frequency in cases with aneuploidy (including trisomy 21) but it is nonspecific and could be observed also in about 0.5% of normal fetuses. In addition, this marker was identified also in other disorders like bowel atresia, congenital infection, meconium ileus secondary and cystic fibrosis. The presence of hyperechoic bowel also represents a risk factor for intrauterine growth retardation, fetal death and placenta-related complications [62]. To standardize this feature, a scale with three values was proposed: grade 1—mildly diffuse echogenic, grade 2—moderately focal echogenic and grade 3—very echogenic (like in a bone). The echogenicity of normal bowel increases with transducer frequency, and to minimize the subjectivity, is preferable to take in consideration only the cases with moderate and markedly hyperechoic bowel. In these situations, the risk for fetal aneuploidy is high, but the sensitivity remains acceptable [89].

3.2.2.6. Skeletal abnormalities

Skeletal abnormalities in trisomy 21 that could be identified in the second trimester of gestation are limb shortening, clinodactyly and widened pelvic angle. The last two are difficult to detect and for this reason are not commonly used in screening protocols [62]. A slightly rhizomelic short stature is characteristic for trisomy 21, with both shortening of femur and shortening of humerus. These features can be detected in some cases with trisomy 21 during the second trimester [90], but a shortened humerus is a slightly more specific indicator than a shortened femur. These markers vary with gestational age, ethnic group and fetal gender. The practical use of these parameters is based on the comparison of measurement of humerus and femur length with expected length of these bones. Optimal results were obtained by using a multiple-of-the median data and corresponding likelihood ratios rather than a single cut-off. However, in a simplified manner a single cut-off of 0.91 multiples of the median for a short femur and 0.89 for a short humerus could be used [62, 90].

3.2.2.7. Renal pyelectasis

Mild pyelectasis (hydronephrosis) is associated with high risk for aneuploidy (especially for trisomy 21). This marker was also detected in about 3% of normal fetuses. The interpretation of this feature is very subjective because its prevalence varies with gestational age and it is influenced also by maternal hydration and degree of fetal bladder distension. Renal pyelectasis is measured as the fluid-filled renal pelvis in an anterior–posterior dimension. The threshold for a positive finding is a dimension ≥3. At this threshold, the risk of trisomy 21 is 1.6-fold over the baseline risk [62, 91].

3.2.2.8. Echogenic Intracardiac foci

Echogenic intracardiac foci (EIF) are marker that are found in 3–4% of normal fetuses, with a three times bigger prevalence in Asian populations [92]. The evaluation of EIF is very subjective and depends on resolution of the sonographic equipment, technique, thoroughness of the examination, the sonographer's experience and fetal position. In normal fetuses, it typically disappears during the third trimester of pregnancy [93]. The EIF is not an efficient marker for detection of trisomy 21 because it occurs only in 16% of fetuses with this anomaly and the false positive rate is 17%. In contrast, EIF is present in 29% of those with trisomy 13% [94, 95]. The likelihood ratio of EIF in trisomy 21 has been estimated in the range of 1.8–4.2 [62]. Usually, the EIF is detected in the left ventricle, but right-sided or bilateral EIF had an approximately twofold greater risk of aneuploidy compared with left-sided foci [96].

3.2.2.9. Mild ventricular dilatation

The lateral cerebral ventricles normally show a mean diameter of 6.1 ± 1.3 mm. The presence of ventriculomegaly is suspected when diameter reaches 10 mm and such change has been associated with trisomy 21 (and also with other aneuploidies) [97]. The prevalence of this marker in trisomy 21 fetuses varies between 2.8 and 5% [98–100]. On the other hand, van der Hof et al. showed that mild ventriculomegaly is present in 0.15% of euploid fetuses compared with 1.4% of the fetuses with trisomy 21, with a likelihood of aneuploidy 9 times greater in aneuploid fetuses versus normal fetuses [101].

3.3. Prenatal diagnosis methods

The prenatal diagnosis is based on the chromosomal or molecular analyses of embryonic or fetal cells obtained using an invasive method.

3.3.1. Invasive methods to obtain embryo-fetal cells

The methods for obtaining embryonic or fetal cells are chorionic villus sampling, amniocentesis and cordocentesis.

Chorionic villus sampling (CVS) is a method that allows prenatal diagnosis in the first trimester of pregnancy, typically at 10–12 weeks of gestation. It is done transabdominal or transcervical, under ultrasound guidance. The samples obtained contain trophoblast cells (derived from fetus) and maternal decidua cells. The last must be removed before analysis. The major advantages of this technique are reduced maternal risk generated by termination of pregnancy and a limited emotional trauma on the patient. The risks of this method are injury of the embryo (especially limb abnormalities in early procedures), miscarriage, bleeding or embryonic infection [102, 103]. The risk of miscarriage after performing chorionic villus sampling was initially estimated at 2–3%. Recent data disproves this risk, showing that the real risk is about 0.22% [104].

Amniocentesis is performed from the 16th week of gestation (rarely sooner) and involves the transabdominal extraction of 10–20 ml of amniotic fluid, under ultrasound guidance. The method has a low risk of miscarriage and other incidents. The risk of miscarriage was initially estimated at 1%, but recent data disproves this risk, showing that the real risk is about 0.11%. There is also a risk of amniotic fluid leakage and some rare complications (placental hemorrhage, intra-amniotic infection, abdominal wall hematoma and fetal lesion). A major disadvantage of this method is that it provides the final results of prenatal diagnosis in the second half of the pregnancy [103–105].

Cordocentesis is a method that consists of transabdominal or transvaginal puncture of the umbilical cord under ultrasound guidance in order to obtain small amounts of fetal blood. The method is performed after week 20 of pregnancy and has a reduced applicability in the diagnosis of chromosomal diseases. It is usually used to diagnose fetal blood diseases. Risk of fetal loss is high, about 3%. The major advantage of the diagnosis of chromosomal disorders is associated with the best results of blood cells culture in comparison with amniotic or chorionic cells [106].

3.3.2. Methods of prenatal diagnosis

The biological material obtained via invasive prenatal diagnosis methods can be used for cytogenetic or molecular assays.

3.3.2.1. Cytogenetic techniques

Cytogenetic techniques require dividing cells. They can be applied directly or after a cell culture.

3.3.2.1.1. First trimester cytogenetic analyses

In the case of trophoblast cells, obtained by chorionic villi sampling, the analysis can be done directly because the rate of division of placental tissue is high. However, even in the case of chorionic tissue, the cell culture is preferable because after harvest the quality is better and the cell number is high. Direct analysis of dividing cytotrophoblast cells is provided after uniform staining or after a chromosome banding procedure. The major advantages of this method are rapid final results (2/3 days) and absence of maternal cell contamination [103, 107].

The culture of chorionic villus cells is done in a special medium, after fragmentation of trophoblast tissue. The culture allows the formation of cell colonies adhering to the surface of the flask culture. At the end of 12–14 days, the cell division is blocked and chromosomal preparations are made. The chromosomes are banded using an R banding protocol because it does not require an aging period. The metaphases are analyzed on an optical microscope in direct illumination, using an immersion objective [103, 107].

The main advantage of cytogenetic diagnosis in the first trimester of pregnancy is achieving final results quickly, which decreases the time of uncertainty, the psychological distress of the parents and allows the end of pregnancy in the first trimester, when methods are easier and less traumatic [103, 107].

The main disadvantages of the chromosomal analysis in cells obtained by CVS are reduced number of mitosis and poor quality of chromosomal preparations which reduces resolution, allowing only the identification of numeric chromosomal abnormalities and those structural abnormalities of large dimensions. Another inconvenience is the possible detection of chromosomal mosaics. This could be real or confined to placenta. The inconsistencies can be explained by possible contamination with maternal cells, a chromosomal abnormality that occurs during the culture or the real existence of a placental mosaicism. In these cases, the karyotype must be repeated after amniocentesis or cordocentesis to determine real fetal chromosomal formula. Another problem associated with CVS is the failure of culture that requires the repeat of CVS or the application of amniocentesis in the second trimester of gestation [103, 107].

3.3.2.1.2. Second-trimester cytogenetic analyses

Fetal karyotype analysis, using cells obtained by amniocentesis, requires a step of 10–14-day cell culture. Culture technique and processing steps are similar to those used in the case of trophoblastic cells. Amniotic cultures can be done in situ (allow differentiation between mosaics and pseudomosaics) or in culture flasks. In the last case, at the end of the cultures, the separation of cells from the vessel is obtained using an enzymatic treatment. The contamination with maternal cells is insignificant and the quality of prepared chromosomes is better in comparison with chorionic villus cells [103, 107].

3.3.2.2. Molecular techniques

Molecular techniques for prenatal diagnosis of chromosomal disorders were introduced in the medical practice in the last 25 years with the aim of improving the resolution of chromosomal detection and to eliminate the major inconvenient of classic cytogenetic techniques—the requirement of cell culture. Such techniques are fluorescence in situ hybridization (FISH), quantitative fluorescent polymerase chain reaction (QF-PCR), multiplex ligation probe amplification (MLPA) and array-comparative genome hybridization (CHG).

3.3.2.2.1. Fish

FISH technique allows a hybridization between a fluorescent probe and a complementary DNA sequence present on the target chromosome. In prenatal diagnosis this method has been developed in order to identify the aneuploidy of chromosomes 21, 18, 13, X and Y (the most common chromosomal abnormalities) (**Figure 7**). The probes for chromosomes 13 and 21 are locus specific while the rest are centromeric. The method is done on uncultivated interphasic amniocytes. The final results are obtained in 24–48 hours after amniocentesis which allows maternal anxiety relief [108–110]. The results are obtained after the evaluation of minimum 50 cells. The main advantages are faster results, high specificity and sensibility (close to 100%) and the absence of cell culture. The inconvenients are impossibility of detection of blood contamination, bad quantification of chromosomal mosaics and impossibility of detection of structural abnormalities of chromosomes investigated. FISH can be done also for the evaluation and elucidation of uncommon structural abnormalities: microdeletion syndromes, cryptic or subtle duplications and translocations, complex rearrangements and marker chromosomes [111].

3.3.2.2.2. QF-PCR

QF-PCR method allows the detection of major prenatal numerical chromosome disorders within 24–48 hours. The method identifies polymorphic chromosomal specific repeat sequences (short tandem repeats—STRs) that are amplified by the PCR using fluorescent

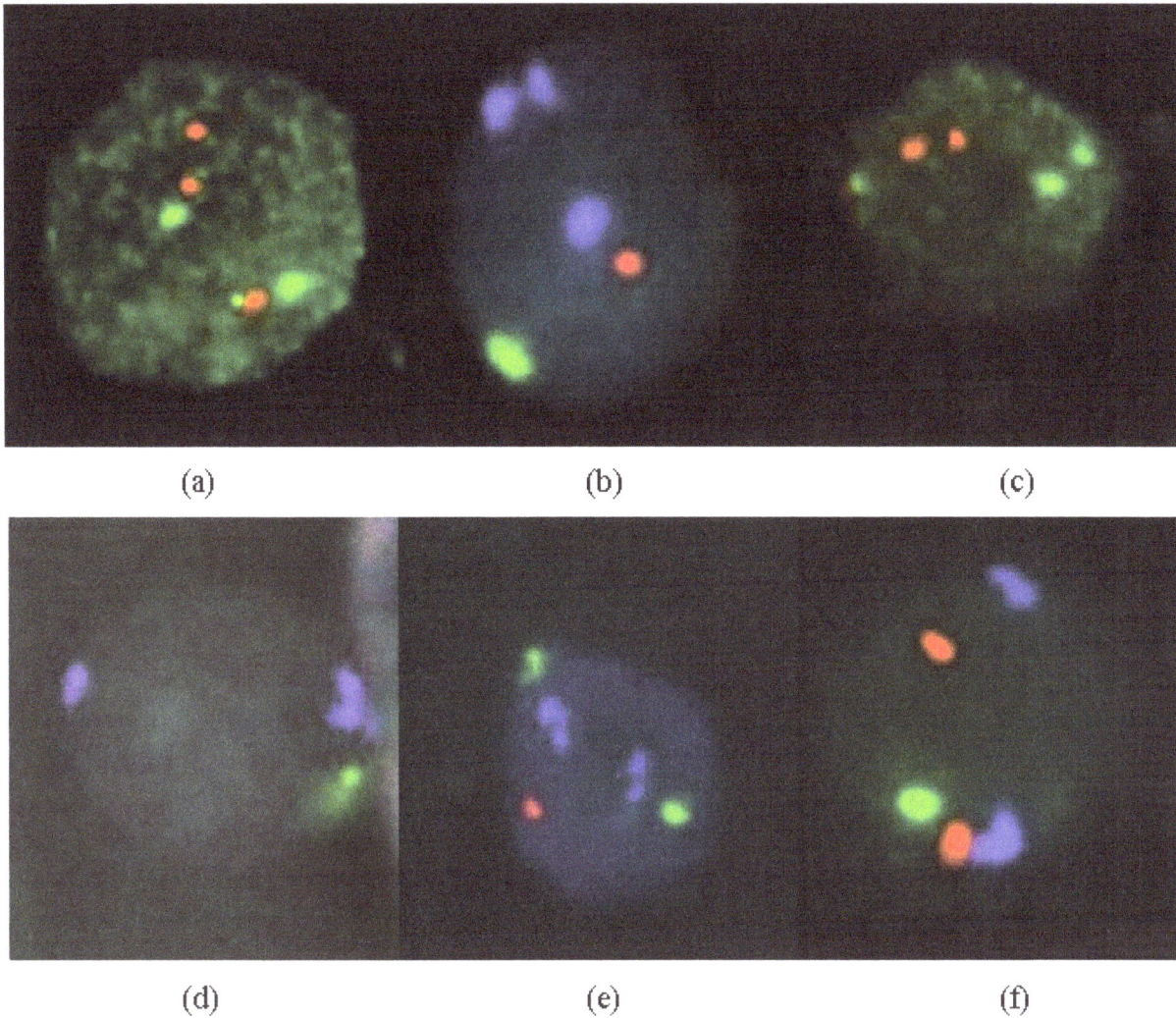

Figure 7. Aneuploidies detected using FISH method. (a) Trisomy 21; (b) Trisomy 13; (c) Trisomy 18; (d) Monosomy X; (e) Trisomy XXY; (f) Trisomy XYY (collection of prenatal diagnosis laboratory of "Cuza Vodă" obstetrics and gynecology hospital, Iaşi, Romania).

primers. The amplification is observed and quantified using a genetic analyzer and appropriate software. In a normal case, two peaks of fluorescence activity were obtained that reflect a normal heterozygous fetus (1:1 diallelic normal ration). Trisomic samples demonstrate either three peaks with a ratio of 1:1:1 (trisomic triallelic) or two peaks with a ratio of 2:1 (trisomic diallelic) for each informative probe. For each chromosome four or more polymorphic STR markers are analyzed, and thus only few fetal samples will remain uninformative. By comparison with FISH, QF-PCR can detect mosaicisms that have a rate of 20–30% and also identify the maternal cell contamination. The main advantage of QF-PCR is that it is considerably more cost-effective particularly when larger sample numbers are processed [111]. The main limitation of assay is the impossibility to detect triploidy [112].

3.3.2.2.3. MLPA

MLPA is a PCR-based method used for quantification of the copy numbers of specific sequences of DNA. This method uses a two-part probe of unique length that, when hybridized to adjacent target sequences on genomic DNA, can be joined together by the DNA ligase. This permits the amplification of all target sites, using a single primer pair that is complementary to the two free ends which are common to all probes. The PCR products are run on a capillary electrophoresis system and MLPA allows relative quantification of up to 50 different target sequences in one reaction. MLPA is a fast method (final results in 2–3 days) and it is less labor intensive and cheaper compared to karyotyping and FISH. The main domain of application of MLPA in prenatal diagnosis is the detection of most common aneuploidies (of chromosomes 21, 18, 13, X and Y) but this technique has some inconvenients associated with the impossibility of detection of triploidy, mosaicisms and maternal contamination. Other applications concern the cases with multiple congenital anomalies and intrauterine growth retardation detected by ultra-sonography. In these situations, using subtelomere probes or specific probes for some specific syndromes (velocardiofacial, Williams, Wolf-Hirschhorn, Prader-Willi, etc.), MLPA could confirm the presence of some subtle unbalanced structural chromosomal anomalies. MLPA can also be used to determine the origin of marker chromosomes, frequently discovered in chromosomal prenatal diagnosis [113, 114].

3.3.2.2.4. Array-CGH

Array CGH is a method that can detect simultaneously sub-microscopic copy number changes across the whole genome, thus overcoming the limitations of karyotyping and locus-specific techniques. Array CGH has become an important tool for clinical diagnostics and gene-identification studies and is having a great impact on the understanding of pathologies, the counseling of families and patient management. Different types of array CGH platforms at an increasingly higher resolution have been developed, differing mainly in the type of the interrogating probes and in their coverage of the genome. The microarray consists of thousands of unlabeled different probes (particular to a specific DNA sequence) fixed on a glass slide or a silicon chip, arranged in orderly rows in the form of a network with a specific density ("DNA chip"). The two samples of DNA (genomic DNA extracted from patient and reference sample) are fragmented and labeled with different fluorochromes (Cy3—green for patient and Cy5—red for test sample), mixed in equal amounts, denatured and co-hybridized on the microarray. The chips are scanned with a microarray scanner and the images obtained are analyzed using a programme that determines the intensities of emissions of both red and green fluorochrome for each spot on the network and calculates their report. This ratio is in proportion to the number of copies of the patient's genome DNA and test sample. If the intensities of the two fluorochromes are equal to a spot (ratio Cy3/Cy5 = 1, or $\log_2 = 0$), this region of the patient's DNA is interpreted as normal. If there is a deletion, the test sample hybridizes preferentially to DNA control, and the ratio Cy3/Cy5 will be smaller than 1 (ex. 1:2, $\log_2 = -1$). On the other hand, if there is a duplication, the patient DNA will hybridize preferentially, and the ratio Cy3/Cy5 will be greater than 1 (ex. 3:2, $\log_2 = 0.58$.) [115].

The application of array CGH eliminates the majority of fetal chromosomal analysis inconveniences: the long period of waiting for the final result, the possible failures of culture, the poor quality of chromosomal preparations and the reduced number of chromosomal bands. The method uses genomic DNA from fetal cells and can be applied on cells in interphase or division. The sensitivity of method is higher than the standard karyotype, and thus array-CGH allows the detection of all unbalanced chromosomal abnormalities (excepting polyploidy), even the smallest such subtelomeric rearrangements. In the prenatal diagnosis, "targeted" arrays are commonly used, containing genomic clones for subtelomeric regions and those that are frequently involved in microdeletion/microduplication syndromes. The major advantage of array-CGH is the very high resolution, this technique allowing the detection of genomic changes of 50–100 kb. The main inconvenient is the possibility of detecting copy number variants (CNVs) with unknown clinical consequences. In this case, with limited possibility of fetal phenotype investigation, the evaluation of functional consequences of genomic changes is very difficult. A CNV discovered in these conditions is most probably pathogen if it is de novo, has a size >1 Mb, contains a deletion rather than a duplication and involves a gene-rich area [116–118].

Nowadays, in developed countries, the array-CGH represents the first option in the prenatal genetic investigation of fetuses with multiple congenital anomalies detected by ultra-sonography.

4. The combined use of biochemical and ultrasound prenatal screening

Each method used in prenatal screening has some inconvenients that can be limited by using a combination of multiple assays. Biochemical and ultrasound screening can be done at the same time or at different times. The first method is called concurrent and the second sequential. The sequential protocol can offer the results when all analyses are complete—non-disclosure method—or at the time when each analysis is finished—step-wise method [119].

The biochemical screening in the first trimester is based on the detection of PAPP-A and ß-hCG. The PAPP-A has a different discriminatory power in a different week of gestation with a decline from the 10th to 13th week. For a predicted detection rate with 5% false positive rate the combination of PAPP-A and ß-hCG has a detection rate of 72% in 10th week, 65% in 11th week, 57% in 12th week and 51% in 13th week. By using a combination between double test (PAPP-A and ß-hCG) with detection of aFP and μE during second trimester, the detection rate increases to 78% (with PAPP-A measured in the 10th week), 72% (with PAPP-A measured in the 11th week), 66% (with PAPP-A measured in the 12th week) and 61% (with PAPP-A measured in 13th week) [119].

Nuchal translucency (NT) is independent for gestational age and its screening can be done at 11–13 weeks, with a detection rate of 73% for a 5% false positive rate. By combining biochemical screening in the first trimester with sonographic examination, the detection rate can increase. The best solution is to apply the biochemical screening in weeks 10–12 and the sonographic examination 1 week later. Using this protocol, the detection rate is 92% with double test done in the 10th week, 89% with double test done in the 11th week and 87% with double test done in the 12th week [119].

The best results are obtained using a non-disclosure protocol that combined NT with double test in the first trimester and detection of aFP and μE in the second trimester. This test, called integrated test, generates a detection rate of 93% (with PAPP-A measured in the 10th week), 92% (with PAPP-A measured in the 11th week), 91% (with PAPP-A measured in the 12th week) and 90% (with PAPP-A measured in the 13th week) for a 5% false positive rate. The use of such an algorithm has the inconvenience of having to wait a long time because the final results are done during the second trimester which increases the anxiety of the couple and limits its reproductive options [119, 120].

5. Conclusions

The chromosomal disorders have an important impact on the health of future infants. For this reason, in the last decade, important efforts were made to improve the prenatal screening and diagnosis. The prenatal screening uses non-invasive methods that allow the detection of pregnancies with risk of chromosomal anomalies. These methods can be done in the first or second trimesters of pregnancy. The first-trimester screening methods are biochemical and sonographic. Biochemical screening for first trimester uses the detection of PAPP-A and β-hCG in the maternal serum. Sonographic examination in the first trimester allows the detection of some markers—nuchal translucency, absence of the nasal bone, tricuspid regurgitation or abnormal blood flow through the ductus venosus—that are associated with high risk for aneuploidy. The prenatal screening during the second trimester of pregnancy can be done by biochemical or sonographic examinations as well. The biochemical screening is based on the detection of aFP, hCG (or β-hCG), μE and inhibin A in maternal serum. The sonographic examinations in the second trimester can identify some structural defects (cardiac, cerebral, renal, etc.) but more frequent are the sonographic markers like nuchal thickening, hyperechoic bowel, shortened limbs, pyelectasis, echogenic intracardiac foci, widened pelvic angle, and so on. The best choice for prenatal screening of aneuploidies is the use of combined biochemical (in the first and second trimesters) and sonographic examination. Such protocol has a detection rate higher than 90% at 5% false positive rate. The prenatal diagnosis requires an invasive procedure (chorionic villus sampling, amniocentesis, cordocentesis) to obtain fetal material. The fetal cells can be used for cytogenetic or molecular analyses. The cytogenetic analyses (fetal karyotype) require a long-time cell culture and have a limited resolution but have the advantage of diagnosis of all chromosomal anomalies. Some molecular analyses (FISH, QF-PCR, MLPA) are targeted methods and can identify only specific anomalies, such as aneuploidies of chromosomes 21, 18, 13 X and Y. Array-CGH (molecular karyotype) eliminates the major inconvenience of karyotype (long-time culture and limited resolution) but is expensive and thus it's use remains prohibitive in countries with limited economical resources. However, the implementation of prenatal screening and diagnosis allows many couples the opportunity to take an informed decision in relation to their baby's future.

Author details

Eusebiu Vlad Gorduza[1]*, Demetra Gabriela Socolov[2] and Răzvan Vladimir Socolov[2]

*Address all correspondence to: vgord@mail.com

1 Medical Genetics Department, "Grigore T. Popa" University of Medicine and Pharmacy, Iaşi, Romania

2 Obstetrics and Gynecology Department, "Grigore T. Popa" University of Medicine and Pharmacy, Iaşi, Romania

References

[1]   Gorduza EV. Compendiu de Genetică umană și medicală. Tehnopres: Iași; 2007

[2]   Hook EB. Prevalence, risks and recurrence. In: Brock DJH, Rodeck CH, FergusonSmith MA, editors. Prenatal Diagnosis and Screening. Edinburgh: Churchill Livingstone; 1992. pp. 351-392

[3]   Gorduza EV, Covic M, Stoica O, Voloşciuc M, Angheloni T, Butnariu L, Studii BE. clinice, epidemiologice și citogenetice pe un lot de 221 pacienți cu sindrom Down. Revista Medico-Chirurgicala a Societatii De Medici Si Naturalisti Din Iasi. 2007;**111**(2):363-372

[4]   Egan JF, Benn P, Borgida AF, Rodis JF, Campbell WA, Vintzileos AM. Efficacy of screening for fetal down syndrome in the United States from 1974 to 1997. Obstetrics and Gynecology. 2000;**96**:979-985

[5]   Aneuploidy SK. Screening in the first trimester. American Journal of Medical Genetics Part C Seminars in Medical Genetics. 2007;**145C**:18-32

[6]   Snijders RJM, Sebire NJ, Nicolaides KH. Maternal age and gestational age specific risks for chromosomal defects. Fetal Diagnosis and Therapy. 1995;**10**:356-357

[7]   Nicolaides KH. Screening for fetal aneuploidies at 11 to 13 weeks. Prenatal Diagnosis. 2011;**31**:7-15

[8]   Nicolaides KH. Turning the pyramid of prenatal care. Fetal Diagnosis and Therapy. 2011;**29**:183-196

[9]   Merkatz IR, Nitowsky HM, Macri JN, Johnson WE. An association between low maternal serum alpha-fetoprotein and fetal chromosomal abnormalities. American Journal of Obstetrics and Gynecology. 1984;**148**:886-894

[10] van Lith JM, Pratt JJ, Beekhuis JR, Mantingh A. Second trimester maternal serum immuno-reactive inhibin as a marker for fetal Down's syndrome. Prenatal Diagnosis 1993;**12**:801-806

[11] Brambati B, Macintosh MCM, Teisner B, Maguiness S, Shrimanker K, Lanzani A, Bonacchi I, Tului L, Chard T, Grudzinskas JG. Low maternal serum level of pregnancy associated plasma protein (PAPP-A) in the first trimester in association with abnormal fetal karyotype. BJOG. 1993;**100**:324-326

[12] Aitken DA, Wallace EM, Crossley JA, Swanston IA, van Pareren Y, van Maarle M, Groome NP, Macri JN, Connor JM. Dimeric inhibin a as a marker for Down's syndrome in early pregnancy. The New England Journal of Medicine. 1996;**334**:1231-1236

[13] Benn PA. Advances in prenatal screening for down syndrome: II first trimester testing, integrated testing, and future directions. Clinica Chimica Acta. 2002;**324**:1-11

[14] Wald NJ, Kennard A, Hackshaw AK. First trimester serum screening for down syndrome. Prenatal Diagnosis. 1995;**15**:1227-1240

[15] Cuckle HS, van Lith JMM. Appropriate biochemical parameters in first trimester screening for down syndrome. Prenatal Diagnosis 1999;**19**:505-512

[16] Spencer K, Souter V, Tul N, Snijders R, Nicolaides KH. A screening program for trisomy 21 at 10-14 weeks using fetal nuchal translucency, maternal serum free bhuman chorionic gonadotropin and pregnancy-associated plasma protein-a. Ultrasound in Obstetrics & Gynecology. 1999;**13**:231-237

[17] Wald NJ, Kennard A, Hackshaw A, McGuire A. Antenatal screening for Down's syndrome. Journal of Medical Screening. 1997;**4**:181-246

[18] Laigaard J, Cuckle H, Wewer UM, Christiansen M. Maternal serum ADAM12 levels in Down's and Edwards' syndrome pregnancies at 9-12 weeks gestation. Prenatal Diagnosis. 2006;**26**:689-691

[19] Laigaard J, Spencer K, Christiansen M, Cowans NJ, Larsen SO, Pedersen BN, Wewer UM. ADAM12 as a first trimester maternal serum marker in screening for Down's syndrome. Prenatal Diagnosis. 2006;**26**:973-979

[20] Biagiotti R, Cariati E, Brizzi L, Cappelli G, D'Agata A. Maternal serum screening for trisomy 18 in the first trimester of pregnancy. Prenatal Diagnosis. 1998;**18**:907-913

[21] Spencer K, Ong C, Skentou H, Liao AW, Nicolaides KH. Screening for trisomy 13 by fetal nuchal translucency and maternal serum free h-hCG and PAPP-A at 10– 14 weeks of gestation. Prenatal Diagnosis. 2000;**20**:411-416

[22] Spencer K, Tul N, Nicolaides KH. Maternal serum free betahCG and PAPP-A in fetal sex chromosome defects in the first trimester. Prenatal Diagnosis. 2000;**20**:390-394

[23] Spencer K, Liao AW, Skentou H, Cicero S, Nicolaides KH. Screening for triploidy by fetal nuchal translucency and maternal serum free beta-hCG and PAPP-A at 10– 14 weeks of gestation. Prenatal Diagnosis. 2000;**20**:495-499

[24] Cuckle H, Benn P, Wright D. Down syndrome screening in the first and/or second trimester: Model predicted performance using meta-analysis parameters. Seminars in Perinatology. 2005;**29**:252-257

[25] Wald NJ, Rodeck C, Hackshaw AK, et al. First and second trimester antenatal screening for Down's syndrome: The results of the serum, urine and ultrasound screening study (SURUSS). Health Technology Assessment. 2003;**7**:1-88

[26] Wald NJ, Huttly WJ, Hackshaw AK. Antenatal screening for Down's syndrome with the quadruple test. Lancet. 2003;**361**:835-836

[27] Benn PA. Advances in prenatal screening for down syndrome: I. General principles and second trimester testing. Clinica Chimica Acta. 2002;**323**:1-16

[28] Palomaki GE, Haddow JE. Maternal serum a-fetoprotein, maternal age, and down syndrome risk. American Journal of Obstetrics and Gynecology. 1987;**156**:460-463

[29] Dimao M, Baumgarten A, Greenstein RM, Saal HM, Mahony MJ. Screening for Down's syndrome in pregnancy by measuring maternal serum alpha-fetoprotein levels. The New England Journal of Medicine. 1987;**317**:342-346

[30] Newby D, Aitken DA, Crossley JA, Howatson AG, Macri JN, Connor JM. Biochemical markers of trisomy 21 and the pathophysiology of Down's syndrome pregnancies. Prenatal Diagnosis. 1997;**17**:941-951

[31] Bogart MH, Pandian MR, Jones OW. Abnormal maternal serum chorionic gonadotropin levels in pregnancies with fetal chromosome abnormalities. Prenatal Diagnosis. 1987;**7**:623-630

[32] Cole LA, Seifer DB, Kardana A, Braunstein GD. Selecting human chorionic gonadotropin immunoassays: Consideration of cross-reacting molecules in first trimester pregnancy serum and urine. American Journal of Obstetrics and Gynecology. 1993;**168**:1580-1586

[33] Benn PA, Egan JFX, Ingardia CJ. Extreme second trimester serum analytes in down syndrome pregnancies with hydrops fetalis. The Journal of Maternal-Fetal & Neonatal Medicine. 2002;**11**:1-4

[34] Benn PA, Gainey A, Ingardia CJ, Rodis JF, Egan JFX. Second trimester maternal serum analytes in triploid pregnancies: Correlation with phenotype and sex chromosome complement. Prenatal Diagnosis. 2001;**21**:680-686

[35] Saller DN, Canick JA, Schwartz S, Blitzner MG. Multiple marker screening in pregnancies with hydropic and non-hydropic turner syndrome. American Journal of Obstetrics and Gynecology. 1992;**67**:1021-1024

[36] Jørgansen PI, Trolle D. Low urinary oestriol excretion during pregnancy in women giving birth to infants with Down's syndrome. Lancet. 1972;**ii**:782-784

[37] Canick JA, Knight GJ, Palomaki GE, Haddow JE, Cuckle HS, Wald NJ. Low second trimester maternal serum unconjugated oestriol in pregnancies with down syndrome. British Journal of Obstetrics and Gynaecology. 1988;**95**:330-333

[38] Wald NJ, Cuckle HS, Densem JW, Nanchahal K, Canick JA, Haddow JE, Knight GJ, Palomaki GE. Maternal serum unconjugated oestriol as an antinatal screening test for Down's syndrome. British Journal of Obstetrics and Gynaecology. 1988;**95**:334-341

[39] Newby D, Aitken DA, Howatson AG, Connor JM. Placental synthesis of oestriol in Down's syndrome pregnancies. Placenta. 2000;**21**:263-267

[40] Petragelia F, Sawchenko P, Lim ATW, Rivier J, Vale W. Localization, secretion and action of inhibin in human placenta. Science. 1987;**237**:187-189

[41] Dalgliesh GL, Aitken DA, Lyall F, Howatson AG, Conner JM. Placental and maternal serum inhibin-a and activin-a levels in Down's syndrome pregnancies. Placenta. 2001;**22**:227-234

[42] Wald NJ, Densem JW, George L, Muttukrishna S, Knight PG. Prenatal screening for Down's syndrome using inhibinA as a serum marker. Prenatal Diagnosis. 1996;**16**:143-152

[43] Watt HC, Wald NJ, Huttly WJ. The pattern of maternal serum inhibin-a concentrations in the second trimester of pregnancy. Prenatal Diagnosis. 1998;**18**:846-848

[44] Mooney RA, Peterson CJ, French CA, Saller DN, Arvan DA. Effectiveness of combining maternal serum alpha-fetoprotein and hCG in a second-trimester screening program for down syndrome. Obstetrics and Gynecology. 1994;**84**:298-303

[45] Wald NJ, Cuckle HS, Densem JW, Nanchahal K, Royston P, Chard T, Haddow JE, Knight GJ, Palomaki GE, Canick JA. Maternal serum screening for Down's syndrome in early pregnancy. BMJ. 1988;**297**:883-887

[46] Reynolds TM, Penny MD. The mathematical basis of multivariate risk screening: With special reference to screening for down syndrome associated pregnancy. Annals of Clinical Biochemistry. 1989;**27**:452-458

[47] Benn PA, Borgida A, Horne D, Briganti S, Collins R, Rodis JF. Down syndrome and neural tube defect screening: The value of using gestational age by ultrasonography. American Journal of Obstetrics and Gynecology. 1997;**176**:1056-1061

[48] Neveux LM, Palomaki GE, Larrivee DA, Knight GJ, Haddow JE. Refinements in managing maternal weight adjustment for interpreting prenatal screening results. Prenatal Diagnosis. 1996;**16**:1115-1119

[49] Watt HC, Wald NJ, Smith D, Kennard A, Densem J. Effect of allowing for ethnic group in prenatal screening for down syndrome. Prenatal Diagnosis. 1996;**16**:691-698

[50] Wald NJ, Watt HC, George L. Maternal serum inhibin-A in pregnancies with insulin dependent diabetus: Implications for screening for Down's syndrome. Prenatal Diagnosis. 1996;**16**:923-926

[51] Neveux LM, Palomaki GE, Knight GJ, Haddow JE. Multiple marker screening for down syndrome in twin pregnancies. Prenatal Diagnosis. 1996;**16**:29-34

[52] Ferriman EL, Sehmi IK, Jones R, Cuckle HS. The effect of smoking in pregnancy on maternal serum inhibin A levels. Prenatal Diagnosis. 1999;**19**:372-374

[53] Wald NJ, White N, Morris JK, Huttly WJ, Canick JA. Serum markers for Down's syndrome in women who have had in vitro fertilisation: Implications for antenatal screening. British Journal of Obstetrics and Gynaecology. 1999;**106**:1304-1306

[54] Spong CY, Ghidini A, Stanley-Christian H, Meck JM, Seydel FD, Pezzullo JC. Risk of abnormal triple screen for down syndrome is significantly higher in patients with female foetuses. Prenatal Diagnosis. 1999;**19**:337-339

[55] Sancken U, Bartels I. Preliminary data on an association between blood groups and serum markers used for the so-called "triple screening": Free oestriol MoM values are decreased in rhesus-negative (Rh-) women. Prenatal Diagnosis. 2001;**21**:194-195

[56] Maymon R, Cuckle H, Sehmi IK, Herman A, Sherman D. Maternal serum human chorionic gonadotrophin levels in systemic lupus erythematosus and antiphospholipid syndrome. Prenatal Diagnosis. 2001;**21**:143-145

[57] Canick JA, Palomaki GE, Osthanondh R. Prenatal screening for trisomy 18 in the second trimester. Prenatal Diagnosis. 1990;**10**:546-548

[58] Benn PA, Ying J, Beazoglou T, Egan JFX. Estimates for the sensitivity and false-positive rates for second trimester serum screening for down syndrome and trisomy 18 with adjustment for cross-identification and double-positive results. Prenatal Diagnosis. 2001;**21**:46-51

[59] Lambert-Messerlian GM, Saller DN Jr, Tumber MB, French CA, Peterson CJ, Canick JA. Second-trimester maternal serum inhibin A levels in fetal trisomy 18 and turner syndrome with and without hydrops. Prenatal Diagnosis. 1998;**18**:1061-1067

[60] Nicolaides KH, Shawwa L, Brizot M, Snijders RJ. Ultrasonographically detectable markers of fetal chromosomal defects. Ultrasound in Obstetrics & Gynecology. 1993;**3**:56-59

[61] Hill LM. The sonographic detection of trisomies 13 18, and 21. Clinical Obstetrics and Gynecology. 1996;**39**:831-850

[62] Nyberg DA, Souter VL. Sonographic markers of fetal Trisomies: Second trimester. Journal of Ultrasound in Medicine. 2001;**20**:655-674

[63] Nicolaides KH, Heath V, Cicero S. Increased fetal nuchal translucency at 11-14 weeks. Prenatal Diagnosis. 2002;**22**:308-315

[64] Nicolaides KH, Azar G, Byrne D, Mansur C, Marks K. Fetal nuchal translucency: Ultrasound screening for chromosomal defects in the first trimester. BMJ. 1992;**304**:867-869

[65] Wald NJ, Hackshaw AK. Combining ultrasound and biochemistry in first-trimester screening for Down's syndrome. Prenatal Diagnosis. 1998;**18**:511-523

[66] von Kaisenberg CS, Brand-Saberi B, Jonat W, Nicolaides K. Pathophysiology of increased nuchal translucency in chromosomally abnormal foetuses. Prenatal and Neonatal Medicine. 1999;**4**:431-440

[67] Cicero S, Avgidou K, Rembouskos G, Kagan KO, Nicolaides KH. Nasal bone in first trimester screening for trisomy 21. American Journal of Obstetrics and Gynecology. 2006;**195**:109-114

[68] Kagan KO, Cicero S, Staboulidou I, Wright D, Nicolaides KH. Fetal nasal bone in screening for trisomies 21, 18 and 13 and turner syndrome at 11-13 weeks of gestation. Ultrasound in Obstetrics & Gynecology. 2009;**33**:259-264

[69] Cicero S, Rembouskos G, Vandecruys H, Hogg M, Nicolaides KH. Likelihood ratio for trisomy 21 in foetuses with absent nasal bone at the 11-14 weeks scan. Ultrasound in Obstetrics & Gynecology. 2004;**23**:218-223

[70] Falcon O, Auer M, Gerovassili A, Spencer K, Nicolaides KH. Screening for trisomy 21 by fetal tricuspid regurgitation, nuchal translucency and maternal serum free β-hCG and PAPP-A at 11 + 0 to 13 + 6 weeks. Ultrasound in Obstetrics & Gynecology. 2006;**27**:151-155

[71] Kagan KO, Valencia C, Livanos P, Wright D, Nicolaides KH. Tricuspid regurgitation in screening for trisomies 21, 18 and 13 and turner syndrome at 11 + 0 – 13 + 6 weeks of gestation. Ultrasound in Obstetrics & Gynecology. 2009;**33**:18-22

[72] Borrell A, Gonce A, Martinez JM, Borobio V, Fortuny A, Coll O, Cuckle H. First trimester screening for down syndrome with ductus venosus Doppler studies in addition to nuchal translucency and serum markers. Prenatal Diagnosis. 2005;**25**:901-905

[73] Abele H, Wagner P, Sonek J, Hoopmann M, Brucker S, Artunc-Ulkumen B, Kagan KO. First trimester ultrasound screening for down syndrome based on maternal age, fetal nuchal translucency and different combinations of the additional markers nasal bone, tricuspid and ductus venosus flow. Prenatal Diagnosis. 2015;**35**:1-5

[74] Maiz N, Valencia C, Kagan KO, Wright D, Nicolaides KH. Ductus venosus Doppler in screening for trisomies 21, 18 and 13 and turner syndrome at 11-13 weeks of gestation. Ultrasound in Obstetrics & Gynecology. 2009;**33**:512-517

[75] Cereda A, Carey JC. The trisomy 18 syndrome. Orphanet Journal of Rare Diseases. 2012;**7**:81

[76] Houlihan OA, O'Donoghue K. The natural history of pregnancies with a diagnosis of trisomy 18 or trisomy 13; a retrospective case series. BMC Pregnancy and Childbirth. 2013;**13**:209

[77] Snijders RJ, Shawa L, Nicolaides KH. Fetal choroid plexus cysts and trisomy 18: Assessment of risk based on ultrasound findings and maternal age. Prenatal Diagnosis. 1994;**14**:1119-1127

[78] Ghidini A, Strobelt N, Locatelli A, Mariani E, Piccoli MG, Vergani P. Isolated fetal choroid plexus cysts: Role of ultrasonography in establishment of the risk of trisomy 18. American Journal of Obstetrics and Gynecology. 2000;**182**:972-977

[79] Yoder PR, Sabbagha RE, Gross SJ, Zelop CM. The second-trimester foetus with isolated choroid plexus cysts: A meta-analysis of risk of trisomies 18 and 21. Obstetrics and Gynecology. 1999;**93**:869-872

[80] Paladini D, Tartaglione A, Agangi A, Teodoro A, Forleo F, Borghese A, Martinelli P. The association between congenital heart disease and down syndrome in prenatal life. Ultrasound in Obstetrics & Gynecology. 2000;**15**:104-108

[81] DeVore GR. Trisomy 21: 91% detection rate using second-trimester ultrasound markers. Ultrasound in Obstetrics & Gynecology. 2000;**16**:133-141

[82] Vintzileos AM, Campbell WA, Guzman ER, Smulian JC, McLean DA, Ananth CV. Second-trimester ultrasound markers for detection of trisomy 21: Which markers are best? Obstetrics and Gynecology. 1997;**89**:941-944

[83] Filly RA. Obstetric sonography: The best way to terrify a pregnant woman. Journal of Ultrasound in Medicine. 2000;**19**:1-5

[84] Bromley B, Lieberman E, Benacerraf BR. The incorporation of maternal age into the sonographic scoring index for the detection at 14-20 weeks of foetuses with Down's syndrome. Ultrasound in Obstetrics & Gynecology. 1997;**10**:321-324

[85] Verdin SM, Economides DL. The role of ultrasonographic markers for trisomy 21 in women with positive serum biochemistry. British Journal of Obstetrics and Gynaecology. 1998;**105**:63-67

[86] Benacerraf B, Gelman R, Frigoletto F. Sonographic identification of second trimester foetuses with down syndrome. The New England Journal of Medicine. 1987;**317**:1371-1376

[87] Benacerraf BR, Frigoletto FD. Soft tissue nuchal fold in the second trimester foetus: Standards for normal measurements compared to the foetus with down syndrome. American Journal of Obstetrics and Gynecology. 1987;**157**:1146-1149

[88] Bahado-Singh RO, Oz AU, Kovanci E, Deren O, Copel J, Baumgarten A, Mahoney J. New down syndrome screening algorithm: Ultrasonographic biometry and multiple serum markers combined with maternal age. American Journal of Obstetrics and Gynecology. 1998;**179**:1627-1631

[89] Nyberg DA, Resta RG, Mahony BS, Dubinsky T, Luthy DA, Hickok DE, Luthardt FW. Echogenic bowel and Down's syndrome. Ultrasound in Obstetrics & Gynecology. 1993;**3**:330-333

[90] Johnson MP, Michaelson JE, Barr M Jr, Treadwell MC, Hume RF Jr, Dombrowski MP, Evans MI. Combining humerus and femur length for improved ultrasonographic identification of pregnancies at increased risk for trisomy 21. American Journal of Obstetrics and Gynecology. 1995;**172**:1229-1235

[91] Wickstrom EA, Thangavelu M, Parilla BV, Tamura RK, Sabbagha RE. A prospective study of the association between isolated fetal pyelectasis and chromosomal abnormality. Obstetrics and Gynecology. 1996;**88**:379-382

[92] Shipp TD, Bromley B, Liberman EP, Benacerraf BR. The frequency of the detection of fetal echogenic intracardiac foci with respect to maternal race. Ultrasound in Obstetrics & Gynecology. 2000;**15**:460-462

[93] Petrikovsky BM, Challenger M, Wyse LJ. Natural history of echogenic foci within ventricles of the fetal heart. Ultrasound in Obstetrics & Gynecology. 1995;**5**:92-94

[94] Shanks AL, Odibo AO, Gray DL. Echogenic intracardiac foci: Associated with increased risk for fetal trisomy 21 or not? Journal of Ultrasound in Medicine. 2009;**28**:1639-1643

[95] Renna MD, Pisani P, Conversano F, Perrone E, Casciaro E, Di Renzo GC, Di Paola M, Perrone A, Casciaro S. Sonographic markers for early diagnosis of fetal malformations. World Journal of Radiology. 2013;**5**(10):356-371

[96] Bromley B, Lieberman E, Shipp TD, Richardson M, Benacerraf BR. Significance of an echogenic intracardiac focus in foetuses at high and low risk for aneuploidy. Journal of Ultrasound in Medicine. 1998;**17**:127-131

[97] Patel MD, Goldstein RB, Tung S, Filly RA. Fetal cerebral ventricular atrium: difference in size according to sex. Radiology. 1995;**194**:713-715

[98] Devaseelan P, Cardwell C, Bell B, Ong S. Prognosis of isolated mild to moderate fetal cerebral ventriculomegaly: A systematic review. Journal of Perinatal Medicine. 2010;**38**:401-409

[99] Melchiorre K, Bhide A, Gika AD, Pilu G, Papageorghiou AT. Counseling in isolated mild fetal ventriculomegaly. Ultrasound in Obstetrics & Gynecology. 2009;**34**:212-224

[100] Pagani G, Thilaganathan B, Prefumo F. Neurodevelopmental outcome in isolated mild fetal ventriculomegaly: Systematic review and meta-analysis. Ultrasound in Obstetrics & Gynecology. 2014;**44**:254-260

[101] van den Hof MC, Wilson RD, Diagnostic Imaging Committee, Society of Obstetricians and Gynaecologists of Canada, Genetics Committee, Society of Obstetricians and Gynaecologists of Canada. Fetal soft markers in obstetric ultrasound. Journal of Obstetrics and Gynaecology Canada. 2005;**27**:592-636

[102] Shim S-S. Chorionic villus sampling. Journal of Genetic Medicine. 2014;**11**(2):43-48

[103] Tabor A, Alfirevic Z. Update on procedure-related risks for prenatal diagnosis techniques. Fetal Diagnosis and Therapy. 2010;**27**:1-7

[104] Akolekar R, Beta J, Picciarelli G, Ogilvie C, D'Antonio F. Procedure-related risk of miscarriage following amniocentesis and chorionic villus sampling: A systematic review and meta-analysis. Ultrasound in Obstetrics & Gynecology. 2015;**45**:16-26

[105] Cruz-Lemini M, Parra-Saavedra M, Borobio V, Bennasar M, Gonce A, Martinez JM, Borrell A. How to perform an amniocentesis. Ultrasound in Obstetrics & Gynecology. 2014;**44**:727-731

[106] Collins SL, Prenatal IL. Diagnosis: Types and techniques. Early Human Development. 2012;**88**:3-8

[107] Gorduza EV, Popovici C, Mixitch F, Burada F, Ştefănescu D, Covic M. Profilaxia bolilor genetice. In: Covic M, Ştefănescu D, Sandovici I, Gorduza EV, editors. Genetică Medicală. 3rd ed. Iaşi: Polirom; 2017. pp. 585-605

[108] Liehr T, Ziegler M. Rapid prenatal diagnostics in the interphase nucleus: Procedure and cut-off rates. The Journal of Histochemistry and Cytochemistry. 2005;**53**(3): 289-291

[109] Nemescu D, Martiniuc V, Gorduza EV, Onofriescu M. Fetal aneuploidy diagnosis through rapid fluorescence in situ hybridization (FISH) on uncultured amniocytes. Revista română de medicină de laborator. 2011;**19**(2/4):161-168

[110] Gorduza EV, Onofriescu M, Martiniuc V, Grigore M, Mihălceanu E, Iliev G. Importanţa tehnicii FISH în diagnosticul prenatal al aneuploidiilor. Revista Medico-Chirurgicală a Societăţii de Medici şi Naturalişti Iaşi. 2007;**111**(4):990-996

[111] Bui T-H. Prenatal cytogenetic diagnosis: gone FISHing, BAC soon! Ultrasound in Obstetrics & Gynecology. 2007;**30**:247-251

[112] Mann K, Mackie Ogilvie C. QF-PCR: Application, overview and review of the literature. Prenatal Diagnosis. 2012;**32**:309-314

[113] Omrani MD, Azizi F, Rajabibazl M, Naini NS, Omrani S, Abbasi AM, Gargari SS. Can we rely on the multiplex ligation-dependent probe amplification method (MLPA) for prenatal diagnosis? Iranian Journal of Reproductive Medicine. 2014;**12**(4):263-268

[114] Massalska D, Bijok J, Jakiel G, Roszkowski T, Zimowski JG, Jóźwiak A. Multiplex ligation-dependent probe amplification (MLPA) – New possibilities of prenatal diagnosis, Ginekologia Polska 2013;**84**:461-464

[115] Sireteanu A, Covic M, Gorduza EV. Hibridizarea genomică comparativă pe microrețele: considerații tehnice și aplicații. Revista Medico-Chirurgicală a Societății de Medici și Naturaliști Iași. 2012;**116**(2):545-551

[116] Bianchi DW. From prenatal genomic diagnosis to fetal personalized medicine: Progress and challenges. Nature Medicine. 2012;**18**:1041-1051

[117] Wapner RJ, Martin CL, Levy B, Ballif BC, Eng CM, Zachary JM, Savage M, Platt LD, Saltzman D, Grobman WA, Klugman S, Scholl T, Simpson JL, McCall K, Aggarwal VS, Bunke B, Nahum O, Patel A, Lamb AN, Thom EA, Beaudet AL, Ledbetter DH, Shaffer LG, Jackson L. Chromosomal microarray versus karyotyping for prenatal diagnosis. The New England Journal of Medicine. 2012;**367**:2175-2184

[118] Fiorentino F, Napoletano S, Caiazzo F, Sessa M, Bono S, Spizzichino L, Gordon A, Nuccitelli A, Rizzo G, Baldi M. Chromosomal microarray analysis as a first-line test in pregnancies with a priori low risk for the detection of submicroscopic chromosomal abnormalities. European Journal of Human Genetics. 2013;**21**:725-730

[119] Cuckle HS. Growing complexity in the choice of Down's syndrome screening policy. Ultrasound in Obstetrics & Gynecology. 2002;**19**:323-326

[120] Wald NJ, Watt HC, Hackshaw AK. Integrated screening for Down's syndrome based on tests performed during the first and second trimesters. The New England Journal of Medicine. 1999;**341**:461-467

8

Neonatal Ebstein's Anomaly

Umar Boston, Ken-Michael Bayle,
TK Susheel Kumar and Christopher Knott-Craig

Abstract

Ebstein's anomaly is a congenital heart disease that results from failure of delamination of the tricuspid valve with resulting apical displacement of the septal and posterior leaflets of the tricuspid valve. Age at presentation can vary greatly but neonatal presentation is associated with extraordinary high mortality rates. Comprehensive multispecialty care is required starting at the time of fetal diagnosis. Fetal echocardiography is vital in monitoring progression of the disease in utero. Fetal echocardiogram can evaluate for complications such as arrhythmias, pericardial effusion, or fetal hydrops. Post-natal evaluation should include evaluation of functional pulmonary atresia or circular shunt. Despite advances in surgical technique for Ebstein's anomaly, mortality for it remains high with early surgical intervention. Aggressive medical management should be used to support patients with Ebstein's anomaly during the neonatal period. Surgical procedures for neonatal Ebstein's vary widely from systemic to pulmonary shunts with or without tricuspid valve closure to tricuspid valve repair.

Keywords: neonatal Ebstein's anomaly, Ebstein's anomaly, tricuspid valve dysplasia, Fetal Ebstein

1. Introduction

Ebstein's anomaly (EA) was first described by Wilhelm Ebstein in 1866 noting the septal and inferior leaflets of the tricuspid valve arose from the right ventricular myocardium [1]. EA is a rare congenital heart disease with a prevalence of 2.4 per 10,000 live births [2]. Embryologically, EA is a result of varying degrees of failure of leaflets to delaminate from the underlying endocardium that results in a number of characteristic features. There are varying degrees of apical displacement of the tricuspid leaflets with the septal leaflet most severely affected followed by the posterior leaflet. Furthermore, the right ventricle (RV) is myopathic and is separated into two zones, with an "atrialized" poorly functional portion between the true annulus and the hinge point of the apically displaced septal leaflet, while the "functional" RV is the portion below the leaflet hinge point. Depending on the degree of leaflet displacement this functional RV volume can be quite diminutive.

The clinical manifestations of EA vary widely from mild forms presenting in adulthood, to severe forms with high mortality in the neonatal period. In utero, EA can result in hydrops and arrhythmia. Furthermore, an in utero diagnosis of EA has an incidence of 48% fetal demise [3]. Mortality rates are highest in the neonatal period ranging from 17 to 56% [4] and poses significant medical and surgical challenges.

2. Associated anomalies and arrhythmias

Ebstein anomaly is known to have several additional cardiac manifestations. A patent foramen ovale or atrial septal defect is normally present. The right to left shunting across the defect accounts for the relative hypoxia exhibited in certain patients. RV outflow tract obstruction in the form of anatomical pulmonary atresia occurs in about half of the symptomatic neonates requiring surgical intervention [5]. In the setting of pulmonary atresia, a patent ductus arteriosus is required as the source of pulmonary blood flow [6–8]. Left ventricular non-compaction cardiomyopathy has been noted to be associated with EA. A retrospective study demonstrated that 10 of 61 patients (16%) with EA also had left ventricular non-compaction [7]. This was associated with a higher mortality risk of 30% in those with LVNC compared to 13% with EA alone. Wolff-Parkinson-White (WPW) is present in about 10–30% of cases. In about 20% of cases with WPW, there may be more than two accessory pathways present. The accessory pathways are usually present on the tricuspid valve annulus [9, 10]. Due to large right atrium, EA patients are at risk for atrial tachycardia, atrial flutter, intra-atrial reentrant tachycardia, atrial fibrillation, AV node reentrant tachycardia, and ventricular arrhythmias.

3. Pathologic anatomy

Carpentier et al. described the characteristic features of this disorder that are relevant to surgical management [11].

1. Failure of delamination of the TV leaflets is the hallmark of EA whereby the leaflets are tethered to the endocardium by fibromuscular attachments or abnormal foreshortened chordae. Each leaflet exhibits varying degrees of apical displacement and tethering with the septal leaflet most severely affected followed by posterior then anterior leaflets. This results in anterior and apical displacement of the functional annulus.

2. The anterior leaflet is attached to the true anatomical annulus but is large or sail like.

3. The portion of the RV above the functional annulus ('atrialized right ventricle') is dilated and thin. The true tricuspid annulus is almost always enlarged. In a neonate this measures approximately 21 mm.

4. The cavity of the effective RV is reduced ('functional right ventricle').

5. The infundibulum of the RV can be obstructed by the redundant tissue of the anterior leaflet and its chordal attachments to the infundibulum.

In addition to the leaflet abnormalities there is a variable degree of ventricular myocardial dysfunction. Morphometric histopathologic studies have demonstrated that there is an absolute decrease in the number of myocardial fibers in addition to thinning of the wall of the dilated RV in EA [12].

Carpentier et al. also described four grades of Ebstein's anomaly [11].

Type A: The anterior leaflet has normal morphology and the RV is adequate.

Type B: The anterior leaflet has abnormal chordae but normal mobility. The RV is reduced in volume but adequate.

Type C: The anterior leaflet is restricted in movement. The RV is small with a large atrialized component.

Type D: Also called 'tricuspide sac' as the leaflets form a complete sac of fibrous tissue adherent to the RV. The only functional part of the RV is the infundibulum.

3.1. Perinatal period

The long term prognosis of a fetus diagnosed with EA is poor and remains one of the highest mortalities amongst congenital heart disease patients. One multicenter study showed that a fetal diagnosis of EA resulted in a 17% fetal demise. Furthermore, there was an additional 32% in-hospital attrition of live-born babies with EA with an overall 45% perinatal mortality [4]. Risk factors for perinatal mortality include lack of antegrade flow across the pulmonary valve, large cardiothoracic ratio, earlier in utero diagnosis, large tricuspid valve annulus, pericardial effusion, and right ventricular dysfunction [13–16]. Pulmonary valve regurgitation may be the most ominous risk factor representing the end result of severe tricuspid regurgitation with resultant volume load on a myopathic right ventricle that has to pump against retrograde flow from the PDA. This triad of diminished preload, increased afterload and a dysfunctional right ventricle leads to inadequate preload to the left ventricle and subsequent heart failure, cardiogenic shock and perinatal demise. These factors in-utero lead to hydrops and arrhythmias and ultimately fetal demise.

4. Pathophysiology of the newborn

Neonates are symptomatic as a result of ineffective RV cardiac output and severe TV regurgitation. There is usually some degree of cardiomegaly which can be quite severe compressing the lungs. Furthermore, cyanosis results from systemic venous return being shunted across the ASD to the left side of the heart. Neonatal pulmonary vascular resistance (PVR) is elevated and this is a major impediment to effective antegrade flow from the diminutive and myopathic RV. In the first week of life when pulmonary vascular resistance is high pulmonary blood flow is dependent upon the PDA. This results in a physiological state referred to as "functional" pulmonary atresia. When the PVR decreases over the first week of life, the RV may then be able to overcome the afterload to establish antegrade flow. True anatomical pulmonary atresia where there is luminal discontinuity between RV and pulmonary artery is also often seen in these symptomatic neonates. These patients will have ductal dependent pulmonary circulation until a surgical procedure is performed to establish pulmonary blood flow. Left ventricular dysfunction can also play a critical role in the development of decompensated heart failure. This is related to left ventricular displacement of the interventricular septum as a result the severely dilated dysfunctional RV. This "pancaking" of the LV cavity impedes filling and diminishes systemic cardiac output. In less severe forms of EA the RV can generate effective antegrade flow especially when the PVR decreases. Antegrade flow across the RV outflow tract is accompanied by clinical improvement in symptoms. Neonates with severe TR or gross cardiomegaly who are otherwise asymptomatic have an associated mortality of 45% within the first year of life without intervention [17, 18]. The natural history of being diagnosed with EA during infancy is sobering [19]. However those who survive early childhood can expect reasonable longevity. When the disease is mild symptoms are not noticed until later in adult life. Symptoms are often related to exercise intolerance or cyanosis from progressive tricuspid regurgitation.

5. Diagnostic evaluation

5.1. Chest X-ray

Depending on the severity of disease, the chest roentgenograms usually demonstrates massive cardiomegaly with decreased pulmonary vascular markings (**Image 1**).

5.2. Electrocardiography

The electrocardiograms for patients with EA are usually abnormal. The most common finding on ECG are tall P waves and right bundle branch block. The tall P waves are indicative of a large right atrium. The right bundle branch block occurs because abnormal development of the right bundle branch which appears to be associated with septal leaflet and medial papillary muscle development on necropsy studies [5]. Some patients may have a prolonged PR interval from long intra-atrial conduction times from a large right atrium. Wolff-Parkinson-White syndrome is associated with EA, thus ventricular pre-excitation may be seen on ECG.

5.3. Echocardiography

Echocardiography is the gold standard for obtaining the diagnosis for EA. Two dimensional (2-D) echocardiography can evaluate the tricuspid valve leaflets and their excursion. The apical four

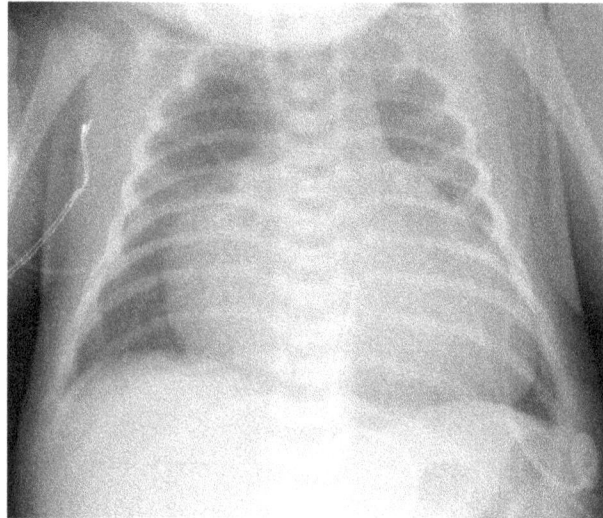

Image 1. Chest x-ray of an infant with EA. there is marked cardiomegaly with a significant cardiothoracic ratio. With marked cardiomegaly lung development can be impaired.

chamber views allow calculation of the displacement index, which measures the distance from the true septal annulus to the level of the apically displaced septal leaflet hinge point (**Image 2**). Distance is indexed to body surface area and values >8 mm/m^2 are consistent with EA [20]. Color Doppler echocardiography can demonstrate the presence and location of tricuspid valve regurgitation (**Image 3**) [21]. However, severity can be difficult to quantitate due to apical displacement. RV dysfunction and functional or anatomic pulmonary atresia can be evaluated by 2-D and color echocardiography [21] **Image 4**. The Great Ormond Street Echocardiogram (G.O.S.E.) score is a mortality risk stratification score for neonates with EA. It is calculated from the apical four chamber view by adding the right atrium and atrialized right ventricular volume and dividing by the sum of the functional right ventricular volume, left atrial and ventricular volumes. (18) A G.O.S.E score of 3 (ratio of 1.1–1.4) with cyanosis or 4 (ratio > 1.5) has a mortality of nearly 100% [18] **Image 5**.

Echocardiography can define other associated abnormalities with EA such as the presence of a patent ductus arteriosus, size and direction of shunting through the atrial septal defect/patent foramen ovale, presence of a ventricular septal defect, and hypertrabeculated left ventricle suggesting left ventricular non-compaction cardiomyopathy.

Fetal echocardiography is a useful diagnostic tool for prenatal diagnosis and monitoring progression of disease in utero. The 4-chamber view of the fetal heart will demonstrate apical displacement of the tricuspid valve annulus, enlarged right ventricular and atrial size, and large tricuspid valve annulus (**Image 6**). Color flow imaging can be used to evaluate the degree of tricuspid valve regurgitation. The pulmonary valve can be evaluated by 2-D and color flow imaging to assess for pulmonary atresia. M-mode assessment can determine any rhythm abnormalities such as supraventricular tachycardia [22]. In addition, signs of hydrops such as pericardial effusions can be visualized (**Image 7**).

Fetal echocardiogram is important for monitoring clinical status of the fetus during pregnancy. A large multicenter study performed by Freud et al. evaluated over 400 fetal echocardiograms of patients with EA. They demonstrated that larger cardiothoracic ratio, more than moderate

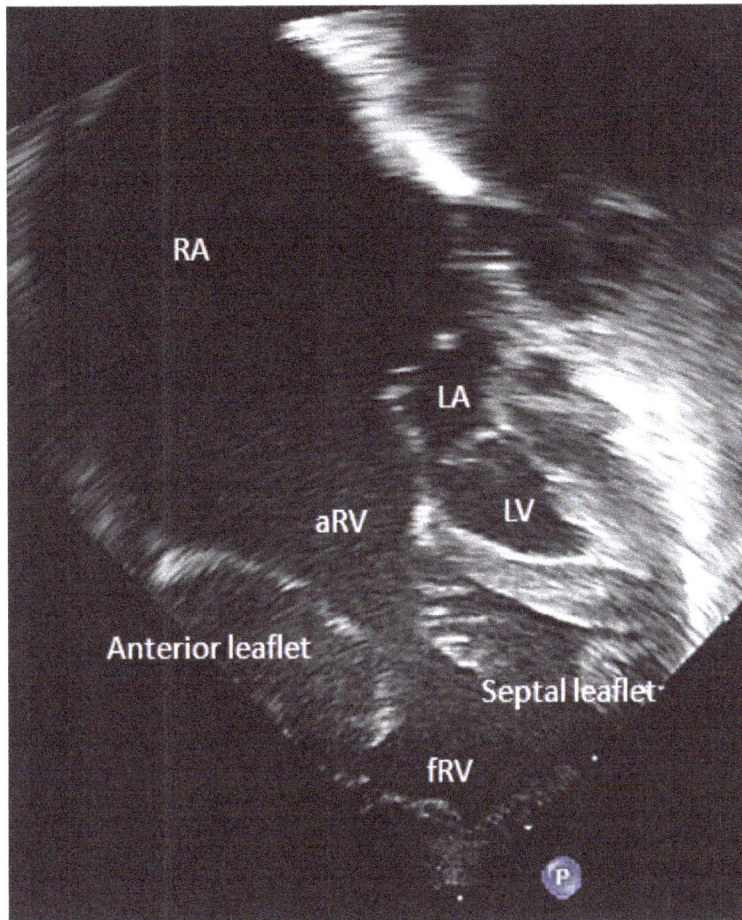

Image 2. Apical 4 chamber view of Ebstein's anomaly with severe enlargement of the right atrium and atrialized portion of the right ventricle. There is apical displacement of the tricuspid valve with tethering of the septal leaflet leading to poor coaptation and tricuspid valve regurgitation. RA: Right atrium. LA: Left atrium. aRV: Atrialized right ventricle. LV: Left ventricle. fRV: Function right ventricle.

tricuspid regurgitation, larger tricuspid annulus diameter z-score, larger diameter vena contracta for tricuspid regurgitation, lack of antegrade pulmonary blood flow, pulmonary regurgitation, and pericardial effusion were associated with increased perinatal mortality [4]. Furthermore, Tierney et al. demonstrated that only 31% of fetuses had no predictive risk factors for poor hemodynamic status at time of diagnosis, and of those, 61% went on to develop one or more signs later in gestation. As such, frequent fetal echocardiograms are necessary to monitor the clinical status of fetuses with EA [23].

5.4. Computed tomography/magnetic resonance imaging

There is limited utility for the use of CT, MRI, or cardiac catheterization in neonatal EA.

5.5. Treatment

5.5.1. Medical

In a study of 415 neonates presenting with symptomatic EA the overall hospital mortality was 24% [19]. Furthermore, surgical intervention in the neonatal period across US hospitals is

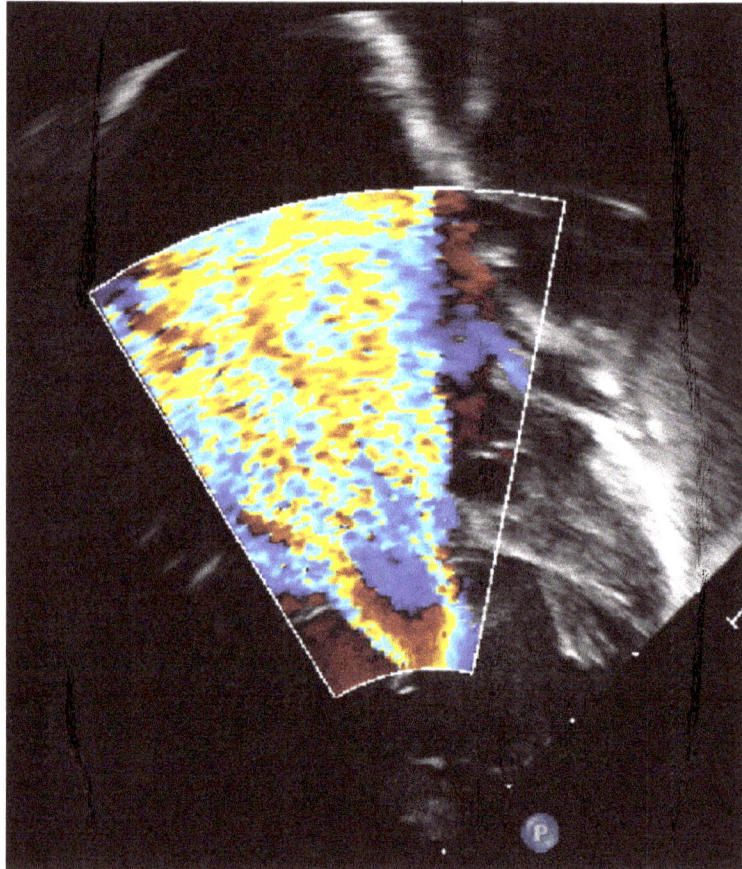

Image 3. Apical 4 chamber with color flow imaging of the tricuspid valve. There is severe tricuspid valve regurgitation due to poor coaptation of the tricuspid valve leaflets.

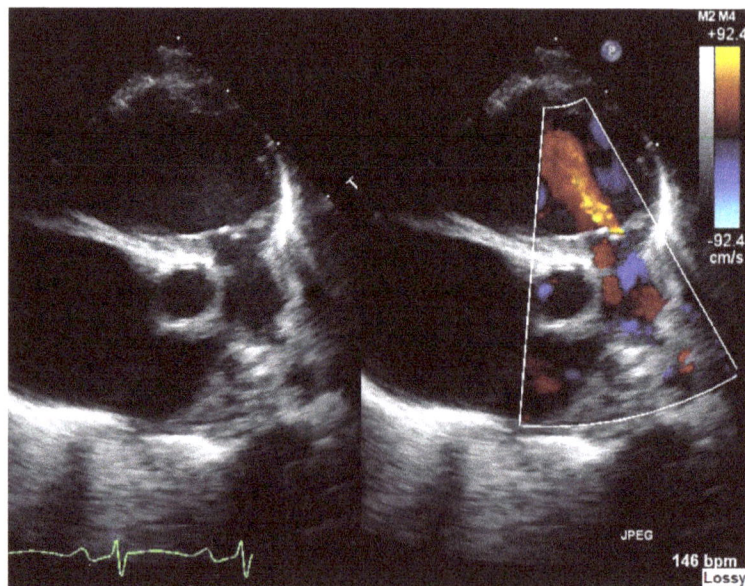

Image 4. Color compare parasternal short axis view demonstrates the small functional right ventricle and pulmonary atresia. The tricuspid valve is rotated in a fashion that the effective orifice opens to the right ventricular outflow tract. Color Doppler demonstrates swirling of blood in the functional right ventricle, tricuspid regurgitation, and no antegrade pulmonary blood flow. aRV: Atrialized right ventricle.

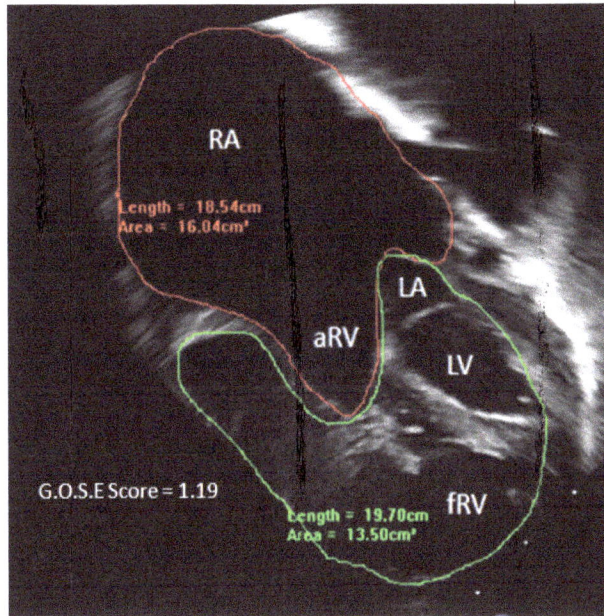

Image 5. Apical four chamber view demonstrating the right atrium, atrialized portion of the right ventricle, functional right ventricle, left atrium and left ventricle. There is a grade 3 GOSE score which correlates with 100% mortality in presence of cyanosis. RA = right atrium. aRV = atrialized right ventricle. fRV = functional right ventricle. LA = left atrium. LV = left ventricle.

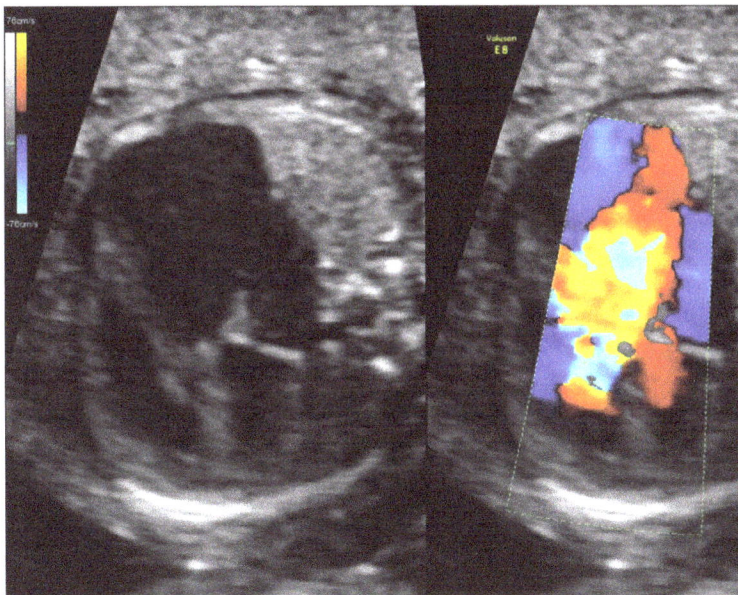

Image 6. Fetal echocardiogram performed at 22 weeks and 3 days gestation. There is severe enlargement of the right atrium with severe tricuspid valve regurgitation demonstrated on color Doppler evaluation. The tricuspid valve annulus dimension is markedly enlarged.

associated with a mortality of 27–36% depending on the procedure performed [19]. There is significant improvement in surgical outcome if the patient can be medically managed out of the neonatal period [24]. As such the best survival rates for EA occurs outside of the neonatal period, thus medical management with supportive care is crucial for improving outcomes.

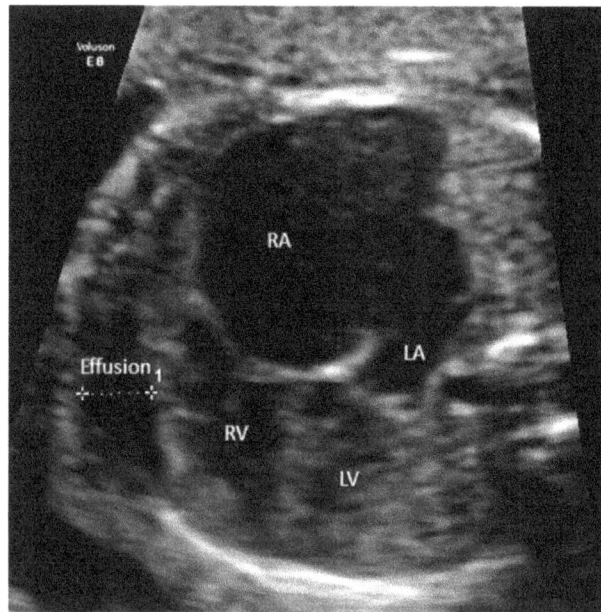

Image 7. Fetal echocardiogram at 22 weeks and 3 days gestation with a four chamber view of the heart. The heart mass takes up the entire thoracic cavity. There is severe enlargement of the right atrium with evidence of a pericardial effusion. RA: Right atrium. RV: Right ventricle. LA: Left atrium. LV: Left ventricle.

Relatively stable but symptomatic patients can be treated with prostaglandin infusion to maintain ductal patency if functional or anatomical pulmonary atresia is evident. Supplemental oxygen should not be greater than 21% fractional inspired oxygen to avoid pulmonary over-circulation and volume loading of the heart. During this phase oxygen saturation should be maintained between 75 and 85%. As the pulmonary vascular resistance decreases, prostaglandin therapy can be discontinued. This will also allow for proper evaluation of antegrade pulmonary blood flow as the ductus closes. If saturations decrease under 80% then agents to lower pulmonary vascular resistance can be administered to promote antegrade flow, these include supplemental oxygen and nitric oxide.

Use of prostaglandins in the presence of pulmonary valve regurgitation may exacerbate heart failure symptoms due to the development of a circular shunt. In this physiology blood flows from left ventricle to aorta, then it is shunted away from the systemic circulation via the large ductus to the pulmonary artery then retrograde via the pulmonary valve into the right ventricle to right atrium via the incompetent tricuspid valve then back to the left side of the heart via the ASD. This creates high output heart failure. Prostaglandins should be stopped if this physiology exists.

Further hemodynamic instability leads to cardiogenic shock. In these situations intubation and mechanical ventilation with large tidal volumes are key to promoting adequate ventilation in patients with massive cardiomegaly. Furthermore, sedation and possible paralysis to limit oxygen requirements may be required. Inotropic support in the form of milrinone complemented with low dose of dopamine or epinephrine may be necessary to assist with cardiac output. Tachyarrhythmias are common in this group of patients so utilization of catecholamine inotropes should be used sparingly.

Milrinone is a very effective drug since it has lusitropic and inotropic effects on the right ventricle. Furthermore, it decreases the pulmonary vascular resistance which promotes antegrade pulmonary blood flow. Frequent echocardiograms during the first week are useful to assess antegrade flow across the RV outflow tract and degree of TV regurgitation. This assessment will help guide weaning prostaglandins, and initiation of nitric oxide and inotropes.

In summary, medical management when pulmonary ductal dependency exists is analogous to single ventricle physiology whereby a balance between systemic and pulmonary circulation needs to be established. This is best done with maintenance of prostaglandins and low oxygen supplementation. Once the pulmonary vascular resistance drops and there is antegrade flow across the pulmonary valve then this management is more analogous to two ventricle physiology with a poor right ventricular pump. As such this is best managed by stopping prostaglandins and allowing for ductal closure. Concomitantly administration of nitric oxide, milrinone and higher oxygen supplementation will augment antegrade flow.

The goal of medical therapy is to avoid an operation particularly during the neonatal period when mortality is highest for any surgical procedure performed.

5.6. Surgical indications

Surgical indications for EA include failure to wean from mechanical ventilator support, failure to wean off prostaglandin with systemic oxygen saturation below 75%, functional or anatomic pulmonary atresia, Great Ormond Street Echocardiography (G.O.S.E.) score of 3 or 4, and patients with right heart failure.

5.7. Surgical procedures

To date there has been many procedures described for the surgical treatment for neonatal EA [11, 25–28, 31–35].

Danielson at the Mayo Clinic first described some of the essential principles for EA repair in any age group [25]. This includes plication of the atrialized RV, posterior tricuspid annuloplasty, closure of ASD and right reduction atrioplasty.

The cone reconstruction first described by da Silva and colleagues has now evolved into the technique of choice when repairing the tricuspid valve for EA [27]. In this procedure, the anterior and posterior leaflets of the tricuspid valve are mobilized from their attachments to the RV endocardium maintaining free edge attachments. The mobilized leaflets are rotated clockwise and then reattached to the true annulus [36]. To date there has been a growing number of reports of utilization of the Cone procedure for neonatal EA [27].

Starnes et al. reported a single ventricle palliation strategy for neonates with good outcome [29]. In the Starnes procedure the RV is excluded by performing a fenestrated patch closure of the tricuspid valve. An atrial septectomy allows for excellent mixing. Finally, a modified Blalock-Taussig-Thomas shunt is performed to establish a regulated source of pulmonary blood flow. Most neonates undergoing a Starnes RV exclusion procedure are then channeled down a single ventricle pathway with a bidirectional Glenn and Fontan procedures.

The two competing strategies for surgical treatment for neonatal EA are whether to perform a biventricular repair or a single ventricle palliative procedure (Starnes Procedure).

The decision for which type of repair is best for neonatal EA is controversial. Mizuno et al. described their center experience with neonatal EA repair. Their results demonstrated greater survival for the biventricular repair group compared to single ventricle palliation, 60 vs. 25% respectively [30]. A recent follow up study by Kumar et al. evaluated the median 7 year follow up for the Starnes procedure in 27 neonatal repairs [29]. Their overall survival for 5 year follow up was 81%. Boston et al. described their outcomes for neonatal biventricular repair for EA. Early survival was 78.1% in their series, while 15 year survival for EA with and without anatomical pulmonary atresia was 40 and 79% respectively. As such caution should be advised for biventricular repairs in EA neonates with anatomical pulmonary atresia [25, 36].

In summary, neonatal EA continues to carry a high perinatal mortality upon fetal diagnosis. A multidisciplinary approach is required for improved outcomes. Fetal echocardiography predicts outcome and is necessary for monitoring progression of EA complications. Comprehensive care with a multi-disciplinary team including high risk obstetrician, pediatric cardiologist, pediatric cardiothoracic surgeon, neonatal intensivist should occur at a tertiary care center. Surgical management during the neonatal period remains high. If possible medical management through the neonatal period improves mortality.

Author details

Umar Boston*, Ken-Michael Bayle, TK Susheel Kumar and Christopher Knott-Craig

*Address all correspondence to: uboston@uthsc.edu

Heart Institute at Le Bonheur Children's Hospital, University of Tennessee Health Science Center, Memphis, United States

References

[1] Ebstein W. Uber einen sehr seltenen fall von insufficienz der valvula tricuspidalis, bedingt durch eine angeborene hochgradige misshildung derselben. Archives of Anatomy and Physiology. 1866;**33**:238-254

[2] Fyler DC, Buckley LP, Hellenbrand WE. Report of the New England regional infant cardiac program. Pediatrics 1980;**65**:375-461

[3] Hornberger LK, Sahn DJ, Dleinman CS, Copel JA, Reed KL. Tricuspid valve disease with significant tricuspid insufficiency in the fetus: Diagnosis and outcome. Journal of the American College of Cardiology. 1991;**17**:167-173

[4] Freud LR, Escobar-Diaz MC, Kalish BT, et al. Outcomes and predictors of perinatal mortality in Fetuses with Ebstein anomaly or tricuspid valve dysplasia in the current era a Multicenter study. Circulation 2015;**132**:481-489

[5] Ho SY, Goltz D, McCarthy K, et al. The atrioventricular junction in Ebstein malformation. Heart 2000;**83**:444-449

[6] Attenhofer Jost CH, Connolly HM, O'Leary PW, Warnes CA, Tajik AJ, Seward JB. Left heart lesions in patients with Ebstein anomaly. Mayo Clinic Proceedings. 2005;**80**:361-368

[7] Pignatelli RH, Texter KM, Denfield SW, et al. LV noncompaction in Ebstein's anomaly in infants and outcomes. JACC. Cardiovascular Imaging. 2014 Feb;**7**(2):207-209

[8] Knott-Craig CJ, Goldberg SP, Ballweg JA, et al. Surgical decision making in neonatal Ebstein's anomaly: An algorithmic approach based on 48 consecutive neonates. World Journal for Pediatric and Congenital Heart Surgery. 2012;**3**(1):16-20

[9] Oh JK, Holmes DR Jr, Hayes DL, Porter CB, Danielson GK. Cardiac arrhythmias in patients with surgical repair of Ebstein's anomaly. Journal of the American College of Cardiology. 1985;**6**:1351-1357

[10] Olson TM, Porter CB. Electrocardiographic and electrophysiologic findings in Ebstein's anomaly: Pathophysiology, diagnosis, and management. Progress in Pediatric Cardiology. 1994;**2**:38-50

[11] Carpentier A, Chauvaud S, Mace L, et al. A new reconstructive operation for Ebstein's anomaly of the tricuspid valve. The Journal of Thoracic and Cardiovascular Surgery. 1988;**96**(1):92-101

[12] Anderson KR, Lie JT. The right ventricular myocardium in Ebstein's anomaly: A morphometric histopathologic study. Mayo Clinic Proceedings. 1979;**54**(3):181-184

[13] McElhinney DB, Salvin JW, Colan SD, Thiagarajan R, Crawford EC, Marcus EN, del Nido PJ, Tworetzky W. Improving outcomes in fetuses and neonates with congenital displacement(ebstein's malformation) or dysplasia of the tricuspid valve. The American Journal of Cardiology 2005;**96**:582-586

[14] Andrews RE, Tibby SM, Sharland GK, Simpson JM. Prediction of outcome of tricuspid valve malformations diagnosed during fetal life. The American Journal of Cardiology. 2008;**101**:1046-1050

[15] Barre E, Durand I, Hazelzet T, David N. Ebstein's anomaly and tricuspid valve dysplasia: Prognosis after diagnosis in utero. Pediatric Cardiology. 2012;**33**:1391-1396

[16] Yu JJ, Yun TJ, Won HS, Im YM, Lee BS, Kang SY, Ko HK, Park CS, Park JJ, Gwak M, Kim EA, Kim YH, Ko JK. Outcome of neonates with ebstein's anomaly in the current ra. Pediatric Cardiology. 2013;**34**:1590-1596

[17] Knott-Craig CJ, Goldberg SP. Management of neonatal Ebstein's anomaly. Seminars in Thoracic and Cardiovascular Surgery. Pediatric Cardiac Surgery Annual. 2007;**112-6**: 101-108

[18] Celermajer DS, Cullen S, Sullivan ID, et al. Outcome in neonates with Ebstein's anomaly. Journal of the American College of Cardiology. 1992;**19**(5):1041-1046

[19] Goldberg SP, Jones RC, Boston US, Haddad LM, Wetzel GT, Chin TK, Knott-Craig CJ. Current trends in the management of neonates with ebstein's anomaly. World Journal of Pediatric and Congenital Heart Surgery. Oct 2011;**2**(4):554-557

[20] Seward JB. Ebstein's anomaly: Ultrasound imaging and hemodynamic evaluation. Echocardiography. 1993;**10**:641-664

[21] Booker OJ, Nanda NC. Echocardiographic assessment of Ebstein's anomaly. Echocardiography. 2015;**32**(S2):S177-S188

[22] Donofrio MT, Moon-Grady AJ, Hornberger LK, et al. Diagnosis and treatment of Fetal cardiac disease a scientific statement from the American Heart Association. Circulation 2014;**129**:00-00

[23] Tierney S, ElifSeda, et al. Asessment of progressive pathophysiology after early Pernatal diagnosis of Ebstein anomaly or tricuspid valve dysplasia. American Journal of Cardiology. 2017;**119**(1):106-111

[24] Boston US, Goldberg SP, Ward KE, et al. Complete repair of Ebstein anomaly in neonates and young infants: A 16-year follow-up. The Journal of Thoracic and Cardiovascular Surgery. 2011;**141**(5):1163-1169

[25] Danielson GK, Maloney JD, Devloo RA. Surgical repair of Ebstein's anomaly. Mayo Clinic Proceedings. 1979;**54**(3):185-192

[26] Knott-Craig CJ. Management of Neonatal Ebstein's anomaly. Operative Techiniques in Thoracic and Cardiovascular Surgery. 101-108

[27] da Silva JP, Baumgratz JF, da Fonseca L, et al. The cone reconstruction of the tricuspid valve in Ebstein's anomaly. The operation: Early and midterm results. The Journal of Thoracic and Cardiovascular Surgery. 2007;**133**(1):215-223

[28] Reemsten BL, Fagan BT, Wells WJ, Starnes VA. Current surgical therapy for Ebstein anomaly in neonates. The Journal of Thoracic and Cardiovascular Surgery. 2006 Dec; **132**(6):1285-1290

[29] Kumar SR, Kung G, Noh N, et al. Single-ventricle outcomes after neonatal palliation of severe Ebstein anomaly with modified Starnes procedure. Circulation. 2016;**134**:1257-1264

[30] Mizuno M, Hoashi T, Sakaguchi H, et al. Application of cone reconstruction for neonatal Ebstein anomaly or tricuspid valve dysplasia. The Annals of Thoracic Surgery. 2016;**101**:1811-1817

[31] Huang SC, Wu ET, Chen SJ, et al. Surgical strategy toward biventricular repair for severe Exstein anomaly in neonates and infancy. The Annals of Thoracic Surgery. 2017 Sep;**104**(3):917-925

[32] Davies RR, Jacobs ML PSK. Current Spectrum of surgical procedures performed for Ebstein's Malformaion: An analysis of the Society of Thoracic Surgeons congenital heart surgery database. The Annals of Thoracic Surgery. 2013;**96**:1703-1710

[33] Dearani J, Bacha E, da Silva JP. Cone reconstruction of the tricuspid valve for Ebstein's anomaly: Anatomic repair. Operative Techniques in Thoracic and Cardiovascular Surgery. 2008;**13**(1):109-125

[34] Sata S, Murin P, Hraska V. Cone reconstruction of Ebstein's anomaly in a neonate. The Annals of Thoracic Surgery. 2012;**94**:e99-100

[35] Knott-Craig CJ, Overholt ED, Ward KE, et al. Repair of Ebstein's anomaly in the symptomatic neonate: an evolution of technique with 7-year follow-up. Annals of Thoracic Surgery. 2002;**73**(6):1786-1792; discussion 1792-3

[36] Boston U, Singh G. Congenital Heart Surgery the Essentials. CVOffice; 2016

9

Management of Pregnancy and Delivery in Prenatally Diagnosed Congenital Anomalies

Diana Ramasauskaite

Abstract

Prenatal diagnosis of congenital anomalies provides valuable information and allows proper management of pregnancy and delivery. The common congenital anomalies are cardiovascular anomalies, congenital anomalies of the central nervous system, fetal thoracic anomalies, abdominal wall defects, kidney and urinary tract defects, and esophageal, gastrointestinal, and anorectal abnormalities. Different defects require particular assessment, evaluation and care. Pregnancy management mainly includes detection of the malformations, genetic assessment, ultrasound follow-ups and evaluation of fetal well-being as well as performing various invasive or non-invasive procedures. Managing delivery is also highly important and fetal anomaly specific. The main aspects of delivery management discussed in this chapter are delivery place, timing, route and delivery room care.

Keywords: congenital anomalies, management, pregnancy, delivery

1. Introduction

Prenatal diagnosis of congenital anomalies provides parents an opportunity to obtain prognostic information prior to birth, learn about treatment options before and after delivery, reach decisions concerning the management approach that is best for their family (e.g., whether to terminate pregnancy or undergo in utero intervention, if available; nonintervention), and plan for specific needs at birth [1].

2. Cardiovascular anomalies

Identification and management of fetal cardiac abnormalities are important because congenital anomalies are the leading cause of infant death and congenital heart disease accounts for 30–50% of these deaths [1]. The best time for evaluating the fetal heart anatomy is 18–22 weeks of gestation, because the fetal cardiac anatomy can be visualized well at this stage of pregnancy, a complete fetal anatomic survey can be performed, and there is time for further evaluation (e.g., echocardiogram, chromosomal microarray), if indicated, while the fetus is still periviable [2]. After 30 weeks of gestation, it can be difficult to obtain good images as the fetus becomes more crowded within the amniotic cavity. Fetal arrhythmias, myocarditis, cardiomyopathy, heart failure, valvular insufficiency or obstruction and cardiac tumors have variable onset. Fetal echocardiography should be performed in fetuses at a higher risk of congenital heart disease (**Table 1**).

Indications with higher risk profile (estimated >2% absolute risk)	Indications with lower risk profile (estimated >1 and <2% absolute risk)
- Maternal pregestational diabetes mellitus or diabetes mellitus diagnosed in the first trimester	- Maternal medications (anticonvulsants, lithium, vitamin A, paroxetine, NSAIDs in first/second trimester)
- Maternal phenylketonuria (uncontrolled)	- Congenital heart disease in second-degree relative of fetus.
- Maternal autoantibodies (SSA/SSB), especially if a previous child had SSA/SSB-related heart disease	- Fetal abnormality of the umbilical cord or placenta (e.g., single umbilical artery, agenesis of the ductus venosus)
- Maternal cardiac teratogens (e.g., thalidomide, angiotensin-converting enzyme [ACE] inhibitor, retinoic acid, nonsteroidal anti-inflammatory drugs [NSAIDs] in the third trimester)	- Fetal intra-abdominal venous anomaly
- Maternal first trimester rubella infection	
- Maternal infection with suspicion of fetal myocarditis because of poor contractility or effusions on standard four-chamber cardiac examination (e.g., coxsackie virus, adenovirus, cytomegalovirus)	
- Pregnancy conceived by assisted reproduction technology (ART)	
- Congenital heart disease in first-degree relative of fetus (maternal, paternal or sibling)	
- Disorder of first- or second-degree relative with Mendelian inheritance with congenital heart disease association (e.g., Noonan, tuberous sclerosis, Holt-Oram, velocardiofacial [DiGeorge] syndrome/22q11 deletion, Alagille syndrome, Williams syndrome)	
- Fetal cardiac abnormality (structural, functional, arrhythmia) suspected on obstetrical ultrasound	
- Fetal noncardiac abnormality suspected on obstetrical ultrasound	
- Fetal chromosome testing reveals a genetic mutation, deletion, rearrangement, or aneuploidy	
- Fetal tachycardia or bradycardia or frequent or persistent irregular heart rhythm	
- Fetal increased nuchal translucency >95 percentile (≥3 mm) on first trimester ultrasound	
- Monochorionic twinning	
- Fetal hydrops or effusions	

Table 1. Indications for fetal echocardiography [2].

2.1. Pregnancy management

When a fetal cardiac abnormality is detected, additional evaluation and follow-up are indicated.

- Assessment for extracardiac anomalies. The extracardiac abnormalities are detected in 20–40% of all fetal cardiac anomalies [1, 3]; the cardiac anomalies are part of numerous fetal syndromes [4]. A systematic review and meta-analysis of studies of prenatal ultrasound and magnetic resonance imaging (MRI) found that brain abnormalities, delay in head growth, and brain-sparing were observed in subgroups of fetuses with congenital heart disease [5] However, the prognostic significance of these findings was unclear.

- Genetic assessment. Fetal genetic assessment is indicated because chromosome abnormalities are common in fetuses with cardiac defects, even when isolated [6]. Forty-one percent of fetuses with prenatally diagnosed structural cardiac defects had an abnormal karyotype [7]. The incidence in infants of congenital heart disease about 15% [6], it is higher because of in utero mortality in many cases, such as the lethal autosomal trisomies (e.g., trisomy 9 or 16). The risk of fetal aneuploidy varies depending on the malformation. For example (risk percent, [2]): atrioventricular septal defect (46–73%), truncus arteriosus (19–78%), double-outlet right ventricle/conotruncal malformations (6–43%), coarctation/arch interruption (5–37%), tricuspid valve dysplasia (including Ebstein malformation, 4–16%), tetralogy of Fallot (7–39 percent), hypoplastic left heart syndrome (HLHS, 4–9%), pulmonic stenosis/atresia with intact septum (1–12%), and transposition of great arteries (0%).

- Ultrasound follow-up. The necessity, timing, and frequency of serial assessment should be guided by the nature and severity of the lesion, presence of heart failure, anticipated timing and mechanism of progression, and the options available for prenatal and postpartum intervention [2]. At least one follow-up examination early in the third trimester is reasonable in order to look for abnormalities that progressed in severity or may not have been detectable earlier in gestation and have peripartum clinical implications. Some causes of progressive fetal cardiac dysfunction include worsening valvular insufficiency or obstruction, increasing obstruction to blood flow in the great arteries, and development or worsening of myocarditis or cardiomyopathy, arrhythmias, or cardiac tumors [2]. Intrauterine fetal growth restriction is more prevalent in these fetuses with congenital heart disease [8].

- Referral to a pediatric cardiologist. The purpose is to educate the patient about the suspected diagnosis and discuss management options before and after delivery, including the preferred site for delivery [1].

- Evaluation of fetal well-being. Fetuses with cardiac structural anomalies, functional disorders, or arrhythmias that have the potential to compromise tissue oxygen delivery are generally followed with antepartum testing, with intervention if results are abnormal. In one retrospective cohort study, fetuses with a genetic syndrome, extracardiac anomaly, or severe valvular regurgitation were at increased risk for fetal demise: 15/197 (7.6%) fetuses with one or more of these risk factors died in utero versus 3/270 (1%) fetuses without any of these risk factors [9]. Six of the 22 fetal deaths occurred at 20–23 weeks and 16 occurred at 26–41 weeks (including three deaths at 37, 39, and 41 weeks). However, there is no strong evidence of the value of this practice and antepartum fetal testing with the nonstress test, biophysical profile, or fetal movement count has not been tested specifically in this clinical setting. The type of test depends on the underlying abnormality; for example, the biophysical profile is particularly useful in fetuses with arrhythmias and provides an opportunity to monitor for development or progression of hydrops in any fetus with severely altered hemodynamics.

- Fetal therapy. Transplacental medical therapy can improve the prognosis of some fetal arrhythmias [1]. Invasive in utero cardiac intervention (aortic or pulmonary balloon valvuloplasty, atrial needle septoplasty) may improve the prognosis of some lesions, such as HLHS or severe valvular abnormalities (severe mitral regurgitation, aortic stenosis, pulmonary atresia). Current evidence on the effectiveness of prenatal intervention for CHD derives mostly from case reports and a few larger series; although the results of the meta-analysis are encouraging in terms of perinatal survival, they should be interpreted with caution when comparing with procedures performed after delivery [10].

2.2. Delivery management

- Delivery place. Delivery should be planned at a facility with the appropriate level of care for the mother and neonate. Neonates with ductal-dependent lesions and most with critical cardiac lesions should be delivered at a facility with a level III NICU and pediatric cardiology expertise. If this is not feasible, transport arrangements should be established in advance of delivery [1].

Specialized delivery room care is recommended for fetuses with:	- d-transposition of the great arteries
	- sustained or uncontrolled tachyarrhythmias with heart failure or hydrops fetalis
Specialized delivery room care planning is reasonable for fetuses with:	- hypoplastic left heart syndrome (HLHS) with restrictive or intact atrial septum and abnormal pulmonary vein flow (pulmonary vein forward/reversed flow ratio < 3) or abnormal hyperoxia test in the third trimester
	- complete heart block and low ventricular rate, cardiac dysfunction, or hydrops fetalis
Specialized delivery room care planning may be considered in fetuses with:	- tetralogy of Fallot with absent pulmonary valve
	- Ebstein anomaly with hydrops fetalis
	- total anomalous pulmonary venous return, obstructed
Specialized delivery room care is not needed for fetuses with:	- mild tetralogy of Fallot, ventricular septal defect, atrioventricular septal defect
	- shunt lesions
	- most ductal-dependent lesions, but initiation of prostaglandin E1 may be indicated in neonatal intensive care unit
	- controlled arrhythmias

Table 2. Need for specialized delivery room care in specific anomalies.

- Timing and route. Cesarean delivery is performed for standard obstetrical indications, as there is no evidence that route of delivery of fetuses with congenital heart disease affects outcome [11]. Based on observational data, induction of labor or scheduled cesarean before 39 weeks of gestation is not recommended in the absence of standard maternal or fetal concerns about well-being, as even early term delivery has been associated with worse outcomes after neonatal cardiac surgery [2, 12]. One exception may be single ventricle defects, where earlier delivery may be beneficial [13].

- Delivery room care. Risk assessment for anticipated compromise in the delivery room or during the first few days of life is disease-specific (**Table 2**, [2]).

3. Congenital anomalies of the central nervous system (CNS)

Malformations of the central nervous system (CNS) are among the most common types of major congenital anomalies. Ultrasound examination is an effective modality for prenatal diagnosis of these anomalies. Poor timing of the examination, rather than poor sensitivity, can be an important factor in failing to detect a CNS abnormality [14]. Ideally, pregnancies at increased risk of fetal CNS anomalies and those with suspicious findings on a basic examination should undergo fetal neurosonography performed by clinicians with expertise in this area. Magnetic resonance imaging (MRI) is an option for further evaluation in cases of diagnostic uncertainty when additional information will influence subsequent management of the pregnancy [15].

3.1. Holoprosencephaly

Holoprosencephaly is a fetal anomaly that cannot be altered or treated. Elective termination of pregnancy is recommended if the diagnosis is made early (till 22–24 weeks of gestation under the pregnancy termination law in different countries). Because approximately 30–50% of fetuses with this anomaly have chromosomal abnormalities, prenatal karyotype is recommended. A family history (the familial recurrences have been reported), the history of current pregnancy (exposure to ethanol, salicylates) should be obtained, the evaluation for cytomegalovirus should be done. If the parents choose the conservative management, there is no fetal intervention for this condition and the cesarean delivery should be considered only for maternal indications [16].

3.2. Agenesis of the corpus callosum

During routine screening for fetal anomalies at 20–22 weeks of gestation, the two most important clues that the corpus callosum needs further assessment to exclude a callosal abnormality are (1) non-visualization of the cavum septi pellucidi and (2) ventriculomegaly (lateral ventricles measuring >10 mm). The cause of this anomaly may be genetic, infectious (TORCH infections and Zika virus), vascular, or toxic (alcohol—fetal alcohol syndrome). Callosal dysgenesis was isolated in only 24% of the fetuses, and isolated callosal abnormalities are associated with normal neurodevelopmental outcome in approximately two-thirds of fetuses [17].

3.2.1. Pregnancy management

- Genetic assessment. Genetic factors are most common. Among the genetic causes, "syndromic" diagnosis is made in 30–45% of cases and a monogenic cause can be identified in 20–35%. Over 200 genetic syndromes, many of which may have variable phenotype, include disorder of the corpus callosum as a feature.

- Magnetic resonance imaging (MRI) is most helpful after the 20th week of gestation, since about 20% of apparently isolated cases diagnosed by ultrasound have associated CNS anomalies on MRI [18].

- Evaluation of fetal well-being. If an isolated agenesis of corpus callosum is detected and the chromosomes are normal, the usual standard pregnancy management should be recommended.

3.2.2. Delivery management

Vaginal delivery is recommended unless is significant hydrocephalus with macrocephaly. Delivery prior to term is not advisable [16].

3.3. Dandy-Walker malformation

'Isolated' Dandy-Walker malformation (DWM) in the light of recent literature, which has demonstrated a potential good clinical and intellectual outcome of fetuses presenting with DWM characterized by partial vermian agenesis and absence of associated anatomical anomalies [19].

3.3.1. Pregnancy management

- Assessment for associated CNS and extra-CNS anomalies. The presence of the additional anomalies adversely affects survival and prognosis for the infant and child with DWM. The risk of associated intracranial anomalies appears to be 20–60%, and in this situation, the mental retardation and perinatal mortality are increased [16].

- Genetic assessment. In the syndromic form of DWM, malformations of the heart, face, limbs, or gastrointestinal or genitourinary system may be present. DWM may occur as part of a Mendelian disorder (e.g., Meckel syndrome), a chromosomal aneuploidy (e.g., 45X, triploidy), environmental exposures (e.g., rubella, alcohol), a multifactorial etiology (e.g., congenital heart defect, neural tube defects), or as a sporadic defect (e.g., holoprosencephaly).

- Evaluation of fetal well-being. The option for elective termination of pregnancy is offered for parents if the diagnosis of DWM with associated CNS anomalies is made early. If the diagnosis is made in the third trimester, conservative management is recommended. In most cases, the cyst, ventricular dilatation, and cisterna magna enlargement occur slowly, rarely severe or rapidly increasing ventriculomegaly needs for obstetrical intervention [16]. There is no fetal intervention for DWM.

3.3.2. Delivery management

The cesarean delivery should be considered only for maternal indications.

3.4. Anencephaly

3.4.1. Pregnancy management

Anencephaly is the most common neural tube defect (NTD) [20]. The anencephalic fetus can be definitively identified by the 12th postmenstrual week by TVS; although in some cases, this diagnosis has been made as early as 9–10 postmenstrual weeks [21]. Early diagnosis can be made if the cranium is examined carefully at the time of nuchal translucency measurement [22].

Up to 75% of anencephalic infants are stillborn. Liveborn infants generally die within hours but occasionally survive for a few days or weeks. There are no neurosurgical management options. In most developed countries where abortion is legal, these pregnancies are interrupted earlier [23]. Because of their poor prognosis, anencephalic infants have been considered as potential organ donors for transplantation. The clinical cases reported that anencephalic infants are not good candidates for organ donation because they do not generally meet criteria for brain death until their clinical condition has declined to the point where the solid organs are damaged [24]. Polyhydramnios develops in up to 50% of the cases during the second and third trimester due to decreased fetal swallowing, but is not present during the first trimester [20].

Prevention is the most important aspect of management of anencephaly. Periconceptional folic acid supplementation is recommended for all women who are pregnant or who may become pregnant. Higher doses of folic acid supplements are usually recommended for women who are taking anticonvulsant drugs or who have had a previous pregnancy affected by a NTD.

3.4.2. Management of labor

Because polyhydramnios is often associated with this condition, the rate of premature labor is increasing. Labor and delivery are frequently associated with an unstable fetal position, dystocia of labor, placental abruption, and postpartum hemorrhage. The cesarean delivery should be considered only for maternal indications.

3.5. Exencephaly

Exencephaly has been detected as early as the 10th postmenstrual week. In the second trimester, the usual appearance of the cranium encasing the brain is lost. The exposed brain has a heterogeneous appearance and is not covered by the cranium. Although the cranial vault is absent, the fetal facial bones can be clearly visualized. Maternal serum alpha-fetoprotein levels are highly elevated.

3.5.1. Pregnancy management

Exencephaly is a lethal condition, the termination of pregnancy should be recommended for parents. Typically, exencephaly is not associated with chromosomal abnormalities, but, because of the severity of the defect, a chromosome analysis should be performed to permit accurate genetic counseling [16].

3.5.2. Delivery management

The cesarean delivery should be considered only for maternal indications. There are no indications for resuscitation of the newborn.

3.6. Encephalocele

3.6.1. Pregnancy management

Encephalocele can be diagnosed at 11–14 weeks during sonographic screening for aneuploidy.

- Genetic assessment. Cephalocele usually occurs as an isolated lesion, but may be a part of a syndrome such as Meckel (or Meckel-Gruber) or Walker-Warburg syndrome in a small percentage of cases. Both syndromes are autosomal recessive.

- Assessment for associated anomalies. Detailed sonography or MRI should be performed to verify the diagnosis and to search for associated anomalies.

Obstetrical management depends on the size of defect, the gestational age at diagnosis, and the presence or absence of associated anomalies. Prognosis depends on (1) the presence and amount of brain in the herniated sac (this is the most important consideration) and (2) the presence or absence of hydrocephalus, microcephaly, and other anomalies. If the encephalocele is diagnosed at less than 22–24 weeks of gestation, the termination of the pregnancy can be offered to the parents. If the pregnancy is not terminated, the consultations of neurosurgeon, neonatologist, and medical genetics are recommended [16].

Fetuses with neural tube defects or central nervous system abnormalities typically remain active; however, the quality of fetal movement is often different from that in normal fetuses [20]. The fetus with an encephalocele did not respond to repeated vibroacoustic stimulation (VAS) with a movement or fetal heart rate (FHR) acceleration [25].

3.6.2. Delivery management

When diagnosed prenatally, vaginal delivery may be safe if the lesion is relatively small. Large encephaloceles require cesarean section. Neonates with encephalocele should be delivered at a facility with a level III NICU. Surgical treatment is appropriate in most cases unless the encephalocele is massive and there is severe microcephaly or other lethal anomalies. The procedure basically consists of removing the overlying sac and closing the defect including the dural defect [26]. In patients with basal encephaloceles or cerebrospinal fluid (CSF) leakage, prompt closure is important to reduce the risk of infection. Patients with hydrocephalus usually undergo ventriculoperitoneal shunt placement prior to encephalocele repair to prevent postoperative CSF leaks.

3.7. Iniencephaly

3.7.1. Pregnancy management

Iniencephaly is a rare, lethal developmental anomaly. Associated malformations occur in up to 84% of cases and include hydrocephaly, microcephaly, ventricular atresia, holoprosencephaly, polymicrogyria, agenesis of the cerebellar vermis, occipital encephalocele, diaphragmatic hernia, thoracic cage deformities, urinary tract anomalies, cleft lip and palate, omphalocele, and polyhydramnios [20]. The sonographic diagnosis has been made as early as 12.5–13 postmenstrual weeks. Detailed sonography or MRI should be performed to verify the diagnosis and to search for associated anomalies. If the iniencephaly is diagnosed at less than 22–24 weeks of gestation, the termination of the pregnancy can be offered to the parents.

3.7.2. Delivery management

The presence of the hyperextended fetal head might cause dystocia. There is no indication for aggressive resuscitation of neonates [16].

3.8. Spinal dysraphism and the Arnold-Chiari malformation

3.8.1. Pregnancy management

Assessment for other abnormalities should be performed by the detailed sonography. Associated brain abnormalities include hydrocephaly, relative microcephaly, agenesis of the corpus callosum, and diastematomyelia. Non-CNS anomalies consist of congenital scoliosis or kyphosis and hip deformities [20]. There is a high prevalence of genetic abnormalities among fetuses with NTDs, especially in the presence of other congenital anomalies so microarray should be offered. The diagnostic sensitivity of prenatal sonography for detection of myelomeningocele in a high risk population is about 97–98% with 100% specificity [27]. Determining the site and extent of the spinal lesion is important because these features correlate with neurologic outcome; more severe neurologic dysfunction is associated with higher and larger lesions. Sonographic diagnosis of open spina bifida typically occurs during the second trimester of the pregnancy.

When the diagnosis of NTD is confirmed, the parents should be offered the opportunity to discuss the long-term prognosis for a child with multidisciplinary team (neonatologist, medical geneticist, pediatric neurologist, pediatric neurosurgeon, pediatric urologist, pediatric orthopedic surgeon). Long-term prognosis is related to the location of the NTD—the lower the defect, the better the prognosis [16]. In fetuses with myelomeningoceles, higher and larger lesions on MRI were significantly associated with full-time wheelchair use. High lesion level was associated with dysphagia. The absence of a covering membrane was associated with scoliosis and high-risk bladder dysfunction [28]. If the diagnosis is at less than 22–24 weeks of gestation, the opportunity of pregnancy termination can be offered to the parents. During prenatal counseling, discussion with the parents includes the natural history of myelomeningocele and the prenatal management decisions, including termination of the pregnancy, pursuit of additional prenatal testing, choice of delivery setting, and, when applicable, the possibility of fetal surgery. The postnatal management choices are also discussed, including surgical closure of the defect and possible need for ventriculoperitoneal shunt placement. Longitudinal follow-up after prenatal diagnosis of myelomeningocele suggests that approximately 60–70% of pregnancies end in termination or fetal demise [29, 30].

- Fetal intervention. Fetal surgery for myelomeningocele can arrest leakage of spinal fluid from the back and might therefore prevent or reverse herniation of the hindbrain (Chiari II malformation) and hydrocephalus [31]. Prenatal surgery for myelomeningocele reduced the need for shunting and improved motor outcomes at 30 months but was associated with maternal and fetal risks [32]. These benefits occurred despite a higher risk of preterm delivery and pulmonary complications among infants undergoing fetal surgery and of obstetrical complications, including placental abruption, dehiscence of the hysterotomy site, and maternal transfusion at delivery [32, 33]. Because fetal surgery is associated with risks of fetal and maternal complications, the family should be informed about the option of prenatal surgery, including the uncertainty regarding whether the risks of the procedure are outweighed by the potential benefits, particularly since long-term outcomes are not clearly known. Women with pregnancies complicated by fetal myelomeningocele who meet established criteria for in utero repair should be counseled in a nondirective fashion regarding all management options, including the possibility of open maternal-fetal surgery. Maternal-fetal surgery for myelomeningocele repair should be offered only to carefully selected patients at facilities with an appropriate level of personnel and resources [34].

3.8.2. Delivery management

For infants with a prenatal diagnosis of myelomeningocele who do not undergo fetal intervention, delivery should occur at a center with a level III NICU, pediatric neurosurgery services, and other personnel experienced in the neonatal management of these infants. Latex-free gloves and equipment should be used during delivery and subsequent care of the infant because patients with myelomeningocele are at risk for developing life-threatening latex allergy.

Term delivery is preferable, but increasing ventriculomegaly with macrocephaly on prenatal ultrasound may necessitate preterm delivery. Fetuses presenting in the breech position are typically delivered by cesarean section. The optimal route of delivery of a fetus presenting in the vertex position is controversial. Vaginal delivery is reasonable if the head is normal size, the meningocele is unlikely to cause dystocia, and there are no obstetrical indications for cesarean [35].

3.9. Fetal cerebral ventriculomegaly

3.9.1. Pregnancy management

Fetal cerebral ventriculomegaly is a relatively common finding on second trimester obstetrical ultrasound examination. Many cases are associated with other abnormal findings, but in some fetuses, ventriculomegaly is the only abnormality [36]. Most children with isolated, mild ventriculomegaly have a normal outcome. The risk of abnormal outcome increases with the severity of ventriculomegaly, progression of ventriculomegaly, and presence of other anomalies. After ventriculomegaly is identified, further management involves identifying whether additional abnormalities (CNS and non-CNS) are present, diagnostic evaluation for the most common causes of ventriculomegaly, and counseling patients about the prognosis and potential pregnancy interventions. If the etiology of ventriculomegaly has been determined (e.g., trisomy, CMV) or associated malformations are identified, the parents can be given more specific information. Before viability, pregnancy termination is an option and should be offered.

- Assessment for associated CNS and extra-CNS anomalies. Associated abnormalities have been reported in 10–76% of cases [36, 37]. Identification of these abnormalities helps in determining the cause of ventriculomegaly and the prognosis. Fetal MRI can be used to identify underlying CNS abnormalities not detected by sonography. Because CNS infection can result in ventriculomegaly, it is important to look for characteristic sonographic findings of fetal infection, such as intracerebral and periventricular calcifications, hepatic calcifications, hepatosplenomegaly, ascites, and polyhydramnios.

- Evaluation for infection. Tests for CMV infection, toxoplasmosis, Zika virus infection, and lymphocytic choriomeningitis virus infection should be recommended. Sporadic cases of ventriculomegaly associated with other viruses have also been reported (mumps enterovirus 71 (EV71), parainfluenza virus type 3, parvovirus B19) [36]. PCR for CMV and toxoplasmosis should also be obtained when amniocentesis is performed. If the patient declines amniocentesis or karyotyping has been done previously, maternal serology is used to identify an infectious etiology. However, serology is neither as sensitive nor as specific as PCR on amniotic fluid, thus amniotic fluid PCR is the preferred method of evaluation for infection [36].

- Genetic assessment. Fetuses with apparently isolated mild ventriculomegaly in 4.7% were found to have an abnormal karyotype [38]. The risk is higher with severe ventriculomegaly or associated abnormalities.

- Follow-up evaluation. Follow-up ultrasound examinations are obtained to look for regression or progression of ventriculomegaly and to re-evaluate for anomalies. Early isolated mild ventriculomegaly may resolve by the third trimester; progression occurs in 16% of cases and has been associated with a worse outcome [36, 39]. Follow-up ultrasounds have detected fetal abnormalities not detected on the initial scan in 13% of cases [36]. Therefore, at least one additional detailed ultrasound examination should be performed between 28 and 34 weeks of gestation to look for CNS and non-CNS abnormalities and regression or progression of dilatation. Antepartum fetal testing has no proven benefit in pregnancies with isolated fetal ventriculomegaly in the absence of other findings, such as intrauterine growth restriction or oligohydramnios.

- Fetal intervention. Intrauterine treatment with ventriculoamniotic shunting was performed in the 1980s. The expert consensus at that time was that these results did not represent an improvement in outcome over expectant management, which led to a de facto moratorium on such procedures [40]. At present, however, such procedures are investigational [36].

3.9.2. Delivery management

Ventriculomegaly may or may not be accompanied by macrocephaly. Most infants with ventriculomegaly have a normal head circumference (HC), there is no increased risk of cephalopelvic disproportion, and cesarean delivery is not required except for standard obstetric complications. When the HC exceeds 40 cm, abdominal delivery should be considered.

Cephalocentesis, which almost always results in fetal death, is rarely used to decompress the head, allow vaginal delivery, and avoid maternal morbidity from cesarean delivery, in cases in which the neurological prognosis is so dismal (trisomy 13 or 18 or lethal co-existent anomalies) [41].

4. Fetal thoracic anomalies

4.1. Congenital diaphragmatic hernia

4.1.1. Pregnancy management

Over the past 20 years, prenatal detection of congenital diaphragmatic hernia (CDH) has improved worldwide, reaching up to 60% in Europe. Pulmonary hypoplasia and persistent pulmonary hypertension are the two main determinants of neonatal mortality and morbidity, so new tools have been focused on their evaluation. Fetal surgery for severe cases requires proper evaluation of the prognosis of fetuses with CDH [42]. After CDH is identified, further management involves referral to a tertiary center for confirmation of the diagnosis, assessment of severity and associated anatomic and genetic abnormalities, multidisciplinary counseling about options and prognosis, and planning further management. Management may be expectant with prenatal referral to a center with expertise in caring for these infants, termination of pregnancy, or fetal intervention [43]. The mean gestational age at diagnosis is about 24 weeks. Polyhydramnios may be present due to esophageal compression. Hydrops fetalis can occur from mediastinal shift and compression of the great vessels.

- Assessment for associated anomalies. Ultrafast fetal MRI to look for associated abnormalities and liver herniation and to estimate lung volumes and fetal echocardiography should be performed.

CDH can be an isolated anomaly, part of a syndrome, or nonsyndromic but associated with other abnormalities. Approximately 50–70% of cases of CDH are isolated. Pulmonary hypoplasia, intestinal malrotation, and cardiac dextroposition are due to the hemodynamic or mechanical consequences of CDH; thus, they are usually considered part of the CDH sequence and do not negate the designation 'isolated CDH.' The other 30–50% of cases are called 'complex', 'nonisolated', or 'syndromic' CDH (CDH+) because they are associated with additional abnormalities, including major structural malformations, chromosomal abnormalities, and/or single gene disorders. Malformations occur in all major organ systems, with no specific pattern [43]. An underlying syndrome is present in approximately 10% of CDH cases occurring with associated anomalies [43]. CDH is a prominent finding in the Fryns phenotype; facial dysmorphology, distal digital hypoplasia, and cardiac/renal/brain anomalies can also occur. CDH and diaphragmatic eventration are also an occasional component of many other syndromes, including Apert, Killian/Teschler-Nicola (Pallister-Killian), CHARGE, Coffin-Siris, Goltz, Perlman, Swyer, Brachmann-Cornelia De Lange, Goldenhar sequence, Beckwith Wiedemann, Simpson-Golabi-Behmel, Donnai-Barrow, Mathew-Wood, Jarcho-Levin, Fraser, Stickler, Pierre Robin, and others [43, 44].

Associated anomalies are most common with bilateral CDH and in stillborn infants with CDH, where the prevalence is as high as 95% [43]. Anomalies in stillborn infants with CDH primarily consist of neural tube defects (anencephaly, myelomeningocele, hydrocephalus, and encephaloceles) and cardiac defects (ventriculoseptal defects, vascular rings, and coarctation of the aorta) [45].

- Genetic assessment. Chromosomal anomalies are identified in 10–20% of prenatally identified cases; the most common diagnoses include trisomies 18, 13, and 21 [43, 46]. Other karyotype abnormalities, such as monosomy X, tetrasomy 12 p (isochromosome 12p), partial trisomy 5, partial trisomy 20, and polyploidies, have also been reported [43, 47].

- Evaluation of prognostic factors for survival. Prognosis is worse in the setting of an abnormal chromosomal microarray, severe associated anomalies, right-sided defect, liver herniation, and lower fetal lung volume [43, 48]. The lung area to head circumference ratio (LHR) is more predictive of morbidity than mortality. A large defect is more likely to result in pulmonary hypoplasia and death than a small defect. The size of the defect is not measurable prenatally, so the presence of liver herniation and fetal lung volume measurements serves as a proxy for defect size [43]. Several other clinical findings for survival have not been confirmed (early gestational age at diagnosis, severe mediastinal shift, polyhydramnios, a small lung-thorax transverse area ratio, left ventricle/right ventricle index, left heart hypoplasia, and the stomach in the chest) [43].

Liver herniation is the most reliable prenatal predictor of postnatal survival. A systematic review of studies that used ultrasound or MRI to evaluate outcome of fetuses with liver herniation included 710 fetuses and reported significantly higher survival rate in fetuses without herniation (74% versus 45% with herniation) [49]. Ultrafast fetal MRI using rapid HASTE technique is the most powerful tool to accurately demonstrate liver herniation [50]. Ultrasound can be useful; in particular, color flow Doppler can visualize bowing of the ductus venosus to the left of the midline or coursing of the portal branches or hepatic veins to the lateral segment of the left lobe above the diaphragm; however, ultrasound has not always accurately demonstrated liver herniation in the fetus with left-sided CDH [43, 50].

Absolute or relative fetal lung volume appears to be useful for predicting survival, but the optimum equation has not been determined [43, 51]. Several small studies have suggested that postnatal survival is poor when fetal lung volume measured by MRI is less than about 30% of expected lung volume for gestational age and especially when <15% [43]. Lung volume can also be assessed using 3D sonography, but MRI may be more reliable.

Right- versus left-sided lesion. Right-sided CDH have a poorer outcome than that reported for fetuses with left-sided CDH with similar lung size before birth [52].

Lung area to head circumference ratio (LHR) is an estimate of contralateral lung size and mediastinal shift at the level of the atria on transverse scan of the fetal thorax. Although there is a significant correlation between LHR and survival, the lower limit of LHR compatible with survival is dropping, so the test is less predictive than in the past [43, 53]. LHR is now more indicative of morbidity than mortality [43]. In left CDH, the LHR is calculated using a two-dimensional perpendicular linear measurement of right lung area (in square millimeters) divided by the head circumference (in millimeters) to minimize lung size differences owing to gestational age [43]. Measurement of fetal lung volume is much more useful than LHR in fetuses without liver herniation [54]. Because lung growth is four times greater than head growth during pregnancy [55], some experts suggest that the LHR should be expressed as a function of gestational age (observed [O]/expected [E] LHR). The O/E LHR can be calculated using a formula specifically developed for this measuring technique and has been validated in fetuses with unilateral isolated CDH in terms of both mortality and morbidity [53]. An online calculator is available (www.totaltrial.eu). O/E LHR is considered extreme if <15%, severe at 15–25%, moderate at 26–35%, and mild if 36–45% [44].

- Fetal interventions. Fetal endoscopic tracheal occlusion (FETO) is an investigational procedure for treatment of isolated severe congenital diaphragmatic hernia to prevent or reverse pulmonary hypoplasia and restore adequate lung growth for neonatal survival. The rationale for this approach is that the dynamics of fetal lung fluid can dramatically affect lung growth [43]. Under normal circumstances, the lungs are net producers of amniotic fluid with lung liquid volume and intratracheal pressure maintained at constant values by fetal laryngeal mechanisms [43]. Prenatal tracheal occlusion (TO) obstructs the normal egress of lung fluid during pulmonary development, increasing transpulmonic pressure and resulting in large fluid-filled lungs. Lack of lung expansion 2 and 7 days after TO is a poor prognostic sign and may indicate that the occlusion is inadequate [56]. Techniques to achieve minimally invasive fetoscopic reversible fetal TO have been developed to decrease the risks of preterm labor and restore surfactant deficiency [43]. A percutaneous procedure under local anesthesia, with fetal pain relief and immobilization, is possible [57]. Fetal TO in severe CDH is associated with a high incidence of PPROM and preterm delivery but a substantial improvement in survival. Smaller and fewer trocars were utilized in another study, resulting in a lower rate of preterm rupture of membranes and preterm delivery [58].

Important factors in offering prenatal therapy continue to be, first and foremost, determining which fetuses have a poor prognosis. The optimal timing, duration, and release of occlusion in humans are not known. The Eurofetus group has had early success with fetal TO [59]. The insertion of the balloon at 26–28 weeks for severe cases and 30–32 weeks for moderate cases is recommended. Ideally, the occlusion is reversed before delivery at 34 weeks, usually by fetoscopy or ultrasound-guided puncture.

The FETO Consortium subsequently reported the outcome of 210 consecutive procedures [57]. Compared with the outcome of expectantly managed cases enrolled in their registry, FETO increased survival in severe cases with left CDH from 24–49% and right CDH from 0–35% (p < 0.001) [57]. However, at least 10 deaths attributed to difficulty with balloon removal before or at the time of emergent delivery have been reported [60]. The Eurofetus consortium also noted that preterm delivery, usually due to premature rupture of membranes, is a common complication and occurred in 17% of cases within 3 weeks of the procedure [43]. FETO has resulted in few clinical side effects on the developing trachea, except in very early occlusions and complications arising at the time of removal [43]. Neonates have tracheomegaly, which does not seem to have a clinical impact other than a barking cough on effort. The Tracheal Occlusion to Accelerate Lung Growth (TOTAL) trial is ongoing in Europe and feasibility studies for FETO are ongoing at several North American fetal centers [43].

- Follow-up assessment. There are no data from well-designed studies on which to base recommendations for antepartum obstetrical management. The intrauterine risk of fetal demise is 2–8%, but higher when other anomalies are present [43]. Twice-weekly nonstress testing or biophysical profile testing at 33–34 weeks should be offered [43]. Ultrasound examinations at 28, 30, 32, and 34–35 weeks of gestation to assess fetal growth and amniotic fluid volume. Polyhydramnios may develop at 28–32 weeks if fetal swallowing is impaired, and oligohydramnios may develop if the fetus is compromised later in gestation. Signs of secondary complications, such as particulate meconium in fluid, dilated stomach in chest, effusions, or ascites, may lead us to deliver the fetus preterm. Fetal growth restriction or oligohydramnios may also lead us to deliver the fetus early. Antenatal glucocorticoids are given, if appropriate, to decrease morbidity from preterm delivery as for standard indication [43].

4.1.2. Delivery management

The optimal mode and gestational age for delivery of an infant diagnosed prenatally with CDH is uncertain [43]. A planned induction of labor between 38 and 39 weeks of gestation is suggested so that the fetus is monitored from the earliest stage of labor and so pediatric surgery and neonatology services are prepared to care for the infant. The fetal lung maturity prior to delivery should not be assessed [43]. Up to 50% of cases require extracorporeal membrane oxygenation (ECMO); therefore, the delivery at a tertiary center with ECMO capability is recommended [43]. Cesarean delivery is performed for standard obstetrical indications [43].

4.2. Congenital pulmonary airway malformation

4.2.1. Pregnancy management

Prenatal diagnosis of congenital pulmonary airway malformation (CPAM) has increased with widespread use of prenatal ultrasonography and magnetic resonance (MR) imaging. When CPAM is diagnosed, the quantitative evaluation helps predict the prenatal course of the disease and should include the following [61]:

1. Congenital pulmonary airway malformation volume ratio (CVR)—Obtained by calculating the volume of the lung mass using the formula for the volume of an oval and normalizing it by gestational age. To normalize by gestational age, the lung mass volume should be divided by the head circumference. CVR = height x anteroposterior diameter x transverse diameter x 0.52 (constant)/head circumference.

2. Mass-to-thorax ratio (MTR)—The ratio between the transverse diameter of the mass and the transverse diameter of the thorax. It is measured on an axial image of the chest, where the four-chamber view of the heart is present.

3. Observed to expected lung-to-head ratio (o/e LHR)—Initially described as a predictor of outcome in congenital diaphragmatic hernia.

The prenatal course depends on the gestational age, size of the mass, amount of mediastinal shift, fetal hemodynamics, and associated anomalies, more than the type of lesion [61]. About 50% of masses persist to delivery [62]. Fifteen percent of these masses decrease in size during the late second and the third trimesters; the majority have a relative decrease in size due to normal fetal thoracic growth, but a few increase in size [61]. It is difficult to predict at the time of the initial ultrasound whether lesions will regress, stabilize, or continue to grow and lead to significant problems, including hydrops, need for surgical intervention or postnatal respiratory assistance, or death. The use of CVR, MTR, and, to a lesser degree, o/e LHR helps better identify patients at risk [61, 63]. A CVR >1.6 is predictive of risk for hydrops, respiratory distress at birth, and probable need for early surgery [61], whereas a CVR <0.91 at presentation predicts a favorable outcome so follow-up examinations can be less frequent [61, 63]. A MTR <0.51 suggests the fetus is at low risk for developing complications [61, 63]. In the absence of hydrops, the prognosis is good with reported live birth rates ≥95% [61].

- Assessment for associated anomalies. A comprehensive fetal survey, including fetal echocardiography, should be performed as 10–20% of fetuses with CPAM have associated congenital abnormalities, such as esophageal atresia with tracheoesophageal fistula, bilateral renal agenesis or dysgenesis, intestinal atresia, other pulmonary malformations, and diaphragmatic, cardiac, central nervous system, and bony anomalies [61]. Fetal echocardiography is recommended in all patients at time of diagnosis to rule out congenital cardiac anomalies.

- Follow-up assessment. All patients should have serial prenatal follow-up examinations every 1 to 4 weeks to assess change in size of the lung mass, change in CVR, and development of polyhydramnios and hydrops [61]. The frequency depends on the gestational age and CVR. Closer follow-up should be performed in those patients at high risk of developing hydrops (CVR ≥1.6, age < 26 weeks), whereas the interval between examinations can be lengthened if the CPAM is very small, CVR is <0.91 [63]. The presence of hydrops is a sign for impending fetal demise and thus it is an indication for fetal intervention [61]. The recommendation of proceeding with fetal intervention is based on results from small case series showing good survival (>90%) if hydrops resolves [61].

For fetuses greater than 32–34 weeks of age, early delivery with immediate postnatal resection is a reasonable option [61]. Ex utero intrapartum therapy (EXIT) has been used to stabilize fetuses with large lesions expected to have difficulty breathing at delivery [64].

For gestations between 20 and 32 weeks, several interventions with the goal of improving fetal hemodynamics and preventing lung hypoplasia have been described and appear to improve survival [61]. Drainage procedures are used for CPAMS with dominant cysts, while solid masses are treated by resection or ablation. Karyotype analysis is recommended prior to initiating fetal therapy [61]. All of the following interventions should be considered investigational.

Antenatal corticosteroids are the only medical treatment of CPAM. They are used primarily for treatment of microcystic CPAM, since these masses cannot be managed by minimally invasive procedures, but have been used for macrocystic disease, as well [61]. In uncontrolled studies, maternal steroid administration appeared to reverse hydrops and improve outcome [61]. Multiple courses of antenatal betamethasone for high-risk fetal CPAMs often result in favorable short-term outcomes without the need for open fetal resection. The fetuses who did not respond to a first course of steroids stabilized or improved (e.g., reduction in lesion size, resolving hydrops) after receiving two to four courses of therapy [65]. The median interval between the first and second courses of steroids was about 2 weeks (range 1–6 weeks) [61].

- Fetal intervention. Successful fetal surgery depends on surgical experience, optimal maternal anesthesia, uterine relaxation, hysterotomy, fetal exposure, and intraoperative fetal monitoring.

4.2.2. Drainage procedures

- Thoracentesis—For fetuses with large pleural effusions, thoracentesis to prevent pulmonary hypoplasia is possible, but rapid reaccumulation of fluid limits its usefulness [61]. The fluid should be sent for cell count to exclude an infectious etiology [61].

- Cyst aspiration should decompress a large macrocyst and reverse the mediastinal shift. Although fluid reaccumulation is common and limits its usefulness [61].

- Thoracoamniotic shunt provides a therapeutic option for select fetuses with large macrocystic lung lesions or pleural effusion at risk for hydrops and/or pulmonary hypoplasia. Survival following shunting depends on gestational age at birth, reduction in mass size, and hydrops resolution [66]. Complications include displacement or malfunction of the catheter, thrombus occlusion of the catheter, fatal fetal hemorrhage, procedure-related abruptio placentae, premature rupture of membranes, and preterm labor [61].

4.2.3. Surgical resection

For solid or mixed solid/cystic CPAM with a large solid component, in-utero open resection has been successfully performed. Following resection, hydrops resolves over 1 to 2 weeks with reversal of the mediastinal shift over 3 weeks [61]. Maternal-fetal surgery requiring hysterotomy appears to be associated with an increased risk of premature labor, premature rupture of membranes, and subsequent pregnancy (uterine dehiscence or rupture) [61]. Percutaneous laser ablation of solid CPAM has been reported in only a few case reports and further research is warranted [61].

4.2.4. Sclerotherapy

A single study described fetal sclerotherapy in three patients under 26 weeks with CPAM and hydrops, severe mediastinal shift, and polyhydramnios [67]. Sclerotherapy was performed with percutaneous injection of Ethamolin (ethanolamine oleate) or Polidocanol (aethoxysklerol) into the mass under ultrasound guidance using a 22-gauge needle [61]. Resolution of hydrops and of the mass effect was observed in all cases. The patients were delivered at term without complications. Further studies are indicated to assess the risks and benefits of this innovative technique [67].

4.2.5. Delivery management

If the lung mass has resolved or is small with no mediastinal shift or hydrops, CPAM itself is not an indication for early delivery or cesarean delivery [61]. Neonatal respiratory problems would be unlikely, but the delivery should be recommended in a tertiary care center. For fetuses with large masses that cause mediastinal shift and/or hydrops, delivery should be planned for a tertiary care center with an intensive care nursery capable of resuscitation of a neonate with respiratory difficulties, including capability of extracorporeal membrane oxygenation (ECMO), and with pediatric surgeons experienced in care of these infants [61]. If hydrops develops after 32 weeks of gestation, early delivery is recommended, possibly with the use of EXIT [61]. In EXIT, the fetus is partially delivered and intubated without clamping the umbilical cord. Uteroplacental blood flow and gas exchange are maintained by using inhalational agents to provide uterine relaxation and amnioinfusion to maintain uterine volume. This provides time for resection of the lung mass prior to complete delivery of the infant in rare instances or, more often, cannulation for extracorporeal membrane circulation, thus creating a controlled situation for delayed removal of the CPAM. Overall fetal survival of 90% has been reported [61].

4.3. Bronchopulmonary sequestration

4.3.1. Pregnancy management

Bronchopulmonary sequestration (BPS) is usually a small lesion and decreases in size in late gestation in about 75% of cases [68].

- Assessment of additional anomalies and genetic evaluation. When a lung mass is first identified, thorough assessment for additional anomalies is necessary. Intralobar sequestration is not associated with an increased risk of additional anomalies [68]. Extralobar BPS is associated with anomalies in up to two-thirds of cases [68]. These anomalies include chest wall and vertebral anomalies hindgut duplications, diaphragmatic hernia, congenital heart disease, and renal and intracranial abnormalities [68]. The incidence of chromosomal abnormalities is not increased above baseline in fetuses with BPS alone [68]. Karyotype analysis is recommended prior to initiating fetal therapy.

Parents should be counseled about the possible course of the BPS during pregnancy. At initial presentation in the early midtrimester, it is difficult to accurately predict what the outcome will be for an individual fetus, but some predictions are possible, e.g., a large BPS with hydrops in the second trimester is likely to do poorly [68].

- Follow-up assessment. All patients should have serial prenatal follow-up examinations to assess change in size of the lung mass and development of hydrops [68]. The frequency depends on the size of the lesion. The larger lesions should be followed more closely. The presence of hydrops is a sign of impending fetal demise and an indication for fetal intervention [68]. This recommendation is based on results from small case series showing higher survival rates if hydrops resolves [68]. Because hydrops is uncommon, fetal intervention is rarely required and is warranted only in cases where the fetus is severely compromised and remote from term. For fetuses greater than 32–34 weeks of age, early delivery with immediate postnatal resection is a reasonable option [68].

For gestations between 20 and 32 weeks, several interventions with the goal of improving fetal hemodynamics and preventing lung hypoplasia have been described and appear to improve survival [69]. These interventions should only be undertaken at centers experienced in fetal surgery. Prenatal intervention requires extensive counseling to the parents on the potential risks versus benefits of surgery.

- Fetal intervention. If the BPS is solid with a large pleural effusion, thoracentesis to prevent pulmonary hypoplasia is possible, but rapid reaccumulation of fluid limits its usefulness. It can be used as a temporizing maneuver to provide prognostic information about the possible result from placement of a thoracoamniotic shunt [68]. The fluid should be sent for cell count to exclude an infectious etiology [68]. Complications of shunts include displacement or malfunction of the catheter, thrombus occlusion of the catheter, fatal fetal hemorrhage, procedure-related abruptio placentae, premature rupture of membranes, and preterm labor [68]. There is also a risk of trauma to the fetal chest wall, especially if the procedure is performed before 20 weeks [68].

- In-utero open resection, percutaneous laser ablation of the feeding vessel has been successfully performed in several small studies [68]. Percutaneous ultrasound-guided fetal sclerotherapy has also been described [68]. Sometimes two procedures were necessary.

4.3.2. Delivery management

If the lung mass has resolved or is small with no mediastinal shift or hydrops, BPS itself is not an indication for early delivery or cesarean delivery [68]. Neonatal respiratory problems would be unlikely. For fetuses with large masses that cause mediastinal shift and/or hydrops, delivery should be planned for a tertiary care center with an intensive care nursery capable of resuscitation of a neonate with respiratory difficulties, including capability of extracorporeal membrane oxygenation (ECMO), and with pediatric surgeons experienced in care of these infants [68]. If hydrops develops after 32 weeks of gestation, early delivery is recommended, possibly with the use of EXIT. In EXIT, the fetus is partially delivered and intubated without clamping the umbilical cord. Uteroplacental blood flow and gas exchange are maintained by using inhalational agents to provide uterine relaxation and amnioinfusion to maintain uterine volume. This provides time for initiating extracorporeal membrane circulation to stabilize the infant, thus creating a controlled situation before resection of BPS in another operating room [68].

4.4. Congenital lobar emphysema

Congenital lobar emphysema (CLE) is a rare congenital malformation and sometimes is detected by prenatal ultrasonography. Lung lesions have increased echogenicity and/or a cystic appearance and usually can be differentiated from other congenital lung lesions [70]. A chest mass may even disappear on prenatal ultrasound and become apparent again on postnatal evaluation [70]. Predictors of severe respiratory distress or mortality include polyhydramnios, fetal hydrops, and lung to thorax transverse area ratio (L/T value) of less than 0.25 [70]. Approximately 25% of cases present at birth, 50% by 1 month of age, and nearly all by 6 months of age. Infants typically have tachypnea and increased work of breathing and often have cyanosis. Recurrent pneumonia or poor feeding with failure to thrive are less frequent presentations that may occur in milder forms [70].

4.5. Pulmonary agenesis

Any fetus with suspected bilateral pulmonary agenesis should have a detailed sonographic assessment to confirm the diagnosis. If the diagnosis is made till periviable pregnancy, the pregnancy termination is an option. If the diagnosis is made at a later gestational age, the delivery should be planned without monitoring for fetal distress [16].

5. Congenital abdominal wall defects

5.1. Gastroschisis

5.1.1. Pregnancy management

There is wide variability in the antenatal management of gastroschisis due to a lack of high-quality evidence to guide clinical practice [71].

- Assessment of associated anomalies. Associated gastrointestinal anomalies and problems (e.g., malrotation, atresia, stenosis, perforation, necrosis, volvulus) occur in up to 25% of cases [72] and may be related to vascular disruption caused by herniated bowel. Disruption of the superior mesenteric artery, for example, may lead to volvulus or to "apple peel" jejunal-ileal lesions. Meckel's diverticulum and gallbladder atresia also occur, but are less common. Bladder herniation has been reported in 6% of cases, with bowel or urinary tract dilation [73]. Most cases have no extraintestinal abnormalities, approximately 10% of gastroschisis cases were associated with major unrelated defects, approximately 2% of cases were part of a recognized syndrome, and cardiac anomalies were detected in 2–3% of cases [74]. Oligohydramnios is the most common amniotic fluid abnormality, but polyhydramnios may occur, particularly in fetuses with reduced bowel motility or obstruction [73].

- Genetic assessment. The prevalence of chromosomal abnormalities in fetuses with isolated gastroschisis is not increased above the baseline population risk, so invasive fetal genetic testing is not routinely offered. The fetal genetic evaluation is suggested if nongastrointestinal structural abnormalities are identified on ultrasound examination. Chromosome abnormalities were detected in 1.2% of the total cases, which included isolated and nonisolated, and the most frequent abnormalities were trisomy 18, trisomy 13, sex chromosome anomalies, and trisomy 21 [73].

- Follow-up assessment. The most common pregnancy complications associated with gastroschisis include development of growth restriction (30–60% of cases), intrauterine fetal demise (3–6%), spontaneous preterm birth (30%), and bowel dilation and wall thickening (common, frequency depends on diagnostic criteria) [73]. The mechanisms causing these adverse outcomes in gastroschisis are unclear. Therefore, pregnancy monitoring is empiric and typically includes serial ultrasound examinations for assessment of fetal growth and fetal bowel abnormality and standard tests for antepartum fetal surveillance [73].

- Assessment of fetal growth and amniotic fluid volume—serial ultrasound examinations every 3 weeks for assessment of fetal growth and amniotic fluid volume (AFV). If growth arrest or oligohydramnios is diagnosed, umbilical artery Doppler flow is evaluated [73]. A systematic error of birth weight underestimation when using the Hadlock formulas in fetuses affected with gastroschisis was found [75]. Siemer and colleagues developed a specific formula for estimating fetal weight in fetuses with abdominal wall defects using the biparietal diameter, occipitofrontal diameter, and femur length measurements [76]. Oligohydramnios may be related to fetal growth restriction and is a risk factor for cord compression and its sequelae. Polyhydramnios is less common, but an important finding because it is often caused by dysfunction of the gastrointestinal tract due to bowel atresia [73].

- Assessment of fetal bowel. Gastric dilatation, bowel dilatation, and bowel wall thickening have been considered poor prognostic signs by several investigators [73]. If these significant changes are observed prior to 34 weeks, a course of glucocorticoids is suggested for fetal maturation [73].

- Antepartum fetal surveillance. Fetal growth restriction and amniotic fluid abnormalities are commonly accepted indications for increased antepartum fetal surveillance. The precise timing and frequency of testing is arbitrary [73].

5.1.2. Delivery management

Gastroschisis increases the risk of preterm delivery; delivery should occur in a facility with appropriate resources for caring for these neonates. Gastroschisis alone is not an indication for preterm intervention or cesarean delivery [73].

The decision on timing of delivery is based on a combination of factors, including gestational age, ultrasound findings (fetal growth profile, AFV, appearance of fetal bowel), and fetal testing results (NST, BPP, umbilical cord Doppler if fetal growth restriction is present). In the absence of standard obstetric indications for abdominal delivery, a trial of labor rather than scheduled cesarean birth for most patients is suggested. Cesarean delivery is reasonable if the liver is significantly herniated because of the theoretic risk of dystocia and trauma. Delivery of pregnancies complicated by fetal gastroschisis at 37 or 38 weeks of gestation is suggested to minimize neonatal morbidity and mortality and avoid the possibility of term (39–40 weeks) stillbirth; however, there is no consensus on the optimum timing of delivery of these pregnancies [73].

5.2. Omphalocele

5.2.1. Pregnancy management

Omphalocele and gastroschisis are the most common fetal abdominal wall defects. By the end of the first trimester (11–14 weeks), almost all omphaloceles can be detected by prenatal ultrasound examination [77].

- Genetic assessment. Multiple chromosomal abnormalities have been reported among fetuses with omphalocele. As many as 60% of omphaloceles not containing liver are associated with fetal aneuploidy, particularly trisomy 18 or 13 [77, 78]. Fetal genetic studies should be offered if omphalocele or related body wall defects are identified prenatally, because of the high risk of aneuploidy. It is reasonable to offer amniocentesis for genetic testing for Beckwith-Wiedemann syndrome, but this testing is complicated and should be discussed with a geneticist [77]. There is a 10–20% risk of Beckwith-Wiedemann syndrome in fetuses with apparently isolated omphalocele on ultrasound.

- Assessment of associated anomalies. Associated abnormalities that occur with increased frequency in these fetuses include additional gastrointestinal abnormalities, cardiac defects (up to 50% of cases), genitourinary anomalies, orofacial clefts, neural tube defects, defects of the diaphragm, polyhydramnios, and growth restriction. Associated syndromes are best categorized by upper, middle, and lower midline omphalocele defects. Omphalocele has been associated with several syndromes, including Pentalogy of Cantrell (upper midline defect), amniotic band sequence, schisis association (at least two of the following defects: neural tube defect, oral cleft, omphalocele, diaphragmatic hernia); lower midline defects are associated with OEIS syndrome (omphalocele, exstrophy of the bladder, imperforate anus, spinal defects), Shprintzen syndrome, Carpenter syndrome, Goltz syndrome, Marshall-Smith syndrome, Meckel-Gruber syndrome, otopalatodigital type II syndrome, CHARGE (coloboma, heart defect, atresia choanae, retarded growth and development, genital abnormality, and ear abnormality) syndrome, and Beckwith-Wiedemann syndrome (hallmark features: macroglossia, gigantism, omphalocele) [77].

- Follow-up obstetrical care. The serial ultrasound examination every 3–4 weeks to evaluate fetal growth is recommended. When growth is appropriate and amniotic fluid volume is normal, weekly nonstress testing or biophysical profile monitoring at 32 weeks of gestation to assess fetal well-being are recommended, as these pregnancies appear to be at increased risk of late fetal death [79]. Fetal growth restriction and preterm delivery are not uncommon in pregnancies complicated by an omphalocele, particularly with associated abnormalities [77]. Nonreassuring fetal testing and/or cessation of fetal growth at or near term is an indication for early delivery. A systematic error of birth weight underestimation in fetuses affected with omphalocele was found, the same situation as discussed in fetuses with gastroschisis. Intrauterine growth restriction in fetuses with abdominal wall defects is predictive of an increased risk of adverse neonatal outcome [77].

5.2.2. Delivery management

Delivery should be planning at a tertiary care center. In the absence of standard indications for early delivery, it is reasonable to await spontaneous labor or achieve 39 weeks of gestation. Preterm birth offers no advantage to affected neonates and is associated with increased morbidity and mortality. There is no evidence that cesarean delivery improves outcome in uncomplicated omphalocele; surgery should be reserved for usual obstetric indications [77]. However, some pediatric surgeons have recommended cesarean delivery for fetuses with giant omphaloceles (defined as an omphalocele containing >75% of the liver and defect greater than 5 cm) in an attempt to avoid dystocia, rupture, infection, and hemorrhage [80]. Visceral trauma has also been reported after cesarean delivery [77].

5.3. Bladder exstrophy

Often the diagnosis of bladder exstrophy is made by prenatal ultrasound and, in some cases, may be confirmed by MRI. In the event that a prenatal diagnosis is not made, the diagnosis should be clinically apparent and recognizable at birth in the delivery room [81]. If a prenatal diagnosis is not made, the diagnosis of bladder exstrophy should be clinically recognizable at delivery. A careful physical examination will differentiate bladder exstrophy from other congenital anomalies that involve abdominal wall defects, such as omphalocele, gastroschisis, and cloacal exstrophy.

Following the prenatal diagnosis of bladder exstrophy, prenatal care includes the following [16, 81]:

1. Education and counseling of the parents, touring the neonatal intensive care unit, meeting the pediatric urologic care team, and allowing the expectant parent(s) the opportunity to interact with other families with a child with bladder exstrophy.

2. Preparation for delivery. In many tertiary centers, one option for planning initial surgical management is an induced vaginal delivery that is scheduled in late gestation with coordination with an on-site pediatric urology service. This approach facilitates bladder closure within 72 hours of life.

The cesarean delivery should be reserved for obstetrical complications.

5.4. Body stalk anomaly and cloacal exstrophy

- Body stalk anomaly (also called limb-body wall complex) is a massively disfiguring and generally lethal malformation of the thorax and/or abdomen, often associated with limb defects. The intrathoracic and abdominal organs lie outside the abdominal cavity and are contained within a sac composed of amnioperitoneal membrane attached directly to the placenta. The umbilical cord may be totally absent or extremely shortened. Severe kyphoscoliosis is often present. Termination of pregnancy is usually offered since the abnormality is generally considered lethal [82]. However, repair has been performed in rare cases [82]. If the pregnancy is continued, vaginal delivery is recommended given the highly lethal nature of this disease, assuming there are no maternal contraindications to vaginal delivery. In this setting, the patient should be extensively counseled on the likelihood of neonatal demise, as well as the severe morbidity associated with a successful repair [82, 83].

- Cloacal exstrophy. The accuracy of sonographic diagnosis appears to be less than 25% due to the rarity of the disorder and the wide spectrum of anatomic variants, which depend upon the degree of cloacal septation completed. Fetal genetic studies during the initial evaluation can be useful, although cloacal exstrophy has not been reported to be associated with specific aneuploidies. The chromosomal findings, which will include gender, may influence the decision to terminate the pregnancy, perform a cesarean delivery for fetal indications, or initiate a series of corrective operations in the newborn period [41]. Although there are no studies of the optimum route of delivery for this rare disorder, cesarean delivery is generally reserved for standard obstetric indications. The umbilical cord should be clamped or ligated carefully to avoid injury to proximate structures. At delivery, saline-soaked sterile dressings should be applied over the exposed bladder and bowel mucosa and covered with plastic wrap to minimize insensible fluid and heat loss. Survival rates of 80–100% have been reported, but quality of life (e.g., bowel, urinary, and sexual function) is a concern [82].

6. Congenital anomalies of the kidney and urinary tract

6.1. Pregnancy management

Congenital anomalies of the kidney and urinary tract (CAKUT) constitute approximately 20–30% of all anomalies identified in the prenatal period [84]. Defects can be bilateral or unilateral, and different defects often coexist in an individual child. In general, the optimal timing recommended for a screening antenatal ultrasound is between 16 and 20 weeks of gestation because of the following factors at this gestational age. Counseling of families with fetuses with CAKUT should be universally available. If the fetal prognosis is poor, as determined by severe bilateral disease, bilateral RA, oligohydramnios, or unfavorable amniotic fluid analysis, legal termination, if possible, can be offered. In all other cases, continued counseling throughout the pregnancy including discussion of postnatal management is required. In particular, discussion with parents regarding their wishes on the level of support given to offspring with severe oligohydramnios, who are at risk for lung hypoplasia that may be incompatible with life, is helpful in establishing guidelines for initial postnatal care [84].

- Assessment of amniotic fluid volume and analysis of biochemical markers are used to evaluate fetal renal function. By 20 weeks of gestation, fetal urine accounts for more than 90% of the amniotic fluid volume. Thus, a decrease in amniotic fluid volume (oligohydramnios) at or beyond the 20th week of gestation is an excellent predictor of abnormal fetal renal function and CAKUT [84]. Severe oligohydramnios due to CAKUT either involves both kidneys or occurs in a solitary kidney in the fetus. Bilateral renal agenesis (RA) or severe dysgenesis, bilateral ureteric obstruction, or obstruction of the bladder outlet or urethra can result in severe oligohydramnios as early as 18 weeks of gestation. Because an adequate amniotic fluid volume is critical for lung development, severe oligohydramnios due to abnormal fetal renal function in the second trimester can result in lung hypoplasia, a potentially fatal disorder.

- Assessment for additional anomalies. Potter's syndrome consists of a typical facial appearance characterized by pseudoepicanthus, recessed chin, posteriorly rotated, flattened ears and flattened nose, decreased fetal movement, musculoskeletal features including clubfoot and clubhand, hip dislocation and joint contractures, and pulmonary hypoplasia.

- Analysis of amniotic fluid. Although oligohydramnios is the most reliable predictor of abnormal fetal renal function, its absence does not assure normal fetal renal function.

Because amniotic fluid is predominantly composed of fetal urine, measurement of biochemical markers contained in amniotic fluid (fetal urine) can be used to assess fetal renal function [84].

- Follow-up assessment. Repeat antenatal ultrasound examinations are performed to help guide management decisions. The timing is dependent on findings on the initial examination. Fetuses with second trimester hydronephrosis (RPD >4 mm) should undergo repeat testing in the third trimester to assess progression and select those who will benefit most from postnatal testing. A repeat examination 2–3 weeks later in fetuses with bilateral involvement (or an affected solitary kidney) and at 32–34 weeks of gestation in those with unilateral involvement is recommended [85].

- In utero intervention. Although there have been case series of antenatal surgery in fetuses with severe hydronephrosis and oligohydramnios, this intervention has not been shown to improve renal outcome. These procedures may increase the amount of amniotic fluid, thus potentially improving lung development and survival rate. In these rare cases, the procedure should only be performed in select centers with expertise and in infants with severe bilateral hydronephrosis, absent of severe renal parenchymal or cystic disease, favorable urinary electrolyte levels and osmolality, and normal karyotype [84]. Data are limited on whether percutaneous vesicoamniotic shunting compared with conservative observation in fetuses with lower urinary tract obstruction improves survival and renal outcome. The percutaneous vesicoamniotic shunting should not be routinely performed in fetuses with lower urinary tract obstruction [85].

6.2. Delivery management

Cesarean delivery should be reserved for obstetrical indications. The time of delivery depends on the fetal well-being and amniotic fluid volume.

7. Esophageal, gastrointestinal, and anorectal atresia

7.1. Pregnancy management

Prenatal sonographic diagnosis of gastrointestinal atresia is challenging since obstruction may not become evident sonographically until the late second trimester, after the typical time of a fetal anatomic survey (18–20 weeks of gestation). It can also be difficult to differentiate dilated small bowel loops from colon or megaureters sonographically [86]. It is unclear whether prenatal diagnosis of esophageal, gastrointestinal, or anorectal atresia improves the prognosis. However, early prenatal diagnosis provides an opportunity for parental counseling and preparation, screening for associated anomalies, and the option for pregnancy termination or delivery at a setting with appropriate personnel and facilities for newborn care [86].

- Indications for magnetic resonance imaging. MRI may be used to confirm or clarify suspected gastrointestinal abnormalities on ultrasound examination if this information is important for managing the pregnancy. Fetal bowel is well visualized by MRI and easily differentiated from adjacent liver, spleen, kidneys, bladder, and gallbladder. Meconium is also well visualized [87]. The normal esophagus, stomach, and duodenum should always be filled with T2 hyperintense fluid (amniotic fluid).

- Assessment of additional anomalies and follow-up assessment. Many of these pregnancies are complicated by polyhydramnios. After diagnosis, the performance of periodic ultrasound examinations to look for any change in the appearance of the atresia or associated anomalies and to assess interval fetal growth and amniotic fluid volume is recommended. Nonstress tests or biophysical profiles are indicated in pregnancies in which the risk of antepartum fetal demise is increased, such as a fetal anomaly associated with growth restriction [86].

7.2. Delivery management

Atresia alone is not an indication for cesarean delivery in the absence of a standard obstetric indication. However, if the abdominal circumference is much larger than the head circumference, cesarean delivery should be considered due to the risk of fetal abdominal dystocia. Delivery should be planned at a center that has an appropriate level of neonatal support.

Author details

Diana Ramasauskaite

Address all correspondence to: diana.ramasauskaite@mf.vu.lt

Vilnius University, Faculty of Medicine, Institute of Clinical medicine, Clinic of Obstetrics and Gynaecology, Vilnius, Lithuania

References

[1] Copel J. Fetal Cardiac Abnormalities: Screening, Evaluation, and Pregnancy Management. Aug 2017. Available rom: www.uptodate.com

[2] Donofrio MT, Moon-Grady AJ, Hornberger LK, Copel JA, Sklansky MS, Abuhamad A, et al. Diagnosis and treatment of fetal cardiac disease: A scientific statement from the American Heart Association. Circulation. 2014;**129**(21):2183

[3] Song MS, Hu A, Dyamenahalli U, Chitayat D, Winsor EJ, Ryan G, et al. Extracardiac lesions and chromosomal abnormalities associated with major fetal heart defects: Comparison

of intrauterine, postnatal and postmortem diagnoses. Ultrasound in Obstetrics & Gynecology. 2009;**33**(5):552

[4] Pajkrt E, Weisz B, Firth HV, Chitty LS. Fetal cardiac anomalies and genetic syndromes. Prenatal Diagnosis. 2004;**24**(13):1104

[5] Jansen FA, Everwijn SM, Scheepjens R, Stijnen T, Peeters-Scholte CM, et al. Fetal brain imaging in isolated congenital heart defects - a systematic review and meta-analysis. Prenatal Diagnosis. Jul 2016;**36**(7):601-613 Epub Jun 19, 2016

[6] Mone F, Walsh C, Mulcahy C, McMahon CJ, Farrell S, MacTiernan A, et al. Prenatal detection of structural cardiac defects and presence of associated anomalies: A retrospective observational study of 1262 fetal echocardiograms. Prenatal Diagnosis. Jun 2015;**35**(6):577-582 Epub Mar 10, 2015

[7] Tuuli MG, Dicke JM, Stamilio DM, Gray DL, Macones GA, Rampersad R et al. Prevalence and likelihood ratios for aneuploidy in fetuses diagnosed prenatally with isolated congenital cardiac defects. American Journal of Obstetrics and Gynecology. 2009;**201**(4): 390.e1

[8] Matthiesen NB, Henriksen TB, Agergaard P, Gaynor JW, Bach CC, Hjortdal VE, et al. Congenital heart defects and indices of placental and fetal growth in a nationwide study of 924 422 liveborn infants. Circulation. 2016;**134**(20):1546 Epub Oct 14, 2016

[9] Divanovic A, Bowers K, Michelfelder E, Jaekle R, Newman T, Marcotte M, et al. Intrauterine fetal demise after prenatal diagnosis of congenital heart disease: Assessment of risk. Prenatal Diagnosis. Feb 2016;**36**(2):142-147 Epub Dec 28, 2015

[10] Araujo Júnior E, Tonni G, Chung M, Ruano R, Martins WP. Perinatal outcomes and intrauterine complications following fetal intervention for congenital heart disease: Systematic review and meta-analysis of observational studies. Ultrasound in Obstetrics & Gynecology. 2016;**48**(4):426 Epub Sep 15, 2016

[11] Peterson AL, Quartermain MD, Ades A, Khalek N, Johnson MP, Rychik J. Impact of mode of delivery on markers of perinatal hemodynamics in infants with hypoplastic left heart syndrome. The Journal of Pediatrics. Jul 2011;**159**(1):64-69 Epub Mar 17, 2011

[12] Costello JM, Pasquali SK, Jacobs JP, He X, Hill KD, Cooper DS, et al. Gestational age at birth and outcomes after neonatal cardiac surgery: An analysis of the society of thoracic surgeons congenital heart surgery database. Circulation. 2014;**129**(24):2511 Epub May 2, 2014

[13] Kipps AK, Feuille C, Azakie A, Hoffman JI, Tabbutt S, Brook MM. Prenatal diagnosis of hypoplastic left heart syndrome in current era. The American Journal of Cardiology. 2011;**108**(3):421

[14] Monteagudo A, Timor-Tritsch IE. Prenatal Diagnosis of CNS Anomalies Other than Neural Tube Defects and Ventriculomegaly. Aug 2017. Available from: www.uptodate

[15] Rossi AC, Prefumo F. Additional value of fetal magnetic resonance imaging in the prenatal diagnosis of central nervous system anomalies: A systematic review of the literature. Ultrasound in Obstetrics & Gynecology. Oct 2014;**44**(4):388-393

[16] Bianchi DW, Crombleholme TM, D'Alton ME. Fetology: Diagnosis and Management of the Fetal Patient. McGraw-Hill; 2000

[17] Li Y, Estroff JA, Khwaja O, Mehta TS, Poussaint TY, Robson CD, et al. Callosal dysgenesis in fetuses with ventriculomegaly: Levels of agreement between imaging modalities and postnatal outcome. Ultrasound in Obstetrics & Gynecology. Nov 2012;**40**(5): 522-529

[18] Sotiriadis A, Makrydimas G. Neurodevelopment after prenatal diagnosis of isolated agenesis of the corpus callosum: An integrative review. American Journal of Obstetrics and Gynecology. Apr 2012:**206**(4);337.e1-337.e5. Epub Dec 27, 2011

[19] Guibaud L, Larroque A, Ville D, Sanlaville D, Till M, Gaucherand P, et al. Prenatal diagnosis of 'isolated' Dandy-Walker malformation: Imaging findings and prenatal counselling. Prenatal Diagnosis 2012;32(2):185

[20] Monteagudo A, Timor-Tritsch IE. Ultrasound Diagnosis of Neural Tube Defects. Aug 2017. Available from: www.uptodate

[21] Blaas HG, Eik-Nes SH. Sonoembryology and early prenatal diagnosis of neural anomalies. Prenatal Diagnosis. Apr 2009;**29**(4):312-325

[22] Fleurke-Rozema JH, van Leijden L, van de Kamp K, Pajkrt E, Bilardo CM, Snijders RJ. Timing of detection of anencephaly in The Netherlands. Prenatal Diagnosis. May 2015; **35**(5):483-485

[23] Tomita T, Ogiwara H. Anencephaly. Aug 2017. Available from: www.uptodate

[24] Peabody JL, Emery JR, Ashwal S. Experience with anencephalic infants as prospective organ donors. The New England Journal of Medicine. 1989;**321**(6):344

[25] van Heteren CF, Boekkooi PF, Jongsma HW, Nijhuis JG. Responses to vibroacoustic stimulation in a fetus with an encephalocele compared to responses of normal fetuses. Journal of Perinatal Medicine. 2000;**28**(4):306

[26] Tomita T, Ogiwara H. Primary (Congenital) Encephalocele. Aug 2017. Available from: www.uptodate

[27] Lennon CA, Gray DL. Sensitivity and specificity of ultrasound for the detection of neural tube and ventral wall defects in a high-risk population. Obstetrics and Gynecology. 1999;**94**(4):562

[28] Chao TT, Dashe JS, Adams RC, Keefover-Hicks A, McIntire DD, Twickler DM. Fetal spine findings on MRI and associated outcomes in children with open neural tube defects. AJR – American Journal of Roentgenology. Nov 2011;**197**(5):W956-W961

[29] Wilson RD. Prenatal screening, diagnosis, and pregnancy management of fetal neural tube defects. Journal of Obstetrics and Gynaecology Canada. 2014;**36**(10):927

[30] Johnson CY, Honein MA, Dana Flanders W, Howards PP, Oakley GP Jr, Rasmussen SA. Pregnancy termination following prenatal diagnosis of anencephaly or spina bifida: A systematic review of the literature. Birth Defects Research. Part A, Clinical and Molecular Teratology. 2012;**94**(11):857 Epub Oct 25, 2012

[31] Sutton LN. Fetal surgery for neural tube defects. Best Practice & Research. Clinical Obstetrics & Gynaecology. 2008;**22**(1):175 Epub Aug 22, 2007

[32] Adzick NS, Thom EA, Spong CY, Brock JW, Burrows PK, Johnson MP, et al. A randomized trial of prenatal versus postnatal repair of myelomeningocele. The New England Journal of Medicine. 2011;**364**(11):993 Epub Feb 9, 2011

[33] Moldenhauer JS, Soni S, Rintoul NE, Spinner SS, Khalek N, Martinez-Poyer J et al. Fetal myelomeningocele repair: The post-MOMS experience at the Children's Hospital of Philadelphia. Fetal Diagnosis and Therapy. 2015;**37**(3):235-240. Epub Aug 15, 2014

[34] Committee on Obstetric Practice, Society for Maternal-Fetal Medicine. Committee Opinion No. 720: Maternal-Fetal Surgery for Myelomeningocele. Obstetrics & Gynecology. 2017;**130**(3):e164

[35] McLone DG, Bowman RM. Overview of the Management of Myelomeningocele (*Spina bifida*). Aug 2017. Available from: www.uptodate

[36] Norton ME. Fetal Cerebral Ventriculomegaly. Aug 2017. Available from: www.uptodate

[37] Hannon T, Tennant PW, Rankin J, Robson SC. Epidemiology, natural history, progression, and postnatal outcome of severe fetal ventriculomegaly. Obstetrics and Gynecology. 2012;**120**(6):1345

[38] Pagani G, Thilaganathan B, Prefumo F. Neurodevelopmental outcome in isolated mild fetal ventriculomegaly: Systematic review and meta-analysis. Ultrasound in Obstetrics & Gynecology. Sep 2014;**44**(3):254-260 Epub Jul 21, 2014

[39] Melchiorre K, Bhide A, Gika AD, Pilu G, Papageorghiou AT. Counseling in isolated mild fetal ventriculomegaly. Ultrasound in Obstetrics & Gynecology. 2009;**34**(2):212

[40] von Koch CS, Gupta N, Sutton LN, Sun PP. Utero surgery for hydrocephalus. Child's Nervous System. 2003;**19**(7-8):574 Epub Jul 25, 2003

[41] Chasen ST, Chervenak FA, McCullough LB. The role of cephalocentesis in modern obstetrics. American Journal of Obstetrics and Gynecology. 2001;**185**(3):734

[42] Benachi A, Cordier AG, Cannie M, Jani J. Advances in prenatal diagnosis of congenital diaphragmatic hernia. Seminars in Fetal & Neonatal Medicine. Dec 2014;**19**(6):331-337 Epub Oct 11, 2014

[43] Hedrick HL, Adzick S. Congenital Diaphragmatic Hernia. Aug 2017. Available from: www.uptodate

[44] Deprest J, Brady P, Nicolaides K, Benachi A, Berg C, Vermeesch J, et al. Prenatal management of the fetus with isolated congenital diaphragmatic hernia in the era of the TOTAL trial. Seminars in Fetal & Neonatal Medicine. Dec 2014;**19**(6):338-348 Epub Nov 11, 2014

[45] Sweed Y, Puri P. Congenital diaphragmatic hernia: influence of associated malformations on survival. Archives of Disease in Childhood. 1993;**69**(1 Spec No):68

[46] Pober BR. Genetic aspects of human congenital diaphragmatic hernia. Clinical Genetics. 2008;**74**(1):1 Epub May 28, 2008

[47] Pober BR, Lin A, Russell M, Ackerman KG, Chakravorty S, Strauss B, et al. Infants with Bochdalek diaphragmatic hernia: Sibling precurrence and monozygotic twin discordance in a hospital-based malformation surveillance program. American Journal of Medical Genetics. Part A. 2005;**138A**(2):81

[48] Mayer S, Klaritsch P, Petersen S, Done E, Sandaite I, Till H et al. The correlation between lung volume and liver herniation measurements by fetal MRI in isolated congenital diaphragmatic hernia: A systematic review and meta-analysis of observational studies. Prenatal Diagnosis. 2011;**31**(11):1086. Epub Sep 14, 2011

[49] Mullassery D, Ba'ath ME, Jesudason EC, Losty PD. Value of liver herniation in prediction of outcome in fetal congenital diaphragmatic hernia: A systematic review and meta-analysis. Ultrasound in Obstetrics & Gynecology. 2010;**35**(5):609

[50] Bebbington M, Victoria T, Danzer E, Moldenhauer J, Khalek N, Johnson M, et al. Comparison of ultrasound and magnetic resonance imaging parameters in predicting survival in isolated left-sided congenital diaphragmatic hernia. Ultrasound in Obstetrics & Gynecology. Jun 2014;**43**(6):670-674 Epub May 5, 2014

[51] Büsing KA, Kilian AK, Schaible T, Endler C, Schaffelder R, Neff KW. MR relative fetal lung volume in congenital diaphragmatic hernia: Survival and need for extracorporeal membrane oxygenation. Radiology. 2008;**248**(1):240

[52] DeKoninck P, Gomez O, Sandaite I, Richter J, Nawapun K, Eerdekens A, et al. Right-sided congenital diaphragmatic hernia in a decade of fetal surgery. BJOG: An International Journal of Obstetrics and Gynaecology. 2015;**122**(7):940

[53] Jani J, Nicolaides KH, Keller RL, Benachi A, Peralta CF, Favre R, et al. Observed to expected lung area to head circumference ratio in the prediction of survival in fetuses with isolated diaphragmatic hernia. Ultrasound in Obstetrics & Gynecology. 2007;**30**(1):67

[54] Sbragia L, Paek BW, Filly RA, Harrison MR, Farrell JA, Farmer DL, et al. Congenital diaphragmatic hernia without herniation of the liver: Does the lung-to-head ratio predict survival? Journal of Ultrasound in Medicine. 2000;**19**(12):845

[55] Peralta CF, Cavoretto P, Csapo B, Vandecruys H, Nicolaides KH. Assessment of lung area in normal fetuses at 12-32 weeks. Ultrasound in Obstetrics & Gynecology. Dec 2005;**26**(7):718-724

[56] Peralta CF, Jani JC, Van Schoubroeck D, Nicolaides KH, Deprest JA. Fetal lung volume after endoscopic tracheal occlusion in the prediction of postnatal outcome. American Journal of Obstetrics and Gynecology. 2008;**198**(1):60.e1. Epub Sep 12, 2007

[57] Jani JC, Nicolaides KH, Gratacós E, Valencia CM, Doné E, Martinez JM et al. Severe diaphragmatic hernia treated by fetal endoscopic tracheal occlusion. Ultrasound in Obstetrics & Gynecology Sep 2009;**34**(3):304-310

[58] Harrison MR, Keller RL, Hawgood SB, Kitterman JA, Sandberg PL, Farmer DL, et al. A randomized trial of fetal endoscopic tracheal occlusion for severe fetal congenital diaphragmatic hernia. The New England Journal of Medicine. 2003;**349**(20):1916

[59] Deprest J, Gratacos E, Nicolaides KH. Fetoscopic tracheal occlusion (FETO) for severe congenital diaphragmatic hernia: Evolution of a technique and preliminary results. Ultrasound in Obstetrics & Gynecology. 2004;**24**(2):121

[60] Jiménez JA, Eixarch E, De Koninck P, Bennini JR, Devlieger R, Peralta CF et al. Balloon removal after fetoscopic endoluminal tracheal occlusion for congenital diaphragmatic hernia. American Journal of Obstetrics and Gynecology. 2017;**217**(1):78.e1. Epub Mar 3, 2017

[61] Egloff A, Bulas DI. Prenatal Diagnosis and Management of Congenital Pulmonary Airway Malformation. Aug 2017. Available from: www.uptodate

[62] Cavoretto P, Molina F, Poggi S, Davenport M, Nicolaides KH. Prenatal diagnosis and outcome of echogenic fetal lung lesions. Ultrasound in Obstetrics & Gynecology. 2008;**32**(6):769

[63] Hellmund A, Berg C, Geipel A, Bludau M, Heydweiller A, Bachour H, et al. Prenatal diagnosis and evaluation of sonographic predictors for intervention and adverse outcome in congenital pulmonary airway malformation. PLoS One. 2016;**11**(3):e0150474 Epub Mar 15, 2016

[64] Liechty KW. Ex-utero intrapartum therapy. Seminars in Fetal & Neonatal Medicine. 2010;**15**(1):34 Epub Aug 15, 2009

[65] Derderian SC, Coleman AM, Jeanty C, Lim FY, Shaaban AM, Farrell JA, et al. Favorable outcomes in high-risk congenital pulmonary airway malformations treated with multiple courses of maternal betamethasone. Journal of Pediatric Surgery. Apr 2015;**50**(4):515-518 Epub Oct 1, 2014

[66] Peranteau WH, Adzick NS, Boelig MM, Flake AW, Hedrick HL, Howell LJ, et al. Thoracoamniotic shunts for the management of fetal lung lesions and pleural effusions: A single-institution review and predictors of survival in 75 cases. Journal of Pediatric Surgery. 2015;**50**(2):301

[67] Bermúdez C, Pérez-Wulff J, Arcadipane M, Bufalino G, Gómez L, Flores L, et al. Percutaneous fetal sclerotherapy for congenital cystic adenomatoid malformation of the lung. Fetal Diagnosis and Therapy. 2008;**24**(3):237 Epub Aug 28, 2008

[68] Bulas DI, Egloff A. Prenatal Diagnosis and Management of Bronchopulmonary Seques-tration. Aug 2017. Available rom: www.uptodate

[69] Lecomte B, Hadden H, Coste K, Gallot D, Laurichesse H, Lemery D, et al. Hyperechoic congenital lung lesions in a non-selected population: From prenatal detection till perina-tal management. Prenatal Diagnosis. 2009;**29**(13):1222

[70] Oermann CM. Congenital Lobar Emphysema. Aug 2017. Available rom: www.uptodate

[71] Overton TG, Pierce MR, Gao H, Kurinczuk JJ, Spark P, Draper ES, et al. Antenatal man-agement and outcomes of gastroschisis in the U.K. Prenatal Diagnosis. 2012;**32**(13):1256 Epub Nov 8, 2012

[72] Abdullah F, Arnold MA, Nabaweesi R, Fischer AC, Colombani PM, Anderson KD, et al. Gastroschisis in the United States 1988-2003: Analysis and risk categorization of 4344 patients. Journal of Perinatology. 2007;**27**(1):50 Epub Oct 12, 2006

[73] Stephenson CD, Lockwood CJ, MacKenzie AP. Gastroschisis. Aug 2017. Available rom: www.uptodate

[74] Mastroiacovo P, Lisi A, Castilla EE, Martínez-Frías ML, Bermejo E, Marengo L, et al. Gastroschisis and associated defects: An international study. American Journal of Medical Genetics. Part A. 2007;**143A**(7):660

[75] Adams SR, Durfee S, Pettigrew C, Katz D, Jennings R, Ecker J, et al. Accuracy of sonog-raphy to predict estimated weight in fetuses with gastroschisis. Journal of Ultrasound in Medicine. 2012;**31**(11):1753

[76] Siemer J, Hilbert A, Hart N, Hoopmann M, Schneider U, Girschick G, et al. Specific weight formula for fetuses with abdominal wall defects. Ultrasound in Obstetrics & Gynecology. 2008;**31**(4):397

[77] Stephenson CD, Lockwood CJ, MacKenzie AP. Omphalocele. Aug 2017. Available rom: www.uptodate

[78] Chen CP. Chromosomal abnormalities associated with omphalocele. Taiwanese Journal of Obstetrics & Gynecology. 2007;**46**(1):1

[79] Deng K, Qiu J, Dai L, Yi L, Deng C, Mu Y, et al. Perinatal mortality in pregnancies with omphalocele: Data from the Chinese national birth defects monitoring network, 1996-2006. BMC Pediatrics. 2014;**14**:160 Epub Jun 23, 2014

[80] Biard JM, Wilson RD, Johnson MP, Hedrick HL, Schwarz U, Flake AW, et al. Prenatally diagnosed giant omphaloceles: Short- and long-term outcomes. Prenatal Diagnosis. 2004;**24**(6):434

[81] Borer JG. Clinical Manifestations and Initial Management of Infants with Bladder Exstrophy. Aug 2017. Available rom: www.uptodate

[82] Stephenson CD, Lockwood CJ, MacKenzie AP. Body Stalk Anomaly and Cloacal Exstro-phy. Aug 2017. Available rom: www.uptodate

[83] Ramasauskaite D, Snieckuviene V, Zitkute V, Vankeviciene R, Lauzikiene D, Drasutiene GA. Rare case report of thoracic Ectopia Cordis: An obstetrician's point of view in multidisciplinary approach. Case Reports in Pediatrics. 2016;**2016**:5097059 Epub Nov 9, 2016

[84] Rosenblum ND. Evaluation of Congenital Anomalies of the Kidney and Urinary Tract (CAKUT). Aug 2017. Available rom: www.uptodate

[85] Baskin LS. Overview of Fetal Hydronephrosis. Aug 2017. Available rom: www.uptodate

[86] Bulas DI. Prenatal Diagnosis of Esophageal, Gastrointestinal, and Anorectal Atresia. Aug 2017. Available rom: www.uptodate

[87] Veyrac C, Couture A, Saguintaah M, Baud C. MRI of fetal GI tract abnormalities. Abdominal Imaging. 2004;**29**(4):411

Permissions

All chapters in this book were first published in CA, by InTech Open; hereby published with permission under the Creative Commons Attribution License or equivalent. Every chapter published in this book has been scrutinized by our experts. Their significance has been extensively debated. The topics covered herein carry significant findings which will fuel the growth of the discipline. They may even be implemented as practical applications or may be referred to as a beginning point for another development.

The contributors of this book come from diverse backgrounds, making this book a truly international effort. This book will bring forth new frontiers with its revolutionizing research information and detailed analysis of the nascent developments around the world.

We would like to thank all the contributing authors for lending their expertise to make the book truly unique. They have played a crucial role in the development of this book. Without their invaluable contributions this book wouldn't have been possible. They have made vital efforts to compile up to date information on the varied aspects of this subject to make this book a valuable addition to the collection of many professionals and students.

This book was conceptualized with the vision of imparting up-to-date information and advanced data in this field. To ensure the same, a matchless editorial board was set up. Every individual on the board went through rigorous rounds of assessment to prove their worth. After which they invested a large part of their time researching and compiling the most relevant data for our readers.

The editorial board has been involved in producing this book since its inception. They have spent rigorous hours researching and exploring the diverse topics which have resulted in the successful publishing of this book. They have passed on their knowledge of decades through this book. To expedite this challenging task, the publisher supported the team at every step. A small team of assistant editors was also appointed to further simplify the editing procedure and attain best results for the readers.

Apart from the editorial board, the designing team has also invested a significant amount of their time in understanding the subject and creating the most relevant covers. They scrutinized every image to scout for the most suitable representation of the subject and create an appropriate cover for the book.

The publishing team has been an ardent support to the editorial, designing and production team. Their endless efforts to recruit the best for this project, has resulted in the accomplishment of this book. They are a veteran in the field of academics and their pool of knowledge is as vast as their experience in printing. Their expertise and guidance has proved useful at every step. Their uncompromising quality standards have made this book an exceptional effort. Their encouragement from time to time has been an inspiration for everyone.

The publisher and the editorial board hope that this book will prove to be a valuable piece of knowledge for researchers, students, practitioners and scholars across the globe.

List of Contributors

Cringu Ionescu
Department of Obstetrics and Gynecology, Clinical Emergency Hospital St Pantelimon, Carol Davila University of Medicine and Pharmacy, Bucharest, Romania

Roxana Cristina Drăgușin, Maria Șorop-Florea, Ciprian Laurențiu Pătru, Lucian Zorilă, Nicolae Cernea and Dominic Gabriel Iliescu
Department of Obstetrics and Gynaecology, University of Medicine and Pharmacy, Craiova, Romania

Cristian Marinaș
Department of Anatomy, University of Medicine and Pharmacy, Craiova, Romania

Cristian Neamțu
Department of Physiopathology, University of Medicine and Pharmacy, Craiova, Romania

Iuliana Ceausu, Cristian Poalelungi, Cristian Posea, Nicolae Bacalbasa and Dragos Dobritoiu
Department of Obstetrics–Gynecology, University of Medicine and Pharmacy "Carol Davila," "Dr. I. Cantacuzino" Hospital, Bucharest, Romania

Dominic Iliescu
Department of Obstetrics–Gynecology, University of Medicine and Pharmacy, Craiova, Romania

Liana Ples
Department of Obstetrics–Gynecology, University of Medicine and Pharmacy "Carol Davila," "Sf. Ioan" Emergency Hospital, Bucharest, Romania

Simona Vlădăreanu, Mihaela Boț, Claudia Mehedințu and Simona Popescu
University of Medicine and Pharmacy "Carol Davila", Bucharest, Romania

Costin Berceanu
University of Medicine and Pharmacy of Craiova, Romania

Sidonia Catalina Vrabie, Liliana Novac, Maria Magdalena Manolea and Lorena Anda Dijmarescu
Department of Obstetrics and Gynecology, University of Medicine and Pharmacy, Craiova, Romania

Marius Novac
Department of Anesthesiology and Intensive Care, University of Medicine and Pharmacy, Craiova, Romania

Mirela Anisoara Siminel
Department of Neonatology, University of Medicine and Pharmacy, Craiova, Romania

Cristian Marinaș
Department of Anatomy, University of Medicine and Pharmacy Craiova, Romania

Virgiliu-Bogdan Șorop
Department of Obstetrics and Gynecology, University of Medicine and Pharmacy "Victor Babeș" Timișoara, Romania

Alina Veduța
Department of Obstetrics and Gynecology, University of Medicine and Pharmacy "Carol Davila" Bucharest, Romania

Nicolae Cernea, Maria Șorop-Florea, Roxana-Cristina Dragușin, Ciprian Laurențiu Pătru, Lucian George Zorilă and Dominic Gabriel Iliescu
Department of Obstetrics and Gynecology, Prenatal Diagnostic Unit, University Emergency County Hospital, University of Medicine and Pharmacy Craiova, Romania

Cristian Neamțu
Department of Pathophysiology, University of Medicine and Pharmacy Craiova, Romania

Eusebiu Vlad Gorduza
Medical Genetics Department, "Grigore T. Popa" University of Medicine and Pharmacy, Iași, Romania

Demetra Gabriela Socolov and Răzvan Vladimir Socolov
Obstetrics and Gynecology Department, "Grigore T. Popa" University of Medicine and Pharmacy, Iași, Romania

Umar Boston, Ken-Michael Bayle, TK Susheel Kumar and Christopher Knott-Craig
Heart Institute at Le Bonheur Children's Hospital, University of Tennessee Health Science Center, Memphis, United States

Diana Ramasauskaite
Vilnius University, Faculty of Medicine, Institute of Clinical medicine, Clinic of Obstetrics and Gynaecology, Vilnius, Lithuania

Index

www.ingramcontent.com/pod-product-compliance
Lightning Source LLC
Chambersburg PA
CBHW080626200326
41458CB00013B/4528